PSYCHOLOGICAL THERAPIES FOR ADULTS WITH AUTISM

"This marvelous book provides a thorough overview of current approaches covering a range of topics and strategies. This book will be greatly appreciated by therapists working to support adults with autism as they increasingly are integrated into communities, families, and the work force. A must have book!"
—Fred R. Volkmar, MD, Irving B Harris Professor, Yale University, Dorothy Goodwin Endowed Chair, Southern Connecticut State University

"A ground-breaking work–likely to be a valuable resource and inspiration to clinicians and researchers alike. This book illuminates the complexities of adulthood for those on the spectrum and offers a diversity of perspectives and approaches to ensure those complexities are better understood and addressed."
—Connor Kerns, PhD, Associate Professor Psychology, Director Anxiety Stress and Autism Program, University of British Columbia

"This much needed compendium overviews a wide range of available treatments for autism. Inclusion of relevant research studies enables readers to evaluate the strength of evidence for each. Case vignettes will be valuable to clinicians engaged in providing services for adults with autism. This volume offers a useful resource for trainees, scholars, and clinicians invested in the well-being of adults with autism."
—James McPartland, PhD, Yale Child Study Center

T0323245

Psychological Therapies for Adults with Autism

EDITED BY DEBBIE SPAIN,

FRANCISCO M. MUSICH, AND

SUSAN W. WHITE

OXFORD
UNIVERSITY PRESS

Oxford University Press is a department of the University of Oxford. It furthers
the University's objective of excellence in research, scholarship, and education
by publishing worldwide. Oxford is a registered trade mark of Oxford University
Press in the UK and certain other countries.

Published in the United States of America by Oxford University Press
198 Madison Avenue, New York, NY 10016, United States of America.

© Oxford University Press 2022

Library of Congress Cataloging-in-Publication Data
Names: Spain, Debbie, editor. | M. Musich, Francisco, editor. |
   W. White, Susan, editor.
Title: Psychological therapies for adults with autism / [edited by] Debbie
   Spain, Francisco M. Musich, and Susan W. White.
Description: New York : Oxford University Press, 2022. |
   Includes bibliographical references and index.
Identifiers: LCCN 2021044629 (print) | LCCN 2021044630 (ebook) |
   ISBN 9780197548462 (paperback) | ISBN 9780197548486 (epub) |
   ISBN 9780197548493
Subjects: LCSH: Autism. | Autism—Treatment. | Psychotherapy.
Classification: LCC RC553.A88 P79 2022 (print) | LCC RC553.A88 (ebook) |
   DDC 616.85/882—dc23/eng/20211019
LC record available at https://lccn.loc.gov/2021044629
LC ebook record available at https://lccn.loc.gov/2021044630

DOI: 10.1093/med-psych/9780197548462.001.0001

9 8 7 6 5 4 3 2 1

Printed by LSC communications, United States of America

CONTENTS

James Acland, PgDip
CBT Therapist
National Adult Autism and ADHD
Psychology Service
South London & Maudsley NHS
Foundation Trust

Arnoud Arntz, PhD
Professor
Programme Group Clinical
Psychology
University of Amsterdam, Faculty of
Social and Behavioural Sciences

Lauren Avellone, PhD
Assistant Professor
Rehabilitation Research and
Training Center
Virginia Commonwealth University

Kelly B. Beck, PhD
Assistant Professor
Department of Rehabilitation Science
and Technology
University of Pittsburgh

Darren Bowring, PhD, MSc, M(Ed)
Honorary Research Fellow
Centre for Educational Development,
Appraisal, and Research (CEDAR)
University of Warwick

Staci Carr, PhD
Technical Assistance Coordinator and
Developmental Psychologist
School of Education Autism Center of
Excellence
Virginia Commonwealth University

Xie Yin Chew, MPsych
Clinical Psychologist
Department of Psychological Medicine
National University Hospital

Caitlin M. Conner, PhD
Research Assistant Professor
Department of Psychiatry
University of Pittsburgh School of
Medicine

Cynthia I. D'Agostino
Licenciate in Psychology/Master
Psychopatology BA/MA
Associate Professor and Coordinator
of Female Autism Program
Department of Psychology and
University Extension
Universidad CAECE

Rudi Dallos, PhD
Emeritus Professor of Clinical
Psychology
Clinical Psychology
University of Plymouth

Caroline van Diest, MSc, RNLD
EMDR Trainer, Consultant and CBT
Therapist
Synthesa Therapy

Thecla Fellas
Chief Executive Officer
Head Office
Asperger East Anglia, Registered
Charity

Naomi Fisher, MA, PhD
Independent Clinical Psychologist,
EMDR Consultant and Facilitator
Hove

Hannie van Genderen, PhD
Clinical Psychologist
Van Genderen Opleidingen

Hilde M. Geurts, PhD
Professor Clinical Neuropsychology
and Head of the Section Brain &
Cognition
Brain & Cognition, Department of
Psychology
University of Amsterdam

Ashleigh Hillier, PhD
Professor
Department of Psychology
University of Massachusetts Lowell

Tomoya Hirota, MD
Assistant Professor
Department of Psychiatry and
Behavioral Sciences
University of California San Francisco

Matthew J. Hollocks, PhD, DClinPsy
Clinical Lecturer and Senior Clinical
Psychologist
Department of Child & Adolescent
Psychiatry
King's College London

Kate Johnston, BSc, MSc, DClinPsy
Consultant Clinical Psychologist
National & Specialist CAMHS
South London & Maudsley NHS
Foundation Trust

Bryan H. King, MD, MBA
Lisa and John Pritzker Family
Distinguished Professor in Child and
Adolescent Psychiatry
Psychiatry and Behavioral Sciences
University of California at San
Francisco

Claire Brito Klein, BA
Graduate Research Assistant
Department of Psychology and
Neuroscience
University of North Carolina at
Chapel Hill

Laura Grofer Klinger, PhD
Executive Director; Associate
Professor
TEACCH Autism Program;
Department of Psychiatry
University of North Carolina at
Chapel Hill

**Peter E. Langdon, BSc (Hons),
PGCertHE, DClinPsy, PhD,
CPsychol, FBPsS**
Professor and Consultant Clinical and
Forensic Psychologist
Centre for Educational Development,
Appraisal, and Research (CEDAR)
University of Warwick
Rainbow Unit
Coventry and Warwickshire
Partnership NHS Trust

Iliana Magiati, DClinPsy, PhD
Associate Professor
School of Psychological Science
University of Western Australia

David Mason, MSc, BSc (Hons)
PhD Student
Social, Genetic, and Developmental
Psychiatry Centre
Institute of Psychiatry, Psychology, and
Neuroscience

David Murphy, PhD
Chartered Forensic and Consultant
Clinical Neuropsychologist
Department of Psychology
Broadmoor Hospital

Francisco M. Musich, PhD
Professor and Head of the Department
of Child and Adolescent Psychology
Department of Children and
Adolescents
Instituto de Neurología Cognitiva and
Fundacion ETCI

Ermione Neophytou, DClinPsy, BSc
Highly Specialist Clinical Psychologist
National & Specialist CAMHS
South London & Maudsley NHS
Foundation Trust

Glenna Osborne, MEd, CESP
Director of Transition Services,
TEACCH Autism Program
Clinical Instructor, Department of
Psychiatry
The University of North Carolina at
Chapel Hill

**Ann Ozsivadjian, BSc (Hons),
DClinPsy**
Independent Clinical Psychologist and
Visiting Senior Lecturer
King's College London

Adam Robertson
BSCeC Politics and History 2:1
Honours, MA International Relations
and European Studies—Distinction
Payroll Officer

Anna Robinson, PhD
Lecturer
School of Education
University of Strathclyde

Carol Schall, PhD
Associate Professor
Rehabilitation Research and Training
Center, School of Education
Virginia Commonwealth University

David Schena
Doctoral Student
Department of Psychology
University of Massachusetts Lowell

Grace Lee Simmons, MA
Graduate Clinician and Researcher
Department of Psychology
The University of Alabama

Debbie Spain, PhD
Visiting Postdoctoral Clinical
Researcher
Institute of Psychiatry, Psychology &
Neuroscience
King's College London

Rebecca Stancer, PhD
Associate Professor
Institute of Education
University of Plymouth

Eloise Stark, DPhil (Oxon)
Postdoctoral Researcher
Department of Psychiatry
University of Oxford

**Lorna Taylor, BSc, MSc, PhD,
DClinPsy**
Principal Clinical Psychologist
National & Specialist CAMHS
South London & Maudsley NHS
Foundation Trust

Brianne Tomaszewski, PhD, MPH
Assistant Professor
TEACCH Autism Program,
Department of Psychiatry
University of North Carolina at
Chapel Hill

**Sandy Toogood, BSc, MA, PhD,
FHEA, BCBA-D**
Professor
School of Education Sciences
Bangor University

Richard Vuijk, PhD
Clinical Psychologist
Sarr Autism Rotterdam
Parnassia Psychiatric Institute

Paul Wehman, PhD
Professor
Department of Special Education and
Counseling
Virginia Commonwealth University,
School of Education

Susan W. White, PhD
Professor
Center for Youth Development and
Intervention
Department of Psychology
University of Alabama

Introduction

SUSAN W. WHITE ■

PREVALENCE OF ASD/AUTISM IN ADULTS

Prevalence of autism spectrum disorder (ASD/Autism) is estimated at one in 54 people (Maenner et al., 2020). Of people diagnosed with ASD/Autism in childhood, 85% continue to meet diagnostic criteria as adults (Billstedt et al., 2005). As with most neurodevelopmental disorders, ASD/Autism has historically been primarily studied as a disorder of childhood. However, this tide is changing. An estimated 50,000 adolescents with ASD/Autism age into adulthood every year (Shattuck et al., 2012). At this rate, we can expect upward of a half-million more adults with ASD/Autism every decade. This reality is inconsistent with the current research focus; only 2% of all ASD/Autism-related research focuses on adult outcomes (U.S. Department of Health and Human Services, 2017).

HISTORY OF WORK IN ADULTS WITH ASD/AUTISM

Although identification of ASD/Autism among people who do not have co-occurring intellectual disability has risen in the last several years, adults with ASD/Autism face worse outcomes than peers without ASD/Autism, as a group. The majority of adults with ASD/Autism are not consistently employed or are underemployed (Engstrom et al., 2003). Young adults with ASD/Autism often lag behind peers in meeting the milestones of this developmental period (e.g., independent living) or experience declines in functioning (Picci & Scherf, 2015; Steinhausen et al., 2016). Adults with ASD/Autism also experience lower quality of life than age- and ability-matched peers (Bishop-Fitzpatrick et al., 2018).

This is not just a problem for people with ASD/Autism and their immediate families. The lack of support for this population, and the suboptimal outcomes experienced by too many with the disorder, is a societal problem. It has been estimated that the lifetime per capita societal cost of ASD/Autism is $3.2 million (USD), with lost productivity and adult care the largest contributors to cost (Ganz, 2007).

CO-OCCURRING CONDITIONS IN ASD/AUTISM AND IN ADULTS

As demonstrated by the chapters in this book, co-occurring mental health problems are very common in adults with ASD/Autism. Using data from Medicaid (which provides health coverage to people who are low-income or have disabilities in the US), and including records of a sample of 1,772 adults with ASD/Autism, Vohra and colleagues determined that 81% had co-occurring psychiatric disorders, relative to 41% of those without ASD/Autism. An earlier large-scale study of 1,507 adults with ASD/Autism on private insurance found that adults with ASD/Autism had higher rates of all major psychiatric disorders relative to non-ASD/Autism adults; 54% of the ASD/Autism sample had comorbid psychiatric conditions (Croen et al., 2015). Conservatively, it is estimated that over half of adults with ASD/Autism are diagnosed with at least one additional psychiatric disorder, a rate that is considerably higher than for the general population (Croen et al., 2015). Although we do not fully understand the reasons underlying the heightened risk for emergence of problems such as anxiety, depression, and suicidality, it is established that people with ASD/Autism face challenges related to access to services and full inclusion in society, a drop in available services around the time of exit from secondary school, and limited mental health services (Laxman et al., 2019; Leno & Simonoff, 2020; Maddox et al., 2019; Smith & White, 2020; Taylor & Seltzer, 2011). All of these factors, along with biological risk factors, likely contribute to heightened risk.

BALANCING THE BRIDGE BETWEEN RESEARCH/ SCIENCE AND PRACTICE

In terms of healthcare utilization, adults with ASD/Autism utilize health care services more often, and at a higher cost, than neurotypical adults and more than adults with attention deficit/hyperactivity disorder (ADHD; Zerbo et al., 2019). With respect to emergency department use, one of the most expensive forms of healthcare, adults with ASD/Autism have 2.3 times more emergency room visits than neurotypical adults, and the reason for the visits is more than three times as likely to be related to a psychiatric disorder, relative to nonautistic peers (Vohra et al., 2016).

The presence of psychiatric, as well as nonpsychiatric, comorbidity among adults with ASD/Autism increases total medical expenses (Vohra et al., 2017). The authors suggested that insufficient availability of, and access to, healthcare providers who are knowledgeable about ASD/Autism and co-occurring conditions could contribute to high services costs, partly because delays in care and prevention could lead to symptom worsening.

As previously stated, most clinical research in ASD/Autism has been with children and adolescents (Howlin, 2008; U.S. Department of Health and Human Services, 2017). Most of the research on treatment for adults with ASD/Autism that does exist has been exclusively focused on people without intellectual disability (Interagency Autism Coordinating Committee, 2016). This state of affairs is unfortunately consistent with the oft-cited gap which spans nearly two decades from research establishing an approach to use in community practice (Atkins et al., 2016). As such, clinical researchers and direct care providers must work together to bridge science and service to address the needs of this growing population. The extant research, in short, is not where we would like it to be (White et al., 2018). However, the need for evidence-based services is too great to simply wait for more research. When we consider treatments for adults with ASD/Autism, we must hasten translation and dissemination. In this volume, we have endeavored for every chapter to distill the existing research as it pertains to the topic at hand, while fully acknowledging that for most of the approaches described herein, much more research is needed. It is our hope that the readers of this volume gain increased skill and confidence in their ability to successfully treat adult patients with ASD/Autism.

Finally, in introducing a book related to adults with ASD/Autism, it is critically important to consider language, specifically the debate over the use of person-first or identity-first language. There are vocal proponents for each approach (Bottema-Beutel et al., 2021; Gernsbacher, 2017; Vivanti, 2020). In this volume, we have opted to let the chapter authors determine the terminology they think best fits the topic covered. This diversity in language reflects the current debate in our field. Indeed, use of person-first language may be, in some ways, more inclusive, as not all people with ASD/Autism prefer identity-first, perhaps especially those who are less verbal. On the other hand, there is evidence that many autistic adults prefer identify-first given the disorder's centrality to identity (Bury, Jellett, Spoort, & Hedley, 2020). Ideally, our terminology is flexible enough to accommodate all preferences and, above all else, reduce ableism and the marginalization of those who have ASD/Autism (Bottema-Beutel et al., 2021). We endeavor to ensure that the diversity of opinions and experiences of adults with ASD/Autism are represented accurately in this volume. All case examples provided are anonymized to protect confidentiality, and all quotes were included only with explicit permission to do so. It is our hope that these lived experiences related to being an adult with ASD/autism, mental health, and treatment inform the work of clinicians and researchers in this area.

REFERENCES

Atkins, M. S., Rusch, D., Mehta, T. G., & Lakind, D. (2016). Future directions for dissemination and implementation science: Aligning ecological theory and public health to close the research to practice gap. *Journal of Clinical Child and Adolescent Psychology, 45*(2), 215–226.

Billstedt, E., Gillberg, C., & Gillberg, C. (2005). Autism after adolescence: Population-based 13-to 22-year follow-up study of 120 individuals with autism diagnosed in childhood. *Journal of Autism and Developmental Disorders, 35*(3), 351–360.

Bishop-Fitzpatrick, L., Mazefsky, C. A., & Eack, S. M. (2018). The combined impact of social support and perceived stress on quality of life in adults with autism spectrum disorder and without intellectual disability. *Autism, 22*(6), 703–711.

Bottema-Beutel, K., Kapp, S. K., Lester, J. N., Sasson, N. J., & Hand, B. N. (2021). Avoiding ableist language: Suggestions for autism researchers. *Autism in Adulthood, 3*(1), 18–29.

Bury, S. M., Jellett, R., Spoort, J. R., & Hedley, D. (2020). "It defines who I am" or "It's something I have": What language do (autistic) Australian adults [on the autism spectrum] prefer? *Journal of Autism and Developmental Disorders.* doi:10.1007/s10803-020-04425-3

Croen, L. A., Zerbo, O., Qian, Y., Massolo, M. L., Rich, S., Sidney, S., & Kripke, C. (2015). The health status of adults on the autism spectrum. *Autism, 19*(7), 814–823.

Engstrom, I., Ekstrom, L., & Emilsson, B. (2003). Psychosocial functioning in a group of Swedish adults with Asperger syndrome or high-functioning autism. *Autism, 7*(1), 99–110.

Ganz, M. L. (2007). The lifetime distribution of the incremental societal costs of autism. *Archives of Pediatrics and Adolescent Medicine, 161*(4), 343–349.

Gernsbacher, M. A. (2017). Editorial perspective: The use of person-first language in scholarly writing may accentuate stigma. *Journal of Child Psychology and Psychiatry, 58*(7), 859–861.

Howlin, P. (2008). Redressing the balance in autism research. *Nature Clinical Practice Neurology, 4*(8), 407.

Interagency Autism Coordinating Committee. (2016). *Strategic Plan for Autism Spectrum Disorder.* U.S. Department of Health and Human Services Interagency Autism Coordinating Committee website. https://iacc.hhs.gov/publications/strategic-plan/2017/

Laxman, D. J., Taylor, J. L., DaWalt, L. S., Greenberg, J. S., & Mailick, M. R. (2019). Loss in services precedes high school exit for teens with autism spectrum disorder: A longitudinal study. *Autism Research, 12*(6), 911–921.

Leno, V. C., & Simonoff, E. (2020). ASD and co-occurring psychiatric conditions: A conceptual framework. In C. A. M. S. W. White & B. M. Maddox (Eds.), *The Oxford Handbook of autism and co-occurring psychiatric conditions* (pp. 3–28). Oxford University Press.

Maddox, B. B., Crabbe, S. R., Fishman, J. M., Beidas, R. S., Brookman-Frazee, L., Miller, J. S., Nicolaidis, C., & Mandell, D. S. (2019). Factors influencing the use of cognitive–behavioral therapy with autistic adults: A survey of community mental health clinicians. *Journal of Autism and Developmental Disorders, 49*(11), 4421–4428.

Maenner, M. J., Shaw, K. A., Baio, J., Washington, A., Patrick, M., DiRienzo, M., Christensen, D. L., Wiggins, L. D., Pettygrove, S., Andrews, J. G., Lopez, M., Hudson, A., Baroud, T., Schwenk, Y., White, T., Rosenberg, C. R., Lee, L.-C., Harrington, R. A., Huston, M., . . . Dietz, P. M. (2020). Prevalence of autism spectrum disorder among children aged 8 years—Autism and Developmental Disabilities Monitoring Network, 11 sites, United States, 2016. *MMWR Surveillance Summaries, 69*(4), 1–12.

Picci, G., & Scherf, K. S. (2015). A two-hit model of autism: Adolescence as the second hit. *Clinical Psychological Science, 3*(3), 349–371.

Shattuck, P. T., Narendorf, S. C., Cooper, B., Sterzing, P. R., Wagner, M., & Taylor, J. L. (2012). Postsecondary education and employment among youth with an autism spectrum disorder. *Pediatrics, 129*(6), 1042–1049.

Smith, I. C., & White, S. W. (2020). Socio-emotional determinants of depressive symptoms in adolescents and adults with autism spectrum disorder: A systematic review. *Autism, 24*(4), 995–1010.

Steinhausen, H. C., Jensen, C. M., & Lauritsen, M. B. (2016). A systematic review and meta-analysis of the long-term overall outcome of autism spectrum disorders in adolescence and adulthood. *Acta Psychiatrica Scandinavica, 133*(6), 445–452.

Taylor, J. L., & Seltzer, M. M. (2011). Employment and post-secondary educational activities for young adults with autism spectrum disorders during transition to adulthood. *Journal of Autism and Developmental Disorders, 41*(5), 566–574.

U.S. Department of Health and Human Services. (2017). *Report to Congress: Young adults and transitioning youth with autism spectrum disorder.*

Vivanti, G. (2020). Ask the editor: What is the most appropriate way to talk about individuals with a diagnosis of autism? *Journal of Autism and Developmental Disorders, 50,* 691–693.

Vohra, R., Madhavan, S., & Sambamoorthi, U. (2016). Emergency department use among adults with autism spectrum disorders (ASD). *Journal of Autism and Developmental Disorders, 46*(4), 1441–1454.

Vohra, R., Madhavan, S., & Sambamoorthi, U. (2017). Comorbidity prevalence, health-care utilization, and expenditures of Medicaid enrolled adults with autism spectrum disorders. *Autism, 21*(8), 995–1009.

White, S. W., Simmons, G. L., Gotham, K. O., Conner, C. M., Smith, I. C., Beck, K. B., & Mazefsky, C. A. (2018). Psychosocial treatments targeting anxiety and depression in adolescents and adults on the autism spectrum: Review of the latest research and recommended future directions. *Current Psychiatry Reports, 20,* 82.

Zerbo, O., Qian, Y., Ray, T., Sidney, S., Rich, S., Massolo, M., & Croen, L. A. (2019). Health care service utilization and cost among adults with autism spectrum disorders in a U.S. integrated health care system. *Autism in Adulthood, 1*(1), 27–36.

2

Experiences of Psychological Therapy as an Autistic Person

DAVID MASON, ELOISE STARK, FRANCISCO M. MUSICH, AND DEBBIE SPAIN ■

KEY CONSIDERATIONS

- Psychological therapies are, by definition, complex interventions, comprised of specific and nonspecific elements. Nonspecific elements of therapy (e.g., the therapeutic relationship, capacity to empathize) are pivotal for the success of specific elements of therapy (e.g., particular interventions and techniques).
- Some autistic adults benefit from adaptations to standard therapeutic work; adaptations may be overarching and general (e.g., a change to the pace or mode of delivery) or highly individual and specific (e.g., accommodating particular sensory or information processing preferences).
- Therapists should think together with autistic clients about how to enhance accessibility of the therapeutic context and interventions used.
- Enhancing resilience is an important aspect of psychological therapy, irrespective of the reason for referral or therapeutic modality offered.

INTRODUCTION

Many autistic adults experience mental health symptoms or conditions at some point in their lives (Lai et al., 2019), often more than one concurrently (Lever & Geurts, 2016). During the past 20 years, there has been an increasing emphasis on developing and evaluating psychological therapies for autistic adults (White et al., 2018). There is now promising evidence of the effectiveness of cognitive behavior therapy (CBT; Spain, 2019); mindfulness (Hartley et al., 2019); social skills interventions (Ke et al., 2018); psychosocial interventions, such as those targeting social cognition (Bishop-Fitzpatrick et al., 2014); and employment-focused interventions (Hedley et al., 2017). However, most research evidence comes from uncontrolled (nonrandomized) studies recruiting, on average, younger autistic adults without a concurrent intellectual disability.

Importantly, clinical and empirical findings indicate that some autistic individuals benefit from adapted psychological therapy (see other chapters in this book). Adaptations may include ensuring that the formulation incorporates autism-relevant aspects and that the environment and therapy process are tailored to the sensory, linguistic, and social preferences of autistic individuals (Adams & Young, 2020; Spain & Happé, 2020; Stark et al., 2021). However, there are several factors that affect the likelihood of suitably adapted input being offered, including a nuanced knowledge about autism and the potential need for adaptations for a wide range of client presentations.

This chapter focuses on the personal experiences of five autistic adults who have had psychological therapy individually and/or in groups; David, Eloise, Jane, Graham, and Miranda. Their narratives provide rich descriptions of the overt and subtle aspects of therapy that have been less or more helpful, and they highlight the centrality of the therapeutic relationship. There are similarities in some of their experiences, despite seeking services for different concerns, having different life stories, and living on three continents. This suggests that there may be key considerations for therapists working with autistic adults, regardless of the setting. Additionally, Jane's and Miranda's mothers offer their perspectives about supporting their grown-up daughters to access strengths-based psychological input.

The decision to place this chapter at the outset of the book is quite deliberate. We invite the reader to reflect on the accounts written by David, Eloise, Jane, Graham, and Miranda; to be curious about how and why some psychological therapy modalities and interventions have seemed more accessible and relevant; to consider which nonspecific elements of the psychological therapy may have enhanced the process for each person; and in turn to consider what this might mean for clinical work going forward.

The first-person accounts that follow are verbatim comments from each contributor.

DAVID

My two experiences of therapy were an 8-week course of counseling when I was around aged 25, and then a 12-week course of behavioural activation when I was around 30 years old. The former was not very effective in a broad sense, but was so in a specific sense. The latter has been genuinely life changing. I can confidently assert I would not be here were it not for the latter treatment.

So, what worked? In the counselling I received, I was encouraged to talk about my situation and reflect on what I was experiencing (at that time I was depressed by my current employment situation). In the specific sense this was helpful, because it helped me realise I could quit my career at the time. (Despite having multiple jobs, quitting a "career" was an option that never occurred to me). In a broader sense it failed to work, as I quickly relapsed into several other bouts of depression—what I experienced did not generalise beyond the situation at hand. This is in spite of how "obvious" it may be to leave a work environment that is unsuitable. Moreover, while it did help me realise I could leave the job I held, it did not help me realise I could entirely change career.

On the other hand, behavioural activation (BA) immediately made sense to me. I often joke it is because it consisted of "boxes and arrows" (of which I am fond). While this may seem to trivialise the approach it was genuinely transformative—these boxes and arrows gave me a framework to organise my behaviours and experiences. The use of Antecedent / Behaviour / Consequence diagrams ("ABC"s) helped me realise that a behaviour could lead me to feel worse, but this behaviour had an antecedent—if the antecedent was an avoidance behaviour I tended to feel worse (and the converse was true for approach behaviours).

I still cannot fully put it into words, but this framework helped me connect internal experiences to internal states or external states. This removed some of the (frustrating) mystery from the world, and why I was responding to events in the way that I was. For example, avoiding doing a task that was aversive—good in the short run, but likely to worsen my mood in the long run. This immediately made an impact on my mood, and my motivation. Once I had learned how to "do the ABCs" in a situation, I became more agentic and able to affect the world around me in the way I wanted. I do flag from time to time—indeed, it might be odd if I did not—however, I have a solid process I can use to analyse a situation and implement behaviours that will help.

Are there other ingredients? Counselling, therapy, behavioural activation . . . while these all have processes or manuals, guidelines, and good practices, there are three extra factors that I think are important, based on my reflections on therapy. First, the patient (in this case me); second, the therapist; third, the interaction. In case one, I was severely underprepared to be counselled. I had no idea what depression was. Consequently, I had no vocabulary or understanding of what depression is like (I only had the diagnostic label from my general practitioner—with no explanation). In fact, at the time, I thought everyone functioned exactly like me (and that they were just more successful); I had no concept that people were different. The counsellor was, as far as I could determine, compassionate and interested in helping me. He was very good at building rapport (indeed, I felt comfortable disclosing my thoughts/feelings etc. despite the novel surroundings which often set me on edge). In sum, I would say that I was not in a position to engage with therapy in an optimal way.

In contrast, with BA, I was more aware of depression and I was tired of being depressed. I remember being asked why I wanted therapy and my response was something like "so that I never have to see someone like you again" (with the required caveat that this was not intended negatively). I went into therapy wanting a toolkit to deal with depression. By this point I had realised that I was likely to be prone to depression, and I guess I was implicitly aware that my previous therapy had not generalised beyond that specific situation. I think I brought a readiness for recovery to the table, and I was prepared to go through a range of experiences to make it happen—over the course of the therapy, I remember facing very aversive experiences, and coming out better for it. The therapist was truly phenomenal. They were attentive, constantly checked in with me, agreed on an agenda for each session, and adapted their practice when we realised that I had a good grasp of BA, but I still needed a few extra skills. Indeed, when I showed a wider interest in BA they provided me with a reading list! Our interaction was really good—I felt able to fully discuss my problems (in so far as I was aware and able to) and the therapist was able to challenge me if I was being reticent or not providing a lot of verbal input. Moreover, they were willing to challenge my interpretations of my experiences and challenged me to consider alternative interpretations. This was vital as I was heavily invested in the rightness of my thoughts, and I found alternative interpretations very challenging to interpret (I still do, but I have managed to relax this a little).

My subsequent thoughts of therapy are largely informed by my positive experiences after case two. The toolkit I built has served me well, and I have managed to add a few extra tools to it. The "boxes and arrows" generalise to pretty much everything I encounter, and that has been a life-changing skill set. I don't think this will apply to every autistic person, but I do think something like this approach could be helpful—some level of abstract rule-based process is great for applying to novel situations. Although we did spend around 8 weeks practicing this and agreeing test scenarios to try it out.

Personally, I also think being challenged in the way I interpreted my thoughts and behaviours was fundamental to getting better. I can get so wrapped up in what I think and really struggle to see an alternative (or, frankly, to consider that an alternative could be right!); the typical "black and white" thinking.

ELOISE

My first experience of psychological therapy was CBT for obsessive compulsive disorder (OCD) during my undergraduate degree. I had been randomly attacked the year earlier by a man who was distressed and unwell and tried to strangle me in the street in broad daylight. I was utterly terrified at the time, and the fear I experienced persisted long beyond the event, morphing into a semblance of OCD. I feared that if I did not keep everything "in its place" and sparklingly clean, it would hurt my family in some way. So, I showered several times a day with harsh cleaning products, kept my room as tidy and clean as possible (a big contrast to my previously messy student bedroom), and spent hours organising items in my room to be "just right" at perfect angles like I was teaching my belongings a geometry lesson.

The way I formulate this presentation with hindsight is that my autistic brain has always experienced the unknown and uncertain as worrisome and potentially threatening. Having something completely uncontrollable and life threatening occur sent my threat system into overdrive. By focusing upon something I felt I could control—danger in the form of "contamination" and "germs"—I was able to regain a felt sense of control over my external world.

The therapist I met was mild and quietly spoken, and listened to me carefully, making detailed notes on everything I said. I had never experienced therapy before and was completely baffled by the new social rules and requirements. I was in such a heightened threat mode that I was constantly hypervigilant and on guard and consequently really struggled to put any of the cognitive-behavioural theory I was learning into practice via the technique of "exposure and response prevention." For example, I knew that my safety behaviour of always carrying antibacterial wipes in my backpack was maintaining the anxiety by preventing me from learning that it would be fine if I did not wipe every surface I touched, but I was unable to test out leaving them at home and not doing so.

I think this fear of exposure techniques and unwillingness to experiment was based upon several factors. First, at this point I did not have my autism diagnosis. The therapist saw my rigidity and deigned me too inflexible for therapy. Actually, I just needed support with the hyperarousal to bring me into a state in which I could react to stimuli more flexibly.

Second, the double empathy problem, by which autistic and nonautistic people both struggle to interpret each other, rather than the lack of empathy being attributed solely to the autistic individual, felt really prominent within our interactions. I did not feel understood by the therapist, although I knew that she was trying her best.

Third, I was trying to camouflage my difficulties like I had always done. When asked "how are you?" I responded with, "fine thank you, how are you?" like a robot. I now know that my authentic, autistic self is perfectly fine and accepted by others. Now, I use mindfulness strategies to prevent myself from slipping into camouflaging autopilot, but then I did not have those skills.

My second experience of psychological input was trauma-focused CBT during my postgraduate years. This time, the therapist knew about my autism as I had now been formally diagnosed prior to starting the therapy, and we built my autistic elements into the formulation. For example, not only did I learn about how the brain responds to trauma with disconnect between the affective regions, hippocampus, and frontal cortex, but we were able to factor in how autism-specific factors such as sensory hypersensitivity and my detail-focused processing fed into the trauma model. I found the CBT model's systematic, scientific approach was helpful for my scientific way of analysing the world. In this course of therapy, I was able to talk about my urge to camouflage, and with this knowledge the therapist was able to bring out my authentic self and I felt able to get things wrong and be myself.

I have also found compassion to be an important ingredient in therapy, as my autistic brain, through no fault of its own, often finds the threat system to be activated more frequently, leading to less relative time for the soothing system to be engaged. Encouraging self-compassion, acting in accordance with my values of kindness, and using my intellect and skills to show compassion to others, has helped rebalance my brain and body to a point where I feel healthy, strong, psychologically minded, and resilient.

I think the most important lesson I learned within therapy and through personal exploration was a sort of cognitive diffusion, an idea encapsulated by the quote often attributed to Viktor Frankl: "Between stimulus and response there is a space. In that space is our power to choose our response. In our response lies our growth and our freedom." I learned that whatever comes into my head, I am in charge of my response and my behaviour. I can choose to worry or ruminate, or I can choose to do something more positive with my time. Similarly, I can appraise something as threatening because it makes me feel slightly anxious, or I can normalise the feelings and appraise it as safe enough. I am grateful to both therapists I had on my journey to well-being, and I hope to use my experiences to help others also benefit from therapy.

JANE

I have attended many therapies in my life. I honestly think that I was able to learn something from each and every one of my previous therapists, but none of them were able to help me with my most important problem: that is, to be on the autism spectrum. One of the therapists helped me with improving my daily living skills and occupying my time, another helped me with finishing secondary school, another with my baking skills and some with my social behaviours, but no one diagnosed me with autism. In total, I went to five or six therapists, until I was referred to my current therapist, who has been really helpful.

I have found it useful to learn how to manage my emotions. One of my previous therapists suggested I learn to knit roses, which I find very relaxing. She also told me that it was good for me to be creative and do manual things. Another therapist told me to focus on baking as I like this a lot, and that I should continue doing it and not be ashamed to charge for the end product. Also, one therapist told me to try to cook something different each day, and she helped me to be more organized in secondary school. What I have found most helpful is when therapists have helped me to be more structured and organized and break things down step by step.

I think therapists should know what affects people with autism daily and how they feel. Also, it would be good for therapists to approach us knowing that we are different than others; that we might struggle sometimes and, at these times, we need to be approached gently. Another important thing is for therapists to give us concrete and tangible steps to follow, to offer practical strategies for us, autistic people, so that we can achieve things that will make us feel good about ourselves, like having more friends and finding a partner. Therapists who work with us should specialize in autism, because despite seeing several professionals, I was diagnosed really late in life and struggled and suffered for a long time throughout my life because of that. One more thing I think it would be good for therapists to do is more surveys and to measure what are the most frequent worries for autistic people.

JANE'S PARENTS

Our 30-year-old daughter has, for many years, attended several different therapies without good outcome. We noticed that she had social difficulties. We were referred to a specialist who diagnosed Jane with autistic at the age of 28. It wasn't easy for us as parents to accept her condition, but with our family and individual meetings with the therapist, we were able to accept, learn, and change our attitudes towards Jane. We feel that a specific approach done by a specialist therapist, combined with CBT, improved her condition and opened up a new path for her.

Finding an adequate therapy tailored for people with autistic is of utmost importance and in our opinion was very useful. Our daughter really benefitted from therapy. Her social interaction improved significantly and her repetitive behaviors, which were very persistent, were less intense and frequent. We think that Jane gained from a structured therapy, and not from unstructured approaches. Therapeutic work needs to involve consistency—even if Jane gets frustrated at times—and progressively, she is helped to acquire tools to improve.

It is important for therapists to know about autism in order to identify the patient's needs, behaviors, and feelings. In addition to a proper assessment and therapy, it is important to address social skills, daily life habits, and disruptive behaviors that might interfere with social integration.

GRAHAM

With my last therapist, I was able to achieve what no previous therapists wanted to believe: that my depression, which lasted for three years, could be treated without medication. In my opinion, there was previously a problem with the method: therapists were unable to find techniques relevant to my functioning and values as a person. When my depression lifted, I was able to find again small old daily things to enjoy. I was able to achieve this without having to use "normalizing" ways that had been proposed to me and were against my core values as a person. Going from one professional to another, without options, only worsened my condition. I would have liked to find an adequate professional sooner.

I found it useful that my therapist was able to understand me, even though I sometimes struggle to talk properly or as "normal people" expect. In our first sessions, he was able to understand my logic and way of processing information. In contrast to working with my previous therapists, we implemented other strategies that had not been suggested before, or had even been vetoed. With my current therapist it was not always easy to understand each other, but it has helped a lot that he can understand how people with autistic "talk": we can sometimes talk without using neurotypical language, like computers using programming language. For me, it was good just to be able to myself. Also, CBT was useful, as this was similar to a scientific method. I was able to change unhelpful beliefs about several topics.

To work effectively with people with autism, therapists should stop trying to "normalize" or expect us to use conventional neurotypical ways. Something I have noticed recently is that people with autism are genuine and like genuineness. We dislike pretending and relying on false interests to reach a goal. We need and must want to do it. When something interests us and it is within our possibilities, we can do it in an obsessive way and not stop. In my case, being tired and experiencing chronic pain has stopped me from dedicating more time to things I want to do more of. It is also important to create and implement alternative ways, to be flexible and innovate, for achieving what one might want at a particular time. One of my mottos is "there is always another way to do things according to functionality." So it is that in this time of pandemic I see this is a time of opportunity, as all interactions are internet-based or remote. Lastly, the therapist needs to be there for when we are facing new challenges and tasks. carefully paying attention to sensory issues and means of escape. Often, we want to achieve many things, but the environment and context can be inappropriate to our senses. Also, it is important to pay attention to how much we can interact socially, without becoming exhausted from the interactions.

MIRANDA

I think that therapists tend to expect their patients to want to be "normal." However, many autistic people do not feel any need to become like allists.[1] We do not see our perceptions of life as inferior or less valid than those of allists. Autism is not a disability. Allists lack some skills that come easily to autists, and vice versa, and that does not mean that either condition is a defect. However, the vast majority of humans are allists, and that means that society in general is tailored to their needs and abilities, so autists need to be able to adapt to a system that was not built for us.

The main thing I have to say about mindfulness therapy is that being aware in one's body is not always as beneficial for autists as it is for allists, considering the various sensory conditions an autist might have. Learning to be present in one's body to calm oneself down is not particularly helpful if one of the stressors that is contributing to the heightened state of arousal is physical stimulation, such as dampness of the skin or unpleasant smells.

1. A person who does not have autism.

Instead, I feel that the opposite strategy might work better for many autists, as it has for me. I withdraw from my senses and my body into my mind, sequestering my presence in my thoughts, to calm myself down and gain control of my emotions. Rejecting sensory data, which often contribute to stress and bind one in the moment, allows me to separate myself from a situation and its emotional accoutrements, leaving me free to calm myself and eventually return to a situation without my previous fervor.

If a patient has a history of psychiatric medication, especially if their prescriptions have changed repeatedly to find an acceptable balance between symptoms, they may have a heightened awareness that emotional states are essentially various chemicals influencing one's brain chemistry and that emotions are not always connected to or caused by the situation to which they are ostensibly reacting to. This means that that patient may recognize that an emotion is part of the circumstances of an incident, rather than part of the patient, and can often be removed by taking the time for it to wear off.

Things I want to say that aren't long enough for a paragraph:

- Your transient emotions are not part of who you are.
- One might use up emotional chemicals without risks or consequences by imagining someone else (a character to whom they relate, perhaps) expressing or experiencing the unwanted emotions ("getting in character").

MIRANDA'S MOTHER, MARION

My daughter is both very autistic, and very articulate. We have been lucky enough to be able to work with a number of highly skilled therapists over the last 15 years. All of them were dedicated, highly trained, and caring. They came from a number of disciplines—traditional therapies focusing on the emotions, pragmatics from the speech therapists and from psychologists, cognitive styles of therapy, exposure therapies for her OCD, and many others.

All of them had one very big difficulty, which has permeated her life elsewhere, as well: translating from the language that most of us speak into "autistic English." If you ask an "allist," as she calls nonautistic people, what was helpful or not in their therapy, they know what you mean, and how to answer the question. If you ask the same question of an autist, it is far too vague and amorphous a question for them, unless you have already translated a dozen similar ones for them.

What does it mean to translate therapy for an autist? First, draw the connection between a person's feelings (acknowledged or unacknowledged) and how they act, how they are perceived, and how this affects their life and their ability to reach their goals. Autists will never instinctively see things that the rest of us come to see when we are ready to see them. They lack the perceptual mechanisms that allow the rest of us to connect those dots. They never get the information that we get if we let ourselves see it. It is not a matter of denial or repression, but of absent information. Just as one would never expect a blind person to understand body language, or a deaf person to interpret meaning from tone of voice, therapists need to work around an autistic person's inability to perceive those things. Then, the autist needs guidance in understanding what these cues say about what the autist is doing and about what results they will get from what they are doing.

Therapy that focuses on emotional insight cannot produce the same results for an autist as it would for an allist without this end-piece that connects it to social interactions in meaningful ways for them. This is a piece that most of us fill in, almost by instinct, but it cannot work that same way for an autist.

On the other hand, my daughter has never been unaware of her own feelings, nor given to hiding them from herself or others. She has a radical honesty that may come from her ongoing inability to see the social pressure exerted on the rest of us to keep certain emotions or states hidden. She sees no point to most of these social conventions and tends to dispense with them as not worth her time. As a result, she has a lot less denial or repression to unravel than you or I would have. She does not need to get in touch with her feelings, because she has never learned to suppress them. This means that a lot of the traditional work of therapy is utterly unnecessary. Trying to do that work has resulted in endless frustration for all parties involved.

I believe that success in therapy for her has resulted when the therapist not only respects her opinion about what is working, what she needs, but also asks for it regularly and responds to that feedback. Every autist is different, perhaps to an even greater degree than the rest of us are. Trying to make the therapist's model of how things should work fit this particular patient has backfired badly.

CONCLUSION

Throughout the narratives in this chapter, we can identify some important considerations for therapists working with autistic clients. We acknowledge that these narratives, despite their enormous value, reflect the views of seven people, and there is a strong case for more systematic research into user perspectives in the future.

It appears that some of the common factors that have contributed to better therapeutic experience and outcomes are a structured, straightforward, tangible, and concrete approach. That is, a more formulaic approach used in several psychological therapies may be more suited for autistic clients who describe an analytical processing style. Additionally, including strategies that are offered visually as well as verbally, as mentioned previously ("boxes and arrows"), may augment understanding of abstract concepts frequently referred to in clinical work. Adapting the therapeutic setting and structure (e.g., amount of time per session, sensory stimuli, and linguistic accommodations) to the specific sensory and cognitive needs of the autistic client also appears fundamental. Potentially, the combination of these factors may be more suited to autistic clients and their processing style.

The clinician's personal style appears to be of great importance; in particular, actively and compassionately engaging in questions and conversation that aim to understand the specific needs, style, and level of functioning of autistic clients. As noted prominently in one narrative, autistic people often hide, or mask, their problems with a veneer of "normality." This could be a significant obstacle to therapy and suggests that a good rapport between client and therapist may help to overcome this issue. Also, in some cases, when providing input for co-occurring conditions rather than core autism traits, adding autism-relevant aspects to the case formulation may enhance outcomes. While not always possible, therapists should consider involving family or significant others in clinical work, subject to client consent. This may provide a better understanding of the autistic adult, as well as their family, environment, and systemic context, thereby improving quality of life for all parties.

The suggested considerations highlighted in this chapter may be useful for clinicians working with autistic adults and may contribute to making therapy more accessible and effective. Overall, we consider one of the most important aspects of therapy is for therapists to maintain a curious and reflective stance toward clients, given the heterogeneity and uniqueness of each individual presenting for therapy. Incorporating the uniqueness of the client into therapeutic work will most likely result in a more beneficial experience, not just for the client but also for the therapist. Ultimately, this attitude toward clients can be thought of as transdiagnostic, as all clients are unique in their presentation. We hope that, in the future, more research will be available, providing a better understanding for therapists on how to improve therapy and meet the needs of autistic adults more adequately.

REFERENCES

Adams, D., & Young, K. (2020). A systematic review of the perceived barriers and facilitators to accessing psychological treatment for mental health problems in individuals on the autism spectrum. *Review Journal of Autism and Developmental Disorders*, 1–18. https://link.springer.com/article/10.1007/s40489-020-00226-7

Bishop-Fitzpatrick, L., Minshew, N., & Eack, S. (2014). A systematic review of psychosocial interventions for adults with autism spectrum disorders. *Journal of Autism and Developmental Disorders*, 43(3), 687–694.

Hartley, M., Dorstyn, D., & Due, C. (2019). Mindfulness for children and adults with autism spectrum disorder and their caregivers: A meta-analysis. *Journal of Autism and Developmental Disorders*, 49(10), 4306–4319.

Hedley, D., Uljarević, M., Cameron, L., Halder, S., Richdale, A., & Dissanayake, C. (2017). Employment programmes and interventions targeting adults with autism spectrum disorder: A systematic review of the literature. *Autism*, 21(8), 929–941.

Ke, F., Whalon, K., & Yun, J. (2018). Social skill interventions for youth and adults with autism spectrum disorder: A systematic review. *Review of Educational Research*, 88(1), 3–42.

Lai, M., Kassee, C., Besney, R., Bonato, S., Hull, L., Mandy, W., Szatmari, P., & Ameis, S. H. (2019). Prevalence of co-occurring mental health diagnoses in the autism population: A systematic review and meta-analysis. *The Lancet Psychiatry*, *6*(10), 819–829.

Lever, A. G., & Geurts, H. M. (2016). Psychiatric co-occurring symptoms and disorders in young, middle-aged, and older adults with autism spectrum disorder. *Journal of Autism and Developmental Disorders*, *46*(6), 1916–1930.

Spain, D. (2019). Cognitive behaviour therapy. In E. Chaplin, D. Spain, & C. McCarthy (Eds.), *A clinician's guide to mental health conditions in adults with autism spectrum disorders: Assessment and interventions* (pp. 290–307). Jessica Kingsley Publishers.

Spain, D., & Happé, F. (2020). How to optimise cognitive behaviour therapy (CBT) for people with autism spectrum disorders (ASD): a delphi study. *Journal of Rational-Emotive & Cognitive-Behavior Therapy*, *38*(2), 184–208.

Stark, E., Ali, D., Ayre, A., Schneider, N., Parveen, S., Marais, K., Holmes, N., & Pender, R. (2021). Psychological therapy for autistic adults (1st digital edition). Authentistic Research Collective. htpps://eloisestark.org/Authentistic.html

White, S., Simmons, G., Gotham, K., Conner, C. M., Smith, I., Beck, K., & Mazefsky, C. (2018). Psychosocial treatments targeting anxiety and depression in adolescents and adults on the autism spectrum: Review of the latest research and recommended future directions. *Current Psychiatry Reports*, *20*(10), 1–10.

3

Systemic Therapy

RUDI DALLOS AND REBECCA STANCER ▪

KEY CONSIDERATIONS

- To what extent do adults with a diagnosis of autism experience differences and similarities in their relationships and families?
- Autism is an extremely diverse condition and how it impacts is unique to each family. Consequently a systemic approach attempts to be flexible and adaptable.
- Adults with a diagnosis of autism may be parents. The focus of systemic work may be with their children and relationships with them.
- Insecure attachment and trauma are common aspects of most clinical presentations and also feature in the development of autism and influence their relationships.
- Systemic therapy attempts to address all relationships in a family and considers how these may impact the well-being and lives of adults with autism.
- Structured and manualized approaches to systemic family therapy (FT) may be compatible with aspects of the autism phenotype which emphasize the need for predictability and clarity.

INTRODUCTION

Arguably, the needs of adults with a diagnosis of autism have been relatively overlooked, leading to legislation in the United Kingdom calling for more services and support (Department of Health 2010a; NHS, 2017; National Autistic Society, "Autism Facts and History," accessed 22 March 2018; NICE guidelines [CG128]). Services continue to be disjointed, however, and many adults find it difficult to access the help they need (McCarthy et al., 2015). Although the legislation was welcomed, our own experience of working with adults suggests that services targeting individuals are not likely to be successful unless they acknowledge the community, family system, strengths, interests, and unique qualities of adults on the autistic spectrum (Warner et al., 2019). In this chapter, we will outline a systemic therapeutic orientation to working with the relational context in which adults with a diagnosis of autism live. There are a number of fundamental features of such an approach: firstly, the focus is on the nature of the relationships between people and how these may serve to exacerbate or alleviate difficulties and challenges. Secondly, there is a recognition that people and problems rarely present as neatly packaged and exclusive, such that "autism" is often accompanied by other issues of living, such as anxieties, traumas, losses, and conflicts (Lever & Geurts, 2016; Manion & Leader, 2013; Strang et al., 2012). Taken together, this may mean that the focus of systemic therapy may not be on the features of autism as such, and in some cases not predominantly on the person with the diagnosis, but on the wider network of their relationships. As an example we have worked with adults with autism who wanted us to assist them with difficulties their child (without a diagnosis) was having at school. It is of course possible that their child's difficulties and their attempts to assist them may have been influenced by the parents' "autism" but in this chapter we want to focus on what they may have in common with other psychological conditions as well as the specific contribution of their autism.

The term autistic adult is also in reality hard to pin down, encompassing a wide range of people with disparate needs and experiences. On the one hand, adults may have multiple and complex needs and be unable to live independently; on the other hand, adults may be living and working independently with specific issues regarding socio-communicative interaction (Crane et al., 2019; Hollocks et al., 2019; Lever & Geurts, 2016; Strang et al., 2012). Adults with autism may be teenagers who are living in their family home, students, parents themselves, or older people living in the community or residential settings. It is commonly overlooked that autistic children will inevitably become autistic adults and that their life cycle, as with most people, involves dynamic and recursive interaction and interdependence with families and communities. It is also worth considering the gray area around individuals with a diagnosis and other family members perceived to have high autistic traits. In many families the person with the diagnosis also has siblings, parents, or grandparents who share many of their qualities, challenges, and beliefs. For all of these reasons our own approach to working with adults with a diagnosis of autism has been to work with the family and community system encompassing children, adults, those with a diagnosis, their families, teachers, and important others. For example, we have worked with autistic parents, their autistic children, their nonautistic siblings, and their child's teachers and family friends. In order to achieve this model of working, we developed a systemic attachment-based intervention called SAFE (systemic autism-related family enabling) and a sister intervention called SAFE with Schools. SAFE is a manualized flexible approach that addresses the unique challenges presented and builds on the strengths and interests characterizing a particular system (McKenzie et al., 2020; Vassallo et al., in press).

Systemic Therapy

One of the core premises of a systemic approach is that problems and difficulties are relational rather than simply residing "within" individuals. This is based on the view that we are mutually influencing each other and problems, and solutions to these problems evolve from the flux of our interactions with each other. In its most radical version a systemic approach holds a formulation of problems, such as depression, anxiety, eating disorders, self-harming, and psychosis, as resulting not from some core genetically inherited abnormality but from adverse events in our lives and relationships (Dallos & Draper, 2015; Crittenden et al., 2014). Systemic approaches typically involve sessions in which all relevant family members are invited to attend to discuss their different views of the difficulties and to reflect on what they have tried to do to resolve the problems. A common feature of sessions is to validate and support the people's intentions and to help them become emotionally calmer in order to be able to explore in detail examples of problematic episodes in their lives. They can then attempt some different ways of acting with each other and consider different ways of understanding their difficulties.

Geoff

As an example, a family may be caught in an unhelpful cycle where the parents try to offer guidance and support to their young adult son with autism, but he experiences it as belittling and being treated as a child (see Figure 3-1). Consequently, he becomes irritated and at times explodes in anger, which leaves the parents both fearful as well as frustrated and feeling they are failing.

In this pattern it may also be the case that the mother Jean tries to "keep the peace" between Geoff and his father Pete who wants to protect the family from Geoff's temper and enforce some rules and discipline regarding his behavior. This can lead to an escalating pattern, including Jean and Pete coming to disagree about the best way to manage Geoff. In the family discussions it may emerge that both

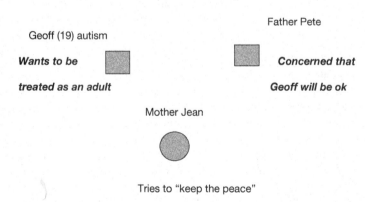

Figure 3-1 Family Triangle—Keeping the Peace

parents are trying to help and prepare Geoff for the outside world which they fear will be difficult for him. It was suggested that the parents retreat a little and allow Geoff to seek support from them when he decides to. Geoff was also invited to understand that his parents were acting out of concern and will welcome assurances from him that he is managing. Visually depicting this process can be helpful to make the processes more concrete, and gradually this can be used to help elaborate how everyone thinks and what their intentions and feelings are.

Evidence in psychiatry increasingly supports the idea that many severe conditions are influenced by events that have occurred in people's lives that have led to traumatic states (Timimi et al., 2011; Van Der Kolk, 2015). More broadly, systemic approaches not only consider the family system, but that of the professional systems, such as mental health, education, and social care services in the developmental trajectory of problems.

In our view, systemic ideas are of particular relevance to the field of autism for a number of reason: adults with autism live within families and communities and many report substantial battles in gaining the support they need in education and social care (Camm-Crosbie et al., 2019). Many adults with autism also recount adverse life events, stress, and mental health problems (Russell et al., 2016) experienced by themselves and their family members impacting their ability to negotiate life's challenges effectively. Consequently, adults with a diagnosis of autism may suffer a range of challenges: the nature of their condition of autism, adverse life events, constraints on the ability of families to cope, and difficulties accessing relevant support. A number of systemic approaches have been developed for assisting families, but these have mainly focused on addressing problems with children (Lewis, 2017; Neely et al., 2012; Smock et al., 2016; Solomon & Chung, 2012; Stoddart, 1999; Parker & Moleni, 2017). Mostly these approaches have concentrated on looking at behavioral sequences, as in the previous example, and on recognizing examples of successes and building on these. Monteiro (2016) has develop a systemic approach which explores the dominant narratives that families hold and, for example, offers the idea of individual "brain styles" as a way of thinking about autism in a more fluid and less diagnostic way. As in the previous example, such approaches suggest that Geoff's autism need not imply that he will "always" be dependent upon them.

Martin

As a further example, Martin was a young man in his 30s who had been diagnosed with autism at the age of 15. He had also experienced considerable anxieties and fears, and as an adult developed an eating disorder which had now become life-threatening. This condition may have been related to fears of contamination connected with his autism, but it had become the primary concern in his family rather than the autism, which had come to be seen by them as less relevant. His parents had both experienced traumatic events in their childhoods and also worked in highly demanding care services resulting in secondary traumatization.

Moreover, Martin was born at a time when his father was suffering with cancer. Unfortunately, Martin and his family fell through the gaps in services available because until recently his eating disorder had not been severe enough to warrant input from psychiatric services, and there were no appropriate services available for adults with a diagnosis of autism. Most relevant to this chapter, there were no services to provide family support/therapy to assist his family, including his brothers who were desperate with anxiety and experiencing a sense of helplessness in how to help him. His parents had worked extremely hard to support Martin and had stretched themselves financially to provide a house for him and his brother.

This is not an uncommon scenario where families take on a long-term caring role for an adult child, but it is unfortunate that their dedication is often not supported by services in terms of recognizing their needs as well as that of the diagnosed adult. Consequently, limited services may be available in terms of support for the adult child in a family but not for the family as a whole. This gap can also be seen to apply more broadly for other adult mental health services (Carr, 2009; Dallos & Draper, 2015).

SAFE

We have developed an approach (McKenzie et al., in press) for families with a child or young adult diagnosed with autism based on attachment narrative therapy (ANT; Dallos, 2006; Dallos & Vetere, 2009), which is a systemic therapy model integrating ideas from attachment theory and aspects of narrative therapy and theory. The core of this model is the idea that the characteristic patterns of interactions that families display are shaped by the attachment experiences that the parents (carers) bring with them from their own childhoods. Systemic therapies focus on identifying current relational dynamics or patterns that are seen to perpetuate difficulties.

SAFE is a manualized implementation of ANT and starts with a multi-family session where parents are invited to act as consultants to each other and share their experiences of autism, including the challenges they have faced and the coping strategies they have evolved. The aim is to offer validation and foster a sense of safety and support to share their difficulties and successes. It has been developed to be compatible with the needs of families with a diagnosis of autism both in its content and focus but also in the structure. We explain that the focus is not simply or predominantly on the person within the family presenting with autistic, but the effects on all of them. As an example, the siblings may feel their needs are being ignored and that their support and the sacrifices they have made are unappreciated. SAFE is a flexible approach with a range of activities, which can be adapted for use with adults, young people, and children within the family.

The sessions are clearly detailed so that the content, timing, and duration of the sessions and activities are clear and expected. There is also an emphasis on visual and action-based techniques and clear information about the verbal content to fit with what is known about the autism phenotype regarding the need for clarity and predictability. There is also an emphasis on continually monitoring the intensity and emotional demands of the session such that feedback is taken at the end and clear plans are stated at the start of each session.

SAFE is a flexible approach. Although we had initially developed it with a child focus, SAFE also addresses all members of the family, including the adults. It includes a range of activities adapted from systemic therapy (Dallos & Draper, 2015), for example mapping genograms, exploring family transitions and perceptions using buttons, tracking repetitive patterns of interactions or circularities, exploring attachment relationships and needs, externalizing using materials to represent the autism and other problems, and exploring areas of special interest. Sculpting with coins consists of inviting family members to represent their relationships with each other by choosing different buttons to represent each of them and placing the buttons spatially to represent closeness and conflicts. This can elicit mutual understanding about the different ways they see their relationships and also consideration of possible changes. Externalizing is another visual technique where families are invited to consider the problem as an external force that has come into their lives. They are invited to draw or make the problem out of clay, give it a name, and consider how it has come to control them and how they may be able to work together to reduce its influence. The aim is to avoid blame and holding each other responsible for the problems and instead focus on how they can work together to resolve their difficulties.

SAFE starts with adults completing the parent development interview (Slade et al., 2004) followed by two 3-hour multi-family sessions and three 3-hour single-family sessions. Prior to the therapy the parents complete the parent development interview with the therapists which explores their attachment relationship with their child and also their own experiences of how they were parented. This provides a platform of shared understanding of their backgrounds and an indication of adverse events and traumatic experiences that may be an influence on their parenting. SAFE was also adapted to address issues arising between families and educational settings (Vassallo et al., in press) by bringing teachers and adults within the family together in two full-day group sessions to build positive relationships and mutual understanding and to effect positive change.

SAFE does not focus specifically on individuals or the symptoms of autism, but on the issues that a relational system views as particularly pressing. For example, emotional aggressive outbursts known as meltdowns or emotional and social withdrawal (shutdowns) trouble many families and education providers. In such cases, a core starting point for assisting the families is to explore in detail these patterns and how the parents' own childhood experiences and attachments were influencing how they respond. For example, one mother described:

> When my son starts screaming it triggers those feelings of stress that I had when my mother used to scream (at me) . . . that kind of brings it all back, it's sort of like triggering, which is why I think that I find it particularly stressful . . . there you know there's a link between the past and the present.

SAFE also seeks to build upon the strengths and preferences that members of the system may have in order to build confidence, coping, and a sense of empowerment. The model strives for collaboration where all concerned are seen as experts in finding solutions and moving forward. For example, discussions may center on areas of special interest and this may be a vehicle for exploring relationships and new avenues of support and understanding.

It has occasionally been surprising for us to find that activities such as exploring areas of special interest, where we ask the children in the family to give a brief presentation to us and their family about something that fascinates them, have been of equal fascination for the parents. One parent who described himself as having autistic traits also talked about his interests. He proceeded to tell us in detail about his interest in astrophysics and, like the children, found it a very positive experience to have an attentive audience rather than feeling it was a burden for his family to hear about his favored topic. Sculpting with coins has also been experienced as helpful for all members of the family. For example, one mother was tearful with joy to see that her children described the period before and after the parents' divorce as one where the buttons representing the children were placed closer by them to their mother after the divorce than before. This is consistent with the practice of systemic therapy in that positive changes in mental health are seen to occur for all family members and can involve positive, mutually beneficial relational cycles so that as the parents feel better, the children feel more secure and the parents are more emotionally available, which in turn leads to further positive changes (see Figure 3-2):

The SAFE program was supported financially by research funding enabling us to work with more than 50 families over the last decade. In this time, we have worked with diverse families, teachers, educational managers, and special educational needs coordinators. The families have included parents, grandparents, adults, and children with and without a diagnosis of autism or perceived autistic traits. Almost all have shared with us substantial challenges, psychological distress, and adverse life events and traumas. We have also been privileged to share the talents, joys, strengths, and dedication of many families. Our research suggests that working systemically with these families has elicited positive change and that

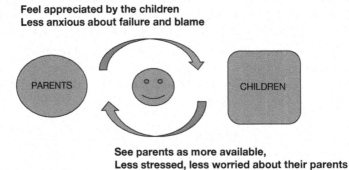

Figure 3-2 Benign Cycle of Positive Change in Families

families and communities experience SAFE as helpful and at times life changing, as one mother expressed (McKenzie et al., in press):

> I have already found these sessions so helpful they have helped me understand what I can do differently to help Joshua, myself and the family and given me confidence to make decisions and changes for the better.

In many cases, families reported to us that they had never been asked to share their life events, interests, and challenges before and that this was a very powerful experience for them. In the following example we describe some key aspects of working with David's family (see Figure 3-3).

David and His Family

David considered himself to have high autistic traits and to share many qualities with his eldest son. David's family consisted of himself, his wife, and their two sons: Malcom, who had a diagnosis of autism, and his younger brother. The family volunteered to take part in the SAFE program in order to obtain help in managing Malcom's behavior. He was intellectually extremely able, but they had become fearful of his "meltdowns," which were especially concerning for David. In working with the family we quickly discovered that when described in detail the "meltdowns" appeared to be relatively mild, but David experienced himself as reacting with considerable anxiety and also described that he was unable to assist his wife Jenny to offer support in setting some rules for Malcom. In David's terms, he felt he was extremely soft on Malcom and let him "get away with anything."

We became curious about why David experienced such anxiety at any form of confrontation with his son. He described a childhood which featured a high level of danger in that his father was an alcoholic and regularly physically attacked his mother and himself and his siblings. He had memories of sleeping with a knife under his pillow, fearing that his father would come and attack them hoping that he could protect his sisters. He had never spoken to anyone about these experiences

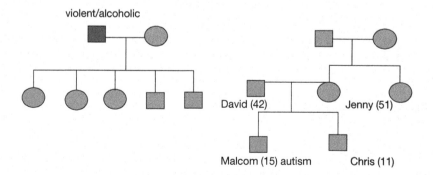

Figure 3-3 David and His Family

and commented that on reflection he realized that he was so determined to be a different, better, and less frightening father than his own that the "corrective pendulum" had maybe swung too far. Exploring such "corrective" scripts revealed this alternative narrative to the family, in contrast to the previous belief that it was because of his own autistic traits that he could not manage difficult relationships. Though the focus of the therapy had not been on David's autistic traits, he stated that he found the family work extremely helpful for himself and the children and that it had also improved his relationship with his wife. In addition, they realized that their other son Chris had been somewhat ignored, and they developed a plan in which they were less organized by their anxieties about David's meltdowns and needs. For example, they decided that they would alternate between Malcom and Chris choosing family outings. Previously they were concerned that Malcom's wishes should always be accommodated to avoid meltdowns. Through discussion of ways forward with the whole family they were able to overcome their worries that Malcom would react badly to this change and reported that Malcom enjoyed the days where his brother led the way and found he was calmer not being the focus of the family's anxieties.

SAFE With Schools (SwiS)

We have adapted the SAFE approach to include a focus on how the family and school systems interact. Sometimes this can be problematic with both sides feeling blamed and criticized by the other. Using many of the formats in SAFE, SwiS invites parent-teacher pairs (where they share a child with an autism spectrum disorder diagnosis) to meet over 2 days in groups of six parent-teacher pairs. The parents and teachers start by describing their typical day with the child and share difficulties and solutions, which is often revealing for both of them since they are not always aware of similarities and differences in the two contexts. Again there is a focus on looking at specific problems, such as meltdowns, and also the needs of parents and teachers in meeting the challenges. There are also opportunities to share successes and positive aspects and for both to feel reassurance of not being blamed or criticized by the other.

As with SAFE, although there is a child focus we have found that the groups are experienced as helpful for the parents who may have a diagnosis or describe themselves as having autistic traits (Vassallo et al., in press). An example of our work with a mother, Sonia, illustrates some features of this approach (see Figure 3-4).

Sonia and Her Family

In working with Sonia's family, we brought her and the school together to explore how relationships could be improved and the family, teacher, and special educational needs coordinator (SENCO) could work together.

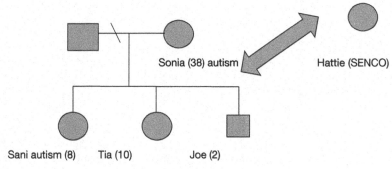

Figure 3-4 Infantilising Parent – Child Cycle

Sonia had a diagnosis of autism, as did one of her daughters, Sani. The other daughter, Tia, had behavior problems, and Sonia also had a toddler to take care of. Her situation was one of instability at home, being in an overcrowded temporary housing situation with three children. Sonia had a difficult childhood being a carer for her alcoholic mother, and in adulthood she had experienced chronic unemployment, substance abuse, and little in terms of a support network. She felt that she was often misunderstood and received a diagnosis of autism in young adulthood. Sonia sought support for her child with behavior problems and felt that Sani was largely unproblematic, as she and Sani understood each other well.

Sonia's relationship with the school had broken down, and her behavior and demands meant she was perceived by the school as being a trouble maker. Sonia felt she wasn't listened to and the school did not know how to support her daughters:

> I didn't have that personal connection with Tia's teacher, and, and from that point onwards I was like, no, this is not working for me, this whole "no conversation, cold shoulder, and out the door" does not work for me as a parent.

She reported that the SwiS sessions particularly helped her in being able to "slow down" and being able to unpack situations rather than getting frustrated with the outcome. She said her brain worked at a "million miles an hour" so she struggled to see *where* and *why* things were going wrong, seeing just that they *were* going wrong. SwiS sessions provided a calm forum to explore unhelpful circularities reflected in her own worries and difficult life events and to discuss her hopes and insights into her children's challenges with the teacher and SENCO. This process made her feel heard by the school and recognized as a parent with something positive to contribute. The experience was powerful for her and her family as she felt the school would subsequently take her seriously and act on her knowledge of her children. Prior to that she felt that she was judged, often as an unfit parent. Sitting with the teacher and talking alleviated some of that feeling and allowed her to work collaboratively with the school to plan a more supportive context for her children. The school was able to understand that she was a caring parent who wished to overcome substantial difficulties and came to appreciate her knowledge of her own life and that of her children, leading to improved channels of communication and support for the children.

Discussion and Conclusion

We have outlined an approach to working with families that we have applied in a variety of clinical settings and presentations. While we recognize the specific needs of adults with a diagnosis of autism, we have also outlined how we consider that they also have much in common with adults living in families presenting with other forms of clinical profiles. In some cases the problems they face are concerned with specific aspects of autism, but as we have suggested in this chapter frequently there are broader issues which have to do with the web of relationships in which they live. Not infrequently there are problems "elsewhere" in their relational systems that are not specific to, or caused by, the autism. A systemic approach can help to assist all of the people involved in a family system, which in turn can be of great benefit to the quality of life of the adult with a diagnosis.

Through these brief snippets of people's stories we hope to convey the importance and power of using a systemic approach that also incorporates aspects of attachment theory. Sonia's children had received interventions at school which were unsupported at home and perceived to be unhelpful. Consequently they were unsuccessful and inappropriate. Similarly limited support for David's son had served to make the family feel anxious and judged for not being able to manage his behavior. They were left helpless in repeated unsuccessful attempts to accommodate his every wish at the expense of their other child. In both cases the substantial needs of the parents were ignored or negatively construed. We have found that adults, young people, and children with a diagnosis of autism benefit enormously, often in surprising ways, from being listened to, supported to find their own solutions, and facilitated to being better understood and connected with important others in their family and community.

We have been granted permission to employ verbatim quotations from our participants in the SAFE and SAFE with Schools research programs.

REFERENCES

Camm-Crosbie, L., Bradley, L., Shaw, R., Baron-Cohen, S., & Cassidy, S. (2019). "People like me don't get support": Autistic adults' experiences of support and treatment for mental health difficulties, self-injury and suicidality. *Autism, 23*(6), 1431–1441.

Carr, A. (2009). The effectiveness of family therapy and systemic interventions for adult-focused problems. *Journal of Family Therapy, 31*(1), 46–74.

Crane, L., Adams, F., Harper, G., Welch, J., & Pellicano, E. (2019). "Something needs to change": Mental health experiences of young autistic adults in England. *Autism, 23*(2), 477–493.

Crittenden, P. M., Dallos, R., Landini, A., & Kozlowska, K. (2014). *Attachment and systemic family therapy*. McGraw-Hill Education.

Dallos, R. (2006). *Attachment narrative therapy*. McGraw-Hill Education.

Dallos, R., & Draper, R. (2015). *An introduction to family therapy: Systemic theory and practice* (4th ed.). McGraw-Hill Education.

Dallos, R., & Vetere, A. (2009). *Systemic therapy and attachment narratives: Applications in a range of clinical settings*. Routledge.

Department of Health. (2010). *Fulfilling and rewarding lives: The strategy for adults with autism in England*. The Stationery Office, London.

Hollocks, M. J., Lerh, J. W., Magiati, I., Meiser-Stedman, R., & Brugha, T. S. (2019). Anxiety and depression in adults with autism spectrum disorder: A systematic review and meta-analysis. *Psychological medicine, 49*(4), 559–572.

Lever, A. G., & Geurts, H. M. (2016). Psychiatric co-occurring symptoms and disorders in young, middle-aged, and older adults with autism spectrum disorder. *Journal of Autism and Developmental Disorders, 46*(6), 1916–1930.

Mannion, A., & Leader, G. (2013). Comorbidity in autism spectrum disorder: A literature review. *Research in Autism Spectrum Disorders, 7*(12), 1595–1616.

McCarthy, J., Chaplin, E., & Underwood, L. (2015). An English perspective on policy for adults with autism. *Advances in Autism, 1*(2), 61–65.

McKenzie, R., Dallos, R., Stedmon, J., Hancocks, H., Vickery, P. J., Barton, A., . . . Ewings, P. (2020). SAFE, a new therapeutic intervention for families of children with autism: a randomised controlled feasibility trial. *BMJ Open, 10*(12), e038411.

Monteiro, M. J. (2016). *Family therapy and the autism spectrum: Autism conversations in narrative practice*. Routledge.

National Autistic Society. (2018). Autism facts and history. http://www.autism.org.uk/about/what-is/myths-factsstats.aspx. Accessed 1 Apr 2018.

NICE: National Institute for Health and Clinical Excellence. Service user experience in adult mental health: improving the experience of care for people using adult NHS mental health services. (Clinical guideline 136.) 2011. http://guidance.nice.org.uk/CG136.

Neely, J., Amatea, E. S., Echevarria Doan, S., & Tannen, T. (2012). Working with families living with autism: Potential contributions of marriage and family therapists. *Journal of Marital and Family Therapy, 38*, 211–226.

NHS England. (2017). *Next Steps on the NHS Five Year Forward View*. NHSE, London.

Parker, M. L., & Molteni, J. (2017). Structural family therapy and autism spectrum disorder: Bridging the disciplinary divide. *American Journal of Family Therapy, 45*(3), 135–148.

Russell, A. J., Murphy, C. M., Wilson, E., Gillan, N., Brown, C., Robertson, D. M., Craig, M. C., Deeley, Q., Zinkstok, J., Johnston, K., McAlonan, G. M., Spain, D., & Murphy, D. G. (2016). The mental health of individuals referred for assessment of autism spectrum disorder in adulthood: a clinic report. *Autism, 20*(5), 623–627.

Slade, A., Aber, J. L., Bresgi, I., Berger, B., & Kaplan, M. (2004). *The parent development interview—revised* [Unpublished protocol]. The City University of New York.

Smock Jordan, S., & Turns, B. (2016). Utilizing solution-focused brief therapy with families living with autism spectrum disorder. *Journal of Family Psychotherapy, 27*(3), 155–170.

Solomon, A. H., & Chung, B. (2012). Understanding autism: How family therapists can support parents of children with autism spectrum disorders. *Family Process, 51*(2), 250–264.

Stoddart, K. P. (1999). Adolescents with Asperger syndrome: Three case studies of individual and family therapy. *Autism, 3*(3), 255–271.

Strang, J., Kenworthy, L., Daniolos, P., Case, L., Wills, M., Martin, A., & Wallace, G. (2012). Depression and anxiety symptoms in children and adolescents with autism spectrum disorders without intellectual disability. *Research in Autism Spectrum Disorders, 6*(1), 406–412.

Timimi, S., Gardner, N., & McCabe, B. (2011). *The myth of autism: Medicalising men's and boys' social and emotional competence.* Palgrave Macmillan.

Van der Kolk, B. A. (2015). *The body keeps the score: Brain, mind, and body in the healing of trauma.* Penguin Books.

Vassallo, T., Dallos, R., & McKenzie, R. (in press). Parent and teacher understandings of the needs of autistic children and the processes of communication between the home and school contexts. *Autism-Open Access.*

Warner, G., Parr, J. R., & Cusack, J. (2019). Workshop report: Establishing priority research areas to improve the physical health and well-being of autistic adults and older people. *Autism in Adulthood, 1*(1), 20–26.

4

Easing the Transition to Adulthood

BRIANNE TOMASZEWSKI, LAURA GROFER KLINGER, GLENNA OSBORNE, AND CLAIRE BRITO KLEIN ∎

KEY CONSIDERATIONS

- Despite increased funding for transition to adulthood services, traditional vocational rehabilitation supports have not improved employment and postsecondary outcomes, even for autistic youth with average or higher intellectual skills.
- There is emerging evidence that targeted interventions focused on autism-specific challenges (e.g., executive function, social skills, emotion regulation, adaptive behavior, self-determination) may ease the transition to adulthood.
- Transition programs have focused on supporting caregivers, creating transition/goal attainment plans to support self-determination, or teaching specific strategies to autistic youth. Few programs combine these three types of transition supports. Transition services may be most effective when provided in community settings where autistic youth are likely to seek support (e.g., community colleges) and when they generalize knowledge to everyday life.

OVERVIEW OF THE PSYCHOLOGICAL APPROACH

History of Transition Services

The increase in the rates of autistic individuals (based on autistic stakeholder preferences, we use identify-first [autistic] language; Bottema-Beutel et al., 2020) has been especially dramatic for those with average or higher intellectual abilities worldwide (Chiarotti & Venerosi, 2020), with current estimates in the United States that only 33% of autistic individuals have an intellectual disability

(Maenner et al., 2020). This is a significant change from the previous generation of adults, when the rate of intellectual disability was estimated to be 75–90%. Given this change in the demographics of autistic transition-aged individuals, there is a growing emphasis on creating evidence-based interventions to support positive adult outcomes, particularly for autistic individuals who have average (or higher) intellectual abilities, who historically have not received transition services.

Currently, autistic young adults with average (or higher) intelligence struggle to transition successfully from high school to postsecondary education and employment settings. Taylor and Seltzer (2011) found that autistic young adults with average intelligence were three times more likely to have no daytime activities after completing high school than autistic individuals with co-occurring intellectual disability. For autistic adults who begin a postsecondary education program or find employment, there are frequent disruptions, job loss, or college expulsion (Flower et al., 2020; Taylor & DaWalt, 2017; Taylor et al., 2015). Newman et al. (2011) reported that only 39% of autistic students who begin a postsecondary education program complete that program, compared to nearly 60% for neurotypical students.

Despite these poor adult outcomes, a decline in services begins in high school for autistic individuals without intellectual disability that persists into adulthood (Laxman et al., 2019). Only 18% of autistic individuals without intellectual disability are reported to receive employment services after leaving school, compared to 86% of those with intellectual disability (Taylor & Seltzer, 2011). However, merely increasing access to services does not seem to be enough to improve outcomes for autistic individuals (Alverson & Yamamoto, 2017; Burgess & Cimera, 2014). From 2003–2012 there was a 571% increase in caseloads of autistic individuals receiving vocational rehabilitation (VR) services. However, this increase in services did not bring an increase in successful employment (i.e., case closures), with only one third of autistic adults achieving successful employment (Alverson & Yamamoto, 2018).

To meet these growing demands for successful transition services, the United States Workforce Innovation and Opportunity Act (WIOA; 2014) mandated that states spend 15% of federal VR funding on Pre-Employment Transition Services (Pre-ETS) for 16- to 21-year-old individuals with a disability. Pre-ETS focuses on transitioning from school to postsecondary education or employment and is considered the first vocational rehabilitation service for high school students and those exiting high school. Pre-ETS includes work-based learning experiences, job exploration counseling, higher education counseling, workplace readiness training, and self-advocacy counseling (WIOA, 2014; see Table 4-1 for definitions of these activities). Activities similar to Pre-ETS have been used in other countries (see the work of Hatfield, Murray, et al., 2017, in Australia). To date, the majority of transition services have focused on providing program supports for youth with intellectual disabilities (e.g., Project SEARCH; see chapter 6) providing work-based learning opportunities for high school students to support a successful transition from school to work. Fewer programs have targeted autistic youth who have average (or higher) intellectual abilities, with no large-scale

Table 4-1 Pre-Employment Transition Services Activities Defined Under the Workforce Innovation and Opportunity Act

Pre-ETS Category	Activities Examples
Job Exploration Counseling	Identifying vocational interests and career pathways; providing information on occupations, local information on the labor market, occupations that match interests, andin-demand occupations.
Work-Based Learning Experiences	Job training, interviewing, work-site tour, job shadowing, or mentoring opportunities and work experiences such as paid and unpaid internships, apprenticeships, short-term employment, fellowships, or on-the-job training.
Higher Education Counseling	Information on the college application and admission processes, completing the Free Application for Federal Student Aid (FAFSA), college course offerings, career options, the types of academic and occupational training needed to succeed in the workplace, postsecondary opportunities associated with career fields or pathways, and resources that may be used to support individual student success in education and training.
Workplace Readiness Training	Programming to develop social skills and independent living, such as communication and interpersonal skills, financial literacy, orientation and mobility skills, job-seeking skills, understanding employer expectations for punctuality and performance, as well as other "soft" skills necessary for employment.
Self-Advocacy Counseling	Instruction on rights, responsibilities, and how to request accommodations or services and supports needed during the transition from secondary to postsecondary education and employment.

randomized controlled trials (RCTs) conducted to date for this group. Given that employment-based transition services for youth with intellectual disabilities are discussed elsewhere in this book (see chapter 6), the focus of this review will be on transition programs targeting autistic individuals who have average or higher intellectual abilities.

AUTISM-SPECIFIC CHALLENGES TARGETED BY TRANSITION SERVICES

Autistic adolescents often experience a combination of learning challenges (e.g., executive function, theory of mind, narrow focus of attention), with 72% of autistic adolescents having two or more of these challenges (Brunsdon et al., 2014). Thus, transition to adulthood programs often target one or more of these cognitive differences or address challenges with everyday life skills, including social skills, daily living skills, and self-determination that may result from these cognitive differences.

Executive Function

Autistic adolescents and adults have challenges with executive functioning (EF), including difficulties with planning, time management, task performance, and flexible thinking (Ambery et al., 2006; Wallace et al., 2016). Impaired EF has been linked to problems in areas that impact health, well-being, and independence in autism, including increased psychiatric symptoms (Lawson et al., 2015; Wallace et al., 2016), quality of life (de Vries & Geurts, 2015), academic achievement (Pellicano et al., 2017; St. John et al., 2018), and adaptive behavior (Kenny et al., 2019; Pugliese et al., 2016; Wallace et al., 2016). These EF impairments often negatively impact success in postsecondary education and employment settings (Hendricks, 2010; McGurk & Mueser, 2003, 2004).

Social Skills

Autistic adolescents and young adults often have difficulties with the social demands of college and employment settings (Hendricks, 2010; Hillier et al., 2018; Sperry & Mesibov, 2005). These social difficulties are associated with underlying cognitive challenges including difficulty with understanding other people's perspectives (i.e., theory of mind; Jones et al., 2018). Autistic transition-aged youth without intellectual disability often appear to be less socially impaired than they are and must simultaneously operate in an environment of more complex social relationships and greater social expectations. This combination frequently leads to awkward, intrusive, or offensive social interactions (Bauminger et al., 2003; Laugeson & Ellingsen, 2014; Sterling et al., 2008). Difficulties understanding colleagues' perspectives can lead to social "faux pas" in work or college settings and difficulty recognizing these "faux pas."

Emotion Regulation

Autistic individuals often experience emotional dysregulation, including co-occurring anxiety and depression, with co-occurring anxiety disorders present in 42% of autistic adults and comorbid depression present in 37% of autistic adults (Hollocks et al., 2019; Kent & Simonoff, 2017). More significant anxiety and depression levels are seen in autistic individuals who have average intelligence (Hallett et al., 2013; Strang et al., 2012). Autistic adults regularly report more significant subjective stress and diminished ability to cope with stressors, relative to neurotypical adults (Bishop-Fitzpatrick et al., 2015). Autistic adults experience exceptionally high levels of stress when there are unexpected changes to plans or routines (Hirvikoski & Blomqvist, 2015), resulting in autistic employees having difficulty coping with criticism and a tendency to dwell on negative experiences (Hillier et al., 2007).

Adaptive Behavior

Adaptive behavior involves everyday skills such as communication, daily living skills, and socialization. Higher adaptive behavior is associated with positive outcomes including employment, independent living, and quality of life during adulthood (Bishop-Fitzpatrick et al., 2016; Farley et al., 2009; Taylor & Mailick, 2014). At a time when adaptive behavior typically shows significant gains, there is evidence of a plateau of adaptive behavior skills in autistic transition-aged youth (Meyer et al., 2018; Smith et al., 2012). Autistic adolescents have significant discrepancies between their intellectual ability and adaptive behavior with almost a three standard deviation difference between IQ and daily living skills for those with above average intellectual abilities (Duncan & Bishop, 2015).

Self-Determination

Self-determination refers to a set of beliefs, knowledge, and skills (e.g., self-awareness, decision making, goal setting) that enable someone to engage in self-directed behavior and pursue their own goals and desires in areas a person feels is important to them (Wehmeyer, 1998). Self-determination theory emphasizes the importance of providing individuals with the opportunity and support to practice self-determined behaviors in their environment. Research on self-determination indicates that autistic adolescents have poorer self-determination abilities than those with intellectual disability or learning disabilities and that self-determination is positively associated with quality of life (Kim, 2019; White et al., 2018). Caregivers rated autistic young adults as having lower capacity than opportunities (Cheak-Zamora et al., 2020; Tomaszewski et al., 2020) in a combined sample of autistic young adults, with and without intellectual disability. Tomaszewski and colleagues (2020) found that in their self-reports, adolescents and young adults reported higher levels of capacity than both caregivers and educators.

SUMMARY OF EMPIRICAL EVIDENCE

Despite a growing consensus on the topics that should be included in transition to adulthood interventions, there are no large-scale RCTs examining the effectiveness of transition intervention programs for autistic youth who have average intellectual skills. However, there have been some promising pilot studies and small RCTs, all in the United States with the exception of one study in Australia, suggesting that interventions can ease the transition from school to adulthood for autistic youth. To date, interventions have either directly targeted caregivers, goal planning with both caregivers and students, or targeted student specific skill development.

Transition Intervention Programs

CAREGIVER-FOCUSED INTERVENTIONS

These interventions typically focus on supporting parent understanding of adult services and effective advocacy for their autistic transition-aged youth. These interventions have included transition-aged youth across a range of intellectual abilities.

Transitioning Together (DaWalt et al., 2018). Transitioning Together is a multi-family group program for autistic high school students and their parents focused on the transition from high school to college. In a preliminary waitlist control RCT, the intervention produced increased parent well-being and improved adolescent social interactions. A preliminary pilot study also demonstrated the feasibility of cultural adaptation of Transitioning Together for Latino families: Juntos en la Transicion (Kuhn et al., 2020).

Volunteer Advocacy Program-Transition (VAP-T; Taylor et al., 2017). Focused on adult service system navigation and disability services advocacy, a waitlist control RCT of VAP-T found that parents receiving the intervention showed increase in empowerment and comfort advocating on behalf of their child, as well as more knowledge about the adult service system.

Goal-Planning Interventions

These interventions focus on collaborating with caregivers and students to develop plans to leave the secondary education setting and include goal setting for a successful transition to adulthood.

Collaborative Model for Promoting Competence and Success for Transition (COMPASS-T; Ruble et al., 2018, Ruble et al., 2019). COMPASS-T is a consultation intervention that aligns the individual, family, and school around Individualized Education Plan (IEP) goal attainment. In COMPASS-T, a consultant works with the teacher, parent, and student (as much as possible) to link IEP social, communication, and work goals to postsecondary goals chosen by the student and parent, identify the student's personal and environmental challenges, and collaboratively develop a plan. In an RCT, COMPASS-T was successfully implemented with autistic transition-age youth with a large effect size for transition IEP goal attainment compared to the control group (Ruble et al., 2018).

Better OutcOmes & Successful Transitions for Autism Spectrum Disorder (BOOST-A; Hatfield, Falkmer, et al., 2017; Hatfield, Murray, et al., 2017). BOOST-A is an online program based in Australia to help initiate the planning process and empower students to develop clear plans for themselves after leaving the secondary education setting. The BOOST-A program consists of four modules: students identify their strengths and interests, identify their team of people supporting their transition, meet with their team to review career options and set goals, and continue these team meetings once per school term to discuss goal progress. A year-long, quasi-RCT of BOOST-A showed preliminary evidence for self-determination outcomes and career exploration outcomes in adolescents (Hatfield, Falkmer, et al., 2017).

Student-Focused Interventions

There is a growing evidence base for transition and support programs for high school and college students focused on supporting autism-specific challenges with a focus on EF, social skills, emotion regulation, daily living skills, and self-determination skills.

Stepped Transition in Education Program for Students with Autism Spectrum Disorder (STEPS; White et al., 2019). Further described in chapter 5, STEPS was designed to support secondary (STEP 1) and postsecondary (STEP 2) autistic adolescents and young adults with average or above average intelligence transition successfully to college. STEPS is a cognitive behavioral approach focused on self-determination and self-regulation skills to improve educational and socioemotional outcomes (White et al., 2017). For high school students (STEP 1), parents and one school personnel (e.g., a teacher) participated in the program along with the student. Postsecondary students (STEP 2) participated in weekly one-on-one counseling sessions and received online content that was also shared with parents. Both STEP 1 and STEP 2 included counseling sessions and community activities (a college immersion day in STEP 1 or outings with a counselor in STEP 2). The purpose of the immersion day was to foster self-determination and independence in a college setting (e.g., reviewing a course syllabus and discussing time management, meeting with the school's disability services office to learn about accommodations). Community outings for postsecondary students (STEP 2) were focused on goal-directed social integration with campus life (e.g., attending a club meeting, finding buildings on campus). Additionally, the counselor in STEP 2 maintained regular communication with the student outside of sessions to monitor and ensure progress toward goals (White et al., 2017). In an RCT of STEPS, high school students showed higher levels of parent-reported transition readiness to enter college (STEP 1) than the control group. College students showed higher levels of adjustment to college (STEP 2) compared to the control group. Further, these gains in adjustment showed increased maintenance after program completion in students with higher self-determination skills. However, both groups showed limited maintenance of skills at a 2-week follow-up, suggesting a need for further investigation into long-term treatment outcomes of transition readiness programs.

McGill Transition Support Program (Nadig et al., 2018). Nadig and colleagues (2018) conducted a small RCT of the McGill Transition Support Program for small groups of four to six autistic young adults without a co-occurring diagnosis of intellectual disability. To promote participant independence, caregivers were not included in the intervention. The program targeted social communication, self-determination, and working with others. Additional aims included improving quality of life and social problem solving. Participants in the intervention group reported increases in self-determination (including self-regulation) and quality of life compared to the control group (Nadig et al., 2018).

Acquiring Career, Coping, Executive Control, and Social Skills Program (ACCESS; Oswald et al., 2018). Another group intervention, the ACCESS Program, aimed to promote adult functioning and independence through social, adaptive, coping, and self-determination skills in autistic adults who had completed high school (Oswald et al., 2018). While participants were not all within the transition age, the curriculum was designed to meet the needs of autistic young adults. This program also included concurrent groups for caregivers to learn to support participants. In a waitlist control RCT, participants showed gains in adaptive skills, self-determination, and ability to access support from family and friends (coping).

The Connections Program (Hillier et al., 2018). This program provides a support group intervention targeting autistic college students (Hillier et al., 2018). Program curriculum included academic skills, interpersonal social skills and group work, future plans, and time and stress management. In a noncontrolled (open) trial, the authors reported that participation in the Connections Program was associated with decreased anxiety and loneliness and increased self-esteem.

TEACCH School Transition to Employment and Postsecondary Education Program (T-STEP; Klinger & Dudley, 2020). The T-STEP program was created as a comprehensive, manualized 12-week intervention program for 16- to 21-year-old autistic transition aged youth. The curriculum is designed to address autism-specific challenges including goal planning and attainment (focused on daily living skills and self-determination), EF (i.e., time management, organization), emotion regulation (i.e., coping with distress, accepting corrective feedback), and social/theory of mind skills (i.e., social niceties, effectively asking for help; see Table 4-2).

The T-STEP was designed to be implemented as a WIOA Pre-ETS program for autistic transition-aged youth currently enrolled in high school or college and includes all five of the Pre-ETS services. Specifically, the T-STEP intervention includes a 24-session work-based readiness class (i.e., a twice-weekly community college class), a work-based learning experience (i.e., a 2-hour per week internship to practice the soft skills learned in the T-STEP class), and weekly counseling services that mirror services typically provided on a college campus (i.e., self-advocacy, career, and higher education/academic counseling). Caregivers participate in initial goal setting sessions and receive regular newsletters throughout the intervention to support generalization of skills. Skills are taught using a variety of evidence-based practices (Hume et al., 2021; see Table 4-3). Because the majority of autistic students begin postsecondary education at a community college (i.e., 88% of young autistic adults attended 2-year colleges or vocational/technical schools; Roux et al., 2015), community colleges were thought to represent an ideal location to provide interventions for autistic transition-aged youth.

Table 4-2 T-STEP DIDACTIC CLASS SESSIONS

Session	Skill Area	Session Content
Pre	Goal planning	Individual goal achievement planning.
1		Introduction to T-STEP.
2		Tools and internships.
3	Executive function	Introduction to time management skills.
4	Executive function	Developing a personal time management system.
5	Social communication	Introduction to asking for help.
6	Social communication	Developing an asking for help routine strategy.
7	Review: Executive function & Social communication	Video modeling: time management and asking for help routine strategies.
8	Review: Executive function & Social communication	Practice: time management and asking for help routine strategies.
9	Emotion regulation	Introduction to distress and coping.
10	Emotion regulation	Developing a calming routine strategy.
11	Emotion regulation	Developing a calming routine strategy (continued).
12	Executive function	Developing a flexibility routine strategy.
13	Executive function	Introduction to organizational skills.
14	Executive function	Developing organizational skills routine strategies.
15	Review: Emotion regulation & Executive function	Video modeling: calming and organizational skills routine strategies.
16	Review: Emotion regulation & Executive function	Practice: calming and organizational skills routine strategies.
17	Social communication	Introduction to professional social skills.
18	Social communication	Developing a professional social skills routine strategy.
19	Emotion regulation	Introduction to dealing with corrective feedback.
20	Emotion regulation	Developing a dealing with corrective feedback routine strategy.
21	Review: Social communication & Emotion regulation	Video modeling: professional social skills and dealing with corrective feedback routine strategies.
22	Review: Social communication & Emotion regulation	Practice: professional social skills and dealing with corrective feedback routine strategies.
23	Review	Summary and review of skills and strategies.
24		Wrap-up and next steps.

Table 4-3 Evidence-Based Practices Integrated Into the T-STEP

Treatment	Description	T-STEP Examples
Cognitive behavioral/ instructional strategies (CBIS)	Teaches explicit strategies to change thinking, behavior, and self-awareness.	Relaxation strategies including deep breathing and muscle relaxation routines, and cognitive restructuring, mantras for challenging irrational thoughts.
Modeling (MD)	Demonstration of a target skill or behavior.	Role-plays of asking for help.
Reinforcement (R)	Consequences following a skill or behavior to promote future use of the skill or behavior.	Self-reinforcement: goal setting and rewards for accomplishment.
Self-management (SM)	Teaches self-management and self-regulation strategies in managing own behaviors and skills.	Use of self-monitoring checklists for organizations.
Social narratives (SN)	Explains social situations to highlight the perspective of others and to suggest appropriate responses.	Social narrative routines for greetings and compliments.
Task Analysis (TA)	Breaks down complex behavioral skills into smaller components. Increases independence in performing the larger behavioral skills over time.	Breaking down goals into action steps. Use of routine strategies to break down complex behavior (e.g., asking for help) into a series of specific steps.
Video Modeling (VM)	Uses video technology to record and show demonstration of a target behavior or skill.	Group videos of managing constructive feedback and asking for help.
Visual Supports (VS)	Concrete cues about an activity, expectation, skill, or routine such as visual schedules, work systems, graphic organizers, and scripts.	Use of visual reminder systems including daily calendar for time management, strategies for organizing study or workplace.

Initial research supports the efficacy of the T-STEP. In an open trial pilot study, 57 students (aged 17–21 years; average age 19.3 years) completed the T-STEP across three community colleges (Klinger & Dudley, 2020). Following student completion of the T-STEP, caregivers reported improved employment readiness skills and daily living skills. Students reported increased self-determination. In focus groups, students reported that the program helped prepare them to learn how to function in the adult world so that they could be successful as a college student and in the workplace. They responded that the program was "definitely" worth the time and that they would recommend it to others. Thus, across qualitative and quantitative assessments, initial results are promising for the T-STEP as an intervention addressing autism specific challenges during the transition to adulthood.

CASE STUDY

Intake Interview and Assessment

Jason is an 18-year-old autistic male who lives at home with his parents. He graduated from high school with a general education diploma and 3.0 GPA. Jason struggled during his first semester at community college and withdrew from all but two classes and earned poor grades in both classes. At intake, Jason had a part-time job at the local home improvement store and was practicing driving to get his driver's license. At home, his parents reported that while Jason could independently complete steps for self-care he needed reminders even for basic skills such as brushing his teeth. Jason and his parents reported that he struggled with time management, including being late to classes and failing to complete or turn in homework. Jason was accustomed to more involved teacher support from his high school setting, and he did not understand how to seek help when he started to struggle at the community college or at work. Jason reported feeling frustrated and anxious most of the time and that he often experienced emotional outbursts at home including crying and yelling at his parents.

Jason showed significant difficulties on the Behavior Rating Inventory of Executive Function-Adult (Gioia et al., 2005), earning an overall score of 57 (77th percentile) on the parent report version. Similarly, his parents reported poor work readiness skills on the Becker Work Adjustment Profile (Becker, 2005), with an overall score of 56 (73rd percentile). Jason obtained a Full-Scale IQ score (Wechsler & Chou, 2011) of 116 in the above average range. In contrast, his Vineland Adaptive Behavior (Sparrow et al., 2016) composite score was much lower at 75.

Case Formulation and Intervention Goals

Without the structure and supports of high school, and with the increased demands of college along with a part-time job, Jason struggled to compensate for problems typically associated with his autism including EF, emotion regulation, social skills, daily living skills, and self-determination. At his local community college, Jason began the T-STEP Program. During the goal planning/attainment module, Jason chose goals related to education (i.e., "I want to make B's in my two classes"), employment (i.e., "I want to increase my hours at work"), and independent living (i.e., "I want to learn to cook different foods").

Strategies and Techniques

Throughout the semester, Jason was given a workbook to support his learning the T-STEP tools (e.g., visual reminders, self-monitoring, self-reward, and routine strategies for time management, professional social skills, and emotion regulation skills). A variety of evidence-based strategies were used to teach Jason these skills (see Table 4-3). During the time management module, Jason was hesitant to try a planner system that incorporated a calendar listing his daily activities as well as self-monitoring of progress toward his goals. However, when the planner was individualized to fit his personal goals (i.e., to write in a time to remember to prepare a snack before work), he began to use the planner more frequently. His program instructor coached him to think about how he could use his planner to prevent most mishaps (e.g., running late to an appointment, not having materials needed for class). He also included self-reward activities in his schedule to reinforce use of time management skills.

During the coping with distress module, Jason created a "calming routine strategy" using a combination of cognitive behavioral intervention strategies (e.g., deep breathing, visualization, mantra) that he could use "in the moment" when he was distressed. He was encouraged to use visual supports to help him remember to use his routine strategies and was particularly enthusiastic about creating a visual reminder for himself that he laminated and kept in his wallet to remind him to use his calming routine strategy. He was also able to use this strategy to manage his anxiety when given corrective feedback at work or school.

Next, Jason and his classmates covered the professional social skills module, including the importance of using an "asking for help routine strategy." The concrete structure of the "asking for help routine strategy" seemed to make sense to Jason and to provide clarity around a confusing process that had seemed obscure to him. He reported that at work he had been worried about asking for help and that he was motivated to use this strategy in the future. When the topic of social niceties (e.g., greetings) was discussed, Jason reported that he knew all of these skills and felt he did not have much room for improvement. However, upon engaging in a video-modeling exercise with his peers in which common social mishaps were enacted, Jason realized that he could make improvements, including greeting his classroom instructors when entering class, telling the instructors "thank you" for the class when leaving, and using greetings at his internship and his part-time work. Jason used a variety of visual reminders to support more frequent use of his new social behaviors. He began smiling more and engaged in more social interaction with peers in class.

Outcomes

At the end of the program, Jason's mother reported improvements in time management ("he doesn't need much prompting to do things when asked"), self-determination ("he's more assertive and has more self-confidence"), and improved social skills ("he's more positive and kinder"). Jason also received a glowing evaluation and recommendation letter from his internship supervisor. Jason left his job at the home improvement store for a job he was excited to get at a local office (similar to his T-STEP internship). He began driving to his job and to classes and continued to improve his study habits and academic performance. Jason reported increases in self-determination and decreases in anxiety, spontaneously telling his T-STEP instructors that the program worked for him because the routine strategies actually taught him how to do the different organization, coping, and social skills rather than just telling him that he needed to improve in these areas. He reported that the "T-STEP gave me the confidence to do things I had been too reserved to do in the past."

CONCLUSIONS

Regardless of cognitive abilities, autistic transition-aged youth have difficulties with EF, social skills, emotion regulation, adaptive behavior, and self-determination, which may lead to increased difficulties in postsecondary and employment settings. There is emerging evidence that targeted interventions focused on these skills may ease the transition to adulthood. However, because of the relative recency of these transition programs for individuals with average or higher intellectual abilities, there is no knowledge about how these interventions lead to long-term outcomes, including employment, postsecondary education, and quality of life. Further, there is no research identifying which transition-aged youth benefit from which of these specific transition supports or a combination of these supports. Thus, further research is needed to recommend a personalized approach for autistic transition-aged youth.

REFERENCES

Alverson, C. Y., & Yamamoto, S. H. (2017). Employment outcomes of vocational rehabilitation clients with autism spectrum disorders. *Career Development and Transition for Exceptional Individuals, 40*(3), 144–155.

Alverson, C. Y., & Yamamoto, S. H. (2018). VR employment outcomes of individuals with autism spectrum disorders: A decade in the making. *Journal of Autism and Developmental Disorders, 48*(1), 151–162.

Ambery, F. Z., Russell, A. J., Perry, K., Morris, R., & Murphy, D. G. M. (2006). Neuropsychological functioning in adults with Asperger syndrome. *Autism, 10*(6), 551–564.

Bauminger, N., Shulman, C., & Agam, G. (2003). Peer interaction and loneliness in high functioning children with autism. *Journal of Autism and Developmental Disorders, 33*(5), 489–507.

Becker, R. L. (2005). *Becker Work Adjustment Profile: 2.* Program Development Associates.

Bellini, S. (2004). Social skill deficits and anxiety in high-functioning adolescents with autism spectrum disorders. *Focus on Autism and Other Developmental Disabilities, 19*(2), 78–86.

Bishop-Fitzpatrick, L., Hong, J., Smith, L. E., Makuch, R. A., Greenberg, J. S., & Mailick, M. R. (2016). Characterizing objective quality of life and normative outcomes in adults with autism spectrum disorder: An exploratory latent class analysis. *Journal of Autism and Developmental Disorders, 46*(8), 2707–2719.

Bishop-Fitzpatrick, L., Mazefsky, C. A., Minshew, N. J., & Eack, S. M. (2015). HHS public access. *Autism Research, 8*(2), 164–173.

Bottema-Beutel, K., Kapp, S. K., Lester, J. N., Sasson, N. J., & Hand, B. N. (2020). Avoiding ableist language: Suggestions for autism researchers. *Autism in Adulthood.*

Brunsdon, V. E. A., Colvert, E., Ames, C., Garnett, T., Gillan, N., Hallett, V., Lietz, S., Woodhouse, E., Bolton, P., & Happ, F. (2014). Exploring the cognitive features in children with autism spectrum disorder, their co-twins, and typically developing children within a population-based sample. *The Journal of Child Psychology and Psychiatry, 56*(8), 893–902.

Burgess, S., & Cimera, R. E. (2014). Employment outcomes of transition-aged adults with autism spectrum disorders: A state of the states report. *American Journal on Intellectual and Developmental Disabilities, 119*(1), 64–83.

Cheak-Zamora, N. C., Maurer-Batjer, A., Malow, B. A., & Coleman, A. (2020). Self-determination in young adults with autism spectrum disorder. *Autism, 24*(3), 605–616.

Chiarotti, F., & Venerosi, A. (2020). Epidemiology of autism spectrum disorders: A review of worldwide prevalence estimates since 2014. *Brain Sciences, 10*(5), 274.

DaWalt, L. S., Greenberg, J. S., & Mailick, M. R. (2018). Transitioning together: A multifamily group psychoeducation program for adolescents with ASD and their parents. *Journal of Autism and Developmental Disorders, 48*(1), 251–263.

de Vries, M., & Geurts, H. (2015). Influence of autism traits and executive functioning on quality of life in children with an autism spectrum disorder. *Journal of Autism and Developmental Disorders, 45*(9), 2734–2743.

Duncan, A. W., & Bishop, S. L. (2015). Understanding the gap between cognitive abilities and daily living skills in adolescents with autism spectrum disorders with average intelligence. *Autism, 19*(1), 64–72.

Farley, M. A., McMahon, W. M., Fombonne, E., Jenson, W. R., Miller, J., Gardner, M., Block, H., Pingree, C. B., Ritvo, E. R., Ritvo, R. A., & Coon, H. (2009). Twenty-year outcome for individuals with autism and average or near-average cognitive abilities. *Autism Research, 2*(2), 109–118.

Flower, R. L., Richdale, A. L., & Lawson, L. P. (2020). Brief report: What happens after school? Exploring post-school outcomes for a group of autistic and non-autistic Australian youth. *Journal of Autism and Developmental Disorders, 51*, 1–7.

Hallett, V., Lecavalier, L., Sukhodolsky, D. G., & Cipriano, N. (2013). Exploring the manifestations of anxiety in children with autism spectrum disorders. *Journal of Autism and Developmental Disorders, 43*(10), 2341–2352.

Hatfield, M., Murray, N., Ciccarelli, M., Falkmer, T., & Falkmer, M. (2017). Pilot of the BOOST-A™: An online transition planning program for adolescents with autism. *Australian Occupational Therapy Journal, 64*(6), 448–456.

Hatfield, M., Falkmer, M., Falkmer, T., & Ciccarelli, M. (2017). Effectiveness of the BOOST-A™ online transition planning program for adolescents on the autism spectrum: A quasi-randomized controlled trial. *Child and Adolescent Psychiatry and Mental Health, 11*(1), 1–13.

Hendricks, D. (2010). Employment and adults with autism spectrum disorders: Challenges and strategies for success. *Journal of Vocational Rehabilitation, 32*, 125–134.

Hillier, A. J., Campbell, H., Mastriani, K., Izzo, M. V., Kool-Tucker, A. K., Cherry, L., & Beversdorf, D. Q. (2007). Two-year evaluation of a vocational support program for adults on the autism spectrum. *Career Development and Transition for Exceptional Individuals, 30*(1), 35–47.

Hillier, A. J., Goldstein, J., Murphy, D., Trietsch, R., Keeves, J., Mendes, E., & Queenan, A. (2018). Supporting university students with autism spectrum disorder. *Autism, 22*(1), 20–28.

Hirvikoski, T., & Blomqvist, M. (2015). High self-perceived stress and poor coping in intellectually able adults with autism spectrum disorder. *Autism, 19*(6), 752–757.

Hollocks, M. J., Lerh, J. W., Magiati, I., Meiser-Stedman, R., & Brugha, T. S. (2019). Anxiety and depression in adults with autism spectrum disorder: a systematic review and meta-analysis. *Psychological Medicine, 49*(4), 559–572.

Hume, K., Steinbrenner, J. R., Odom, S. L., Morin, K. L, Nowell, S. W., Tomaszewski, B., Szendrey, S., McIntryre, N., Yucesoy-Ozkan, S., & Savage, M. (2021). Evidence-based practices for children, youth, and young adults with autism: Third generation review. *Journal of Autism and Developmental Disorders.* https://doi.org/10.1007/s10803-020-04844-2

Jones, C. R. G., Simonoff, E., Baird, G., Pickles, A., Marsden, A. J. S., Tregay, J., Happé, F., & Charman, T. (2018). The association between theory of mind, executive function, and the symptoms of autism spectrum disorder. *Autism Research, 11*(1), 95–109.

Kenny, L., Cribb, S. J., & Pellicano, E. (2019). Childhood executive function predicts later autistic features and adaptive behavior in young autistic people: A 12-year prospective study. *Journal of Abnormal Child Psychology, 47*(6), 1089–1099.

Kent, R., & Simonoff, E. (2017). Prevalence of anxiety in autism spectrum disorders. In C. M. Kerns, P. Renoo, E. A. Storch, P. C. Kendall, & J. J. Wood (Eds.), *Anxiety in Children and Adolescents with Autism Spectrum Disorder: Evidence-Based Assessment and Treatment* (pp. 5–32).

Kim, S. Y. (2019). The experiences of adults with autism spectrum disorder: Self-determination and quality of life. *Research in Autism Spectrum Disorders, 60*, 1–15.

Klinger, L. G., & Dudley, K. M. (2020). Interventions to support transition to adulthood for individuals with autism spectrum disorder. In F. Volkmar (Ed.), *Encyclopedia of autism spectrum disorders* (pp. 1–7). Springer.

Kuhn, J. L., Vanegas, S. B., Salgado, R., Borjas, S. K., Magaña, S., & Smith DaWalt, L. (2020). The cultural adaptation of a transition program for Latino families of youth with autism spectrum disorder. *Family Process, 59*(2), 477–491.

Laugeson, E. A., & Ellingsen, R. (2014). Social skills training for adolescents and adults with autism spectrum disorder. In F. Volkmar, B. Reichow, & J. McPartland (Eds.), *Adolescents and adults with autism spectrum disorders* (pp. 61–85). Springer.

Lawson, R. A., Papadakis, A. A., Higginson, C. I., Barnett, J. E., Wills, M. C., Strang, J. F., Wallace, G. L., & Kenworthy, L. (2015). Everyday executive function impairments predict comorbid psychopathology in autism spectrum and attention deficit hyperactivity disorders. *Neuropsychology, 29*(3), 445–453.

Laxman, D. J., Taylor, J. L., DaWalt, L. S., Greenberg, J. S., & Mailick, M. R. (2019). Loss in services precedes high school exit for teens with autism spectrum disorder: A longitudinal study. *Autism Research, 12*(6), 911–921.

Maenner, M. J., Shaw, K. A., Baio, J., Washington, A., Patrick, M., DiRienzo, M., Christensen, D. L., Wiggins, L. D., Pettygrove, S., Andrews, J. G., Lopez, M., Hudson, A., Baroud, T., Schwenk, Y., White, T., Rosenberg, C. R., Lee, L.-C., Harrington, R. A., Huston, M., . . . Dietz, P. M. (2020). Prevalence of autism spectrum disorder among children aged 8 years—Autism and Developmental Disabilities Monitoring Network, 11 sites, United States, 2016. *MMWR Surveillance Summaries, 69*(4), 1–12.

McGurk, S. R., & Mueser, K. T. (2003). Cognitive functioning and employment in severe mental illness. *The Journal of Nervous and Mental Disease, 191*(12), 789–798.

McGurk, S. R., & Mueser, K. T. (2004). Cognitive functioning, symptoms, and work in supported employment: A review and heuristic model. *Schizophrenia Research, 70*(2–3), 147–173.

Meyer, A. T., Powell, P. S., Butera, N., Klinger, M. R., & Klinger, L. G. (2018). Brief report: Developmental trajectories of adaptive behavior in children and adolescents with ASD. *Journal of Autism and Developmental Disorders, 48*(8), 2870–2878.

Nadig, A., Flanagan, T., White, K., & Bhatnagar, S. (2018). Results of a RCT on a transition support program for adults with ASD: Effects on self-determination and quality of life. *Autism Research, 11*(12), 1712–1728.

Newman, L., Wagner, M., Knokey, A.-M., Marder, C., Nagle, K., Shaver, D., & Wei, X. (2011). The post-high school outcomes of young adults with disabilities up to 8 years after high school: A report from the National Longitudinal Transition Study-2 (NLTS2) (NCSER 2011-3005). SRI International. https://ies.ed.gov/ncser/pubs/20113005/pdf/20113005.pdf

Oswald, T. M., Winder-Patel, B., Ruder, S., Xing, G., Stahmer, A., & Solomon, M. (2018). A pilot randomized controlled trial of the ACCESS Program: A group intervention to improve social, adaptive functioning, stress coping, and self-determination outcomes in young adults with autism spectrum disorder. *Journal of Autism and Developmental Disorders, 48*(5), 1742–1760.

Pellicano, E., Kenny, L., Brede, J., Klaric, E., Lichwa, H., & McMillin, R. (2017). Executive function predicts school readiness in autistic and typical preschool children. *Cognitive Development, 43*, 1–13.

Pugliese, C., Anthony, L., Strang, J., Dudlley, K., Wallace, G., & Kenworthy, L. (2015). Increasing adaptive behavior skill deficits from childhood to adolescence in autism spectrum disorder: Role of executive function. *Journal of Autism and Developmental Disorders, 45*(6), 1579–1587.

Pugliese, C. E., Anthony, L. G., Strang, J. F., Dudley, K., Wallace, G. L., Naiman, D. Q., & Kenworthy, L. (2016). Longitudinal examination of adaptive behavior in autism spectrum disorders: Influence of executive function. *Journal of Autism and Developmental Disorders, 46*(2), 467–477.

Roth, R. M., Isquith P. K., & Gioia G. A. (2005). *Behavior Rating Inventory of Executive Function—Adult Version (BRIEF-A)*. Psychological Assessment Resources.

Roux, A. M., Shattuck, P. T., Rast, J. E., Rava, J. A., & Anderson, K. A. (2015). National autism indicators report: Transition into young adulthood. Life Course Outcomes Research Program, A. J. Drexel Autism Institute, Drexel University.

Ruble, L., McGrew, J. H., Snell-Rood, C., Adams, M., & Kleinert, H. (2019). Adapting COMPASS for youth with ASD to improve transition outcomes using implementation science. *School Psychology Quarterly, 34*(2), 187–200.

Ruble, L. A., McGrew, J. H., Toland, M., Dalrymple, N., Adams, M., & Snell-Rood, C. (2018). Randomized control trial of COMPASS for improving transition outcomes of students with autism spectrum disorder. *Journal of Autism and Developmental Disorders, 48*(10), 3586–3595.

Smith, L. E., Maenner, M. J., & Seltzer, M. M. (2012). Developmental trajectories in adolescents and adults with autism: The case of daily living skills. *Journal of the American Academy of Child and Adolescent Psychiatry, 51*(6), 622–631.

Sparrow, S. S., Cicchetti, D. V., & Saulnier, C. A. (2016). *Vineland Adaptive Behavior Scales, Third Edition (Vineland-3)*. Pearson.

Sperry, L. A., & Mesibov, G. B. (2005). Perceptions of social challenges of adults with autism spectrum disorder. *Autism, 9*(4), 362–376.

St. John, T., Dawson, G., & Estes, A. (2018). Brief report: Executive function as a predictor of academic achievement in school-aged children with ASD. *Journal of Autism and Developmental Disorders, 48*(1), 276–283.

Sterling, L., Dawson, G., Estes, A., & Greenson, J. (2008). Characteristics associated with presence of depressive symptoms in adults with autism spectrum disorder. *Journal of Autism and Developmental Disorders, 38*(6), 1011–1018.

Strang, J. F., Kenworthy, L., Daniolos, P., Case, L., Wills, M. C., & Wallace, G. L. (2012). Depression and anxiety symptoms in children with autism spectrum disorders without intellectual disability. *Research in Autism Spectrum Disorders, 6*(1), 406–412.

Taylor, J. L., & DaWalt, L. S. (2017). Brief report: Postsecondary work and educational disruptions for youth on the autism spectrum. *Journal of Autism and Developmental Disorders, 47*(12), 4025–4031.

Taylor, J. L., Henninger, N. A., & Mailick, M. R. (2015). Longitudinal patterns of employment and postsecondary education for adults with autism and average-range IQ. *Autism, 19*(7), 785–793.

Taylor, J. L., Hodapp, R. M., Burke, M. M., Waitz-Kudla, S. N., & Rabideau, C. (2017). Training parents of youth with autism spectrum disorder to advocate for adult disability services: Results from a pilot randomized controlled trial. *Journal of Autism and Developmental Disorders, 47*(3), 846–857.

Taylor, J. L., & Mailick, M. R. (2014). A longitudinal examination of 10-year change in vocational and educational activities for adults with autism spectrum disorders. *Developmental Psychology, 50*(3), 699–708.

Taylor, J. L., & Seltzer, M. M. (2011). Employment and post-secondary educational activities for young adults with autism spectrum disorders during the transition to adulthood. *Journal of Autism and Developmental Disorders, 41*(5), 566–574.

Tomaszewski, B., Kraemer, B., Steinbrenner, J. R., Smith DaWalt, L., Hall, L. J., Hume, K., & Odom, S. (2020). Student, educator, and parent perspectives of self-determination in high school students with autism spectrum disorder. *Autism Research, 13*(12), 2164–2176.

Wallace, G. L., Kenworthy, L., Pugliese, C. E., Popal, H. S., White, E. I., Brodsky, E., & Martin, A. (2016). Real-world executive functions in adults with autism spectrum disorder: Profiles of impairment and associations with adaptive functioning and comorbid anxiety and depression. *Journal of Autism and Developmental Disorders, 46*, 1071–1083.

Wechsler, D., & Chou, H. (2011). *Wechsler Abbreviated Scale of Intelligence (WASI-II)*. Pearson.

Wehmeyer, M. L. (1998). Self-determination and individuals with significant disabilities: examining meanings and misinterpretations. *Journal of the Association for Persons with Severe Handicaps, 23*(1), 5–16.

White, K., Flanagan, T. D., & Nadig, A. (2018). Examining the relationship between self-determination and quality of life in young adults with autism spectrum disorder. *Journal of Developmental and Physical Disabilities, 30*(6), 735–754.

White, S. W., Elias, R., Capriola-Hall, N. N., Smith, I. C., Conner, C. M., Asselin, S. B., Howlin, P., Getzel, E. E., & Mazefsky, C. A. (2017). Development of a college transition and support program for students with autism spectrum disorder. *Journal of Autism and Developmental Disorders, 47*(10), 3072–3078.

White, S. W., Smith, I. C., Miyazaki, Y., Conner, C. M., Elias, R., & Capriola-Hall, N. N. (2019). Improving transition to adulthood for students with autism: A randomized controlled trial of STEPS. *Journal of Clinical Child and Adolescent Psychology, 50*(2), 187–201.

Workforce Innovation and Opportunity Act (WIOA), Publ. L. No. 113-118, 128 Stat. 1425, 29 U.S.C. § 3101-3361 (2014) https://www.congress.gov/113/bills/hr803/BILLS-113hr803enr.pdf

5

University-Focused Interventions

DAVID SCHENA, GRACE LEE SIMMONS,
ASHLEIGH HILLIER, AND SUSAN W. WHITE ◼

KEY CONSIDERATIONS

The majority of programs that serve young adults with autism (YAA) do not have empirical support.

1. Programs that serve YAA in postsecondary education tend to either assist transition into college or help with individual goal achievement while in college.
2. These programs tend to target college-specific needs (such as academic success, adjusting to college daily living, and accessing disability support services) in place of operating as direct therapy providers.
3. Empirical support for these programs tends to be based on a moderate sample size (average of 27 participants), using a mixture of pre-post studies and interviews over the courses of service delivery. Only one reviewed program has been evaluated with a randomized design.
4. Individualized mentorship was the primary component of the majority (six out of seven) of reviewed programs. This method may be especially useful given the highly diverse nature of abilities and symptoms in YAA.

OVERVIEW

Based on current Centers for Disease Control (CDC) estimates, approximately 1 in 54 youth have a diagnosis of autism/ASD; Maenner et al., 2020). Autism/ASD

In this chapter, we aim to be inclusive and respectful to all stakeholders. Terms such as *college*, *university*, and *postsecondary* are used interchangeably.

rates of diagnosis began to rise in the 1990s, coinciding with heightened recognition of autism/ASD in more cognitively able individuals. The children from this generation are now young adults. Given that 50,000 teens with autism/ASD enter adulthood every year (Shattuck et al., 2012), there will be upwards of 500,000 *more* adults with autism/ASD each decade. Moreover, the estimated societal cost of supporting a single individual with autism/ASD, without co-occurring intellectual disability, across their lifetime has been found to approach $1.5 million (Buescher et al., 2014). Considering this in the context of the fact that just 2% of all autism/ASD-related research focuses on transition and adult outcomes (U.S. Department of Health and Human Services, 2017), the inadequacies of our current support systems and the resulting strain on service delivery systems will grow more problematic.

Recent literature has called for increased focus on evidence-based programming to address barriers that inhibit healthy adult transitions and improve outcomes for youth with autism spectrum disorders (YAA), a growing, high-needs population (Chancel et al., 2020). Unfortunately, YAA frequently experience poor outcomes related to independent living. The adaptive skills of YAA stall or decline as young adults (Taylor & Seltzer, 2011) as opportunities for continued skill development dwindle (Mazefsky & White, 2014). The first 2 years after high school completion are characterized by low rates of paid employment relative to peers with speech and language impairment, learning disability, or intellectual disability (Shattuck et al., 2012), with only about half of YAA stably employed (Roux et al., 2013). Support systems, such as employment supports, can therefore be of great importance for many YAA (McDonough & Revell, 2010). This chapter will focus primarily on university-based supports for YAA.

A large proportion of YAA desire to earn a postsecondary degree (White et al., 2011). The proportion of YAA enrolled is still lower than expected, however, with notably fewer YAA attending college (32%; Wei et al., 2016) than the U.S. average (70%; U.S. Dept. of Health and Human Services, 2017). Those who do enter college may face a wide variety of obstacles; caregivers report concerns about social involvement, academic underachievement, and campus living (Hillier et al., 2020), which are often reflected in YAA self-reported struggles as college students (McLeod et al., 2019). Accordingly, support systems for college students with autism/ASD are of great importance, especially programs which have empirical support. In this chapter, we describe available services and interventions developed specifically for YAA who are in postsecondary settings, including colleges and universities. We acknowledge that there are many programs housed within institutions of higher learning that are dedicated to promoting the academic and social success of enrolled students with autism/ASD. However, the research base on these programs is small. Most support programs for YAA in college exist without any research to support their use. As such, we endeavored to focus on programs that have published data to support their use.

TRANSITION INTO COLLEGE

Beginning a college education can be a significant transition for anyone, but some common symptoms and co-occurring problems can make this transition especially difficult for YAA. Impairments in executive functioning (EF) can make keeping on top of assignments and deadlines challenging, or lead to an inflexible schedule (Alverson et al., 2019), while social and communication difficulties can make connecting with collegiate peers quite difficult (Dipeolu et al., 2014). Individuals and families also need to weigh potential benefits and problems of attending a larger university or a smaller community college, such as living arrangements and mastery of independent living skills (Adreon & Durocher, 2007). Necessary tasks such as navigating the college or university grounds can also be aggravated by the presence of, for example, a co-occurring anxiety disorder (White et al., 2011). In a large-scale, mixed methods needs analysis, White and colleagues (2016) found that primary challenges identified by parents, educators, and YAA included limited interpersonal competence, managing competing demands, and poor emotion regulation.

The Horizons college preparation mentoring program, offered by the University of Massachusetts Lowell (Hillier et al., 2019), aims to alleviate many of the previously listed potential problems via a mentorship program. This program has been in effect since 2009, and since Spring 2018 has been offered both in-person and online. Participants are randomly assigned to the online or in-person version, except during the COVID-19 pandemic when all mentors and mentees met online. Participants were eligible regardless of where they planned to attend college and did not need to be planning to attend UMass Lowell. The primary method of service delivery is through trained university students who provide service to aspiring postsecondary students with autism/ASD over the course of the six-week program. The Horizons mentors use a curriculum covering a broad range of topics designed to help prepare the participants for college life and ease anxiety around this transition.

Hillier and colleagues (2019) found that, at the conclusion of the Horizons program, participants felt better prepared for college life, had a better understanding of how college works, were more familiar with the structure of college lectures, and were increasingly aware of how to access support on campus compared to the beginning of the program. When asked, most participants were very positive about the program model and almost all reported they would recommend the program to others. Participants were particularly enthusiastic about the opportunity to meet one-on-one with a peer who was currently in college,—a highly valuable resource. The flexibility of the program model, which allows the curriculum to be tailored to the needs of individual participants, was also praised for providing an authentic approach where the students' own preferences and priorities are at the center of the program.

The Stepped Transition in Education Program for Students with autism/ ASD (STEPS; White et al., 2017) also provides support to high school students transitioning into adulthood. Unlike Horizons, which aims to improve performance through familiarity, STEPS highlights self-knowledge, self-regulation, and self-determination as targets for the program (White et al., 2017). Development of STEPS included a participatory process approach: developers integrated feedback from focus groups (e.g., college students with autism/ASD, parents of students with autism/ASD, educators and school personnel) as well as results from a nationwide online survey and consultation with a panel of clinical scientists and educators (White et al., 2017). The STEPS curriculum includes two distinct "levels": STEP 1 provides support for high school students planning the transition to college (six biweekly therapy sessions, parent coaching, and an immersion experience); STEP 2 is designed for YAA who have exited secondary school and have enrolled in college or not yet matriculated into secondary education (described in the following section). Students may participate in one or both STEPS levels. Initial findings from the STEPS randomized controlled trial (RCT) with 59 YAA indicated a significant treatment effect, where participants randomly assigned to participate in STEPS 1 demonstrated significant differences in transition readiness compared to those assigned to transition as usual (TAU; White et al., 2019). Specifically, high school students who participated in STEPS 1 were noted by their parents to be more prepared for the transition into college (White et al., 2019). Findings from this RCT suggest STEPS 1 offers demonstrable clinical utility in increasing high school students' transition readiness as they prepare for adulthood.

SUPPORTS WHILE IN COLLEGE

Once enrolled in college, students with autism/ASD can access universal student supports such as academic advising, tutoring, counseling, and careers services. If they register with the disability services office, they may be able to access academic accommodations and other supports. However, availability of services varies across institutions and factors such as self-regulation and self-advocacy may continue to be problems for some students (Adreon & Durocher, 2007; White et al., 2011). Navigating the social world of college may become more important as YAA seek to make friends and join groups. The fast-paced and somewhat unpredictable college lifestyle may prove difficult for some students to navigate, which may co-occur with the potential to experience stigmatization (Cox et al., 2020). Increasingly, universities are focusing on the retention and success of students with autism and many have developed tailored programming to address their specific needs. These supports continue to be of great importance, especially with respect to promoting social growth and development and buffering against executive functioning challenges.

Findings from the STEPS RCT with 59 YAA (described previously) indicated a nonsignificant treatment effect of STEPS 2 at follow up (i.e., two weeks after completion of the STEPS 2 program); however, a significant immediate treatment effect (i.e., while enrolled in STEPS 2, $p = .02$) was noted (White et al., 2019).

Specifically, university students who participated in STEPS 2 were noted to adapt more readily to the demands of college compared to those assigned to TAU, per their own self-report, while enrolled in STEPS 2 (White et al., 2019). Additional analyses of this cohort suggested that participants in the STEPS program experienced a significant reduction in depressive symptoms compared to those in TAU, though significant differences between the groups were not noted across measures of anxiety or loneliness (Capriola-Hall et al., 2020). Findings suggest STEPS offers clinical utility not only in improving YAA-perceived adjustment to college, but also in its mitigation of internalizing symptoms often experienced by YAAs during this transition period.

The Connections program is a support group model designed to address common challenges seen among YAA in a university setting. Aiming to promote friendship, mutual support, and connection between students with autism/ASD, Connections was in place at the University of Massachusetts Lowell from 2011–2018. This program was subsequently merged into a support group tailored for a broader population of students experiencing social challenges and anxiety, with the Connections structure forming the foundation of this and future services. Participants in Connections enrolled in a 7-week curriculum designed to address topics including social life on campus, academic skills, managing group work, and time and stress management. Retrospective data from nine separate cohorts seen over a period of 6 years (n = 52) were analyzed. Results indicated an increase in self-esteem, reduced loneliness, and lower generalized anxiety at the end of the support group program compared to the beginning (Hillier et al., 2018). Academic outcomes were also positive, with the majority (n = 41; 79%) having either graduated or being currently enrolled at the time of data collection (Hillier et al., 2018), impressive when compared to a graduation rate of 63% across the university (University of Massachusetts Lowell, 2018). Social validity was also high with participants indicating they had enjoyed the program, had made friends, and would recommend the program. When examined, a participant sample described improved postsecondary skills, such as study skills, knowledge of how to access resources and supports, goal-setting skills, and stress-coping skills. Previous work has indicated that many of these areas are challenges for students with autism/ASD (Alverson et al., 2019; Van Hees et al., 2015), so it is significant that the participants mentioned these as areas of improvement following the group intervention.

The Autism Mentorship Initiative (AMI) also aims to serve YAA during their college careers (Roberts & Birmingham, 2017; Trevisan et al., 2020). Offered through Simon Frasier University in British Columbia, Canada, AMI is a program encompassing the entirety of the traditional school year, beginning in September and terminating in May. Participants in this program are assigned to a mentor who is also a Simon Frasier student. The mentors receive initial and on-going training in order to best serve program participants. Within this mentoring system, AMI is individually directed and focused, such that every participant could be working on a different skill at the same time. Participants are encouraged to articulate their goals and difficulties in order to work with their mentor toward an improved outcome. AMI's home page describes some potential goals, such as improving academic skills, increasing knowledge of campus life, and becoming familiar with the availability of support (Centre for Accessible Learning, 2020). Other skills may include more familiar goals for people with autism/ASD (such as "improving communication ability"), but with a distinctive college flair; as opposed to working on communication as a whole, participants may seek to improve at talking to professors. Finally, in the event that participants wish to continue in the program, involvement is renewable after the termination of each year's services. AMI was evaluated by Trevisan and colleagues (2020) in a multiple time-point survey study; 19 students and 21 mentors consented to participate in the study, which consisted of pre-post participation comparison of scores on a variety of topics, collectively described as "college adjustment" and grade-point average. Researchers found that participants' academic performance did not differ significantly from September to May; however, they did note that participants made significant gains in all aspects of "college adjustment," including social functioning and emotional adjustment.

York University in Ontario, Canada offers a somewhat different program known as the autism/ASD Mentorship Program (AMP). Within AMP, mentors aim to provide participating YAA with skills necessary to succeed in college. AMP exclusively employs graduate students as mentors and uses a combination of individual meetings and group sessions (Children's Learning Projects, 2014) to teach these goals. The method of goal selection is also somewhat unique to this program; AMP presents potential goals which address academic domains (e.g., "Improve study skills and grades") social domains (e.g., "Develop or improve romantic relationships") and self-regulatory domains (e.g., "Better understand and cope with my feelings"; Ames et al., 2016). Participants select one of these goal categories and develop a specific goal or set of goals based on their desires and individual circumstances: while two participants might select "Improve study skills and grades," one participant might focus on setting aside dedicated study time, while another may strive to use a better study method. Between weekly or biweekly individual meetings and monthly or semimonthly group meetings, AMP aims to provide a supportive environment in which students can prioritize skill development. Ames and colleagues (2016) followed 15 participants through the program, as well as summarizing the growth of the program itself. Students tended to work on an average of six goals during their time with AMP, with 80% of students reporting that they achieved all or most of their goals. These goals tended to target social skills as a whole, improving emotional coping, and developing and improving both friendships and romantic relationships. Dating, romance, and sexual health were also particularly commonly appreciated topics as discussion topics during group meetings (Ames et al., 2016). Finally, the program itself reported a growth of 200% in its first 4 years of existence, though the exact number of participants yearly is unclear.

Inspired by AMP, researchers at Curtin University in Western Australia developed the Curtin Specialist Mentoring Program (CSMP) for university students with autism/ASD (Siew et al., 2017). Students with autism/ASD have the opportunity to register and receive mentoring from a peer, who is either a graduate student or an honors psychology student in their final year (Curtin University, 2020). CSMP primarily offers support through individual, weekly, 60-minute meetings over the course of one academic semester. Qualitative data collected from mentors indicated that mentees most frequently discussed time management, communication with professors and peers, and academic support in these one-on-one meetings (Hamilton et al., 2016). Participants and their mentors also participated in weekly social groups designed to facilitate social interaction and provide opportunities to practice social skills. Results from an initial pilot study of the program are promising; in addition to high rates of program satisfaction, all CSMP participants re-enrolled in the second semester of college. Additionally, a sample of 10 participants reported feeling significantly more supported and had significantly reduced communication anxiety after completion of CSMP (Siew et al., 2017). Qualitative results emphasized a number of positive outcomes including assistance with the transition to college, preparation for self-advocacy in communicating with college staff, and improved ability to manage emotions (Siew et al., 2017).

Finally, researchers at the City University of New York designed Project REACH, a group-based intervention for college students with autism/ASD which focuses on co-primary goals of improving self-advocacy and developing social skills (Gillespie-Lynch et al., 2017). The semester-long program was implemented twice, with two different groups of students who either self-identified as autistic and/or received services in high school for autism, based on review of their individual education plans. Participants were paired with a trained mentor (undergraduate and graduate students) who provided weekly, one-on-one counseling for the semester (14 weeks). Additionally, participating students attended weekly, hour-long, mentor-led group sessions with up to eight other students for approximately 10 weeks. The first program curriculum (spring semester) focused largely on social skills, while the second program (fall semester) focused more explicitly on developing self-advocacy, based on feedback provided during focus groups where students reported themes of self-advocacy after participating in the spring program (e.g., continued reliance on others to advocate for them; Gillespie-Lynch et al., 2017). When piloted with 28 participants, findings indicated that participants reported significantly increased perceived social support from friends after completing the self-advocacy focused program, though this was not noted in the social-skill focused program. Furthermore, the integration of self-advocacy content into the standardized curriculum resulted in participants' report of significantly increased academic self-advocacy skills at the end of the fall semester (Gillespie-Lynch et al., 2017). The authors' integration of student feedback in tailoring the curriculum to their participants' needs highlights the importance of using stakeholder perspectives to shape intervention work and maximize therapeutic gains.

CASE STUDY

Philip is an 18-year-old White male who was diagnosed with autism/ASD at age 2. Philip wanted to study biology, engineering, or a combination of the two disciplines. To best achieve this goal, he entered the Horizons program in spring 2020 (aged 17). He was matched with a mentor from the University of Massachusetts Lowell, a female senior psychology major, and they met during Philip's senior year of high school in spring 2020. Philip completed the program despite the onset of the COVID-19 pandemic; his mentor described him as an "attentive listener," "very engaged," and "advanced in his knowledge about college."

At the end of his time with Horizons, Philip reported being eager to take on increased responsibility, having a clearer understanding of college coursework, and feeling more content with his decision to go to college than he had reported at the beginning of the program. He especially appreciated that Horizons "takes into account individual students" and educates on the individual level. When asked about his least favorite aspect of the program, he described that it was "not fully prepared for students that are ahead" and suggested that the program could "make a schedule for students who are already accepted or have chosen their college."

Philip also participated in a 1-year follow-up interview to describe his college experience and to further discuss his experiences in the Horizons program. He had completed his fall semester at a local 4-year private university where he took five classes and earned a GPA of 3.48. At this time, he was taking four classes, a workload which he reported was harder than that in his first semester. Philip is commuting to campus each day. He is connecting with others on campus, particularly through a weekly radio sports show he hosts. While he felt there were fewer social opportunities due to COVID-19, he has made friends through classes and clubs. He plans to seek out an internship in his field the following year. When asked, he described his primary challenge as the timely completion of assignments and had grown to dislike how many classes assigned work at the same time. He also described how the ever-changing pace of college life had proven to be difficult to adjust to. However, Philip had accessed accommodations through Disability Services, including extra time on tests, use of a smart pen, permission to type notes in class, accessing copies of professors' notes, personally recording lectures, and sometimes testing in a distraction-free environment. Finally, concerning Horizons, he described the meetings with his mentor as helpful and was glad he took part.

OVERALL DISCUSSION

Certain commonalities run through the previously mentioned programs, regardless of whether they target transitioning students or students established in collegiate life. These programs tend to operate on the individual level or in small groups augmented by frequent individual sessions. Horizons and STEPS, for example, make use of individual meetings, while AMP and Project REACH combine this individual approach with regular group sessions. This is an interesting trend and a practical response to the famous heterogeneity of symptoms, abilities, and needs within the autistic population (Hollander et al., 2011). Connections, in contrast, prioritizes group meetings and discussions over individual goal completion in service to the primary goal of promoting friendship and support between students with autism/ASD.

It is also interesting that most reviewed programs contain an element of "mentorship." Exactly whom this mentorship is coming from varies slightly from program to program. Horizons and AMI both use undergraduates as mentors, while STEPS and AMU recruit graduate student mentors. The exact sources of mentors may be indicative of a variety of factors, such as mentorship philosophy (e.g., whether the influence of a peer or a professional may be superior) and pragmatic considerations (e.g., availability of doctoral students). However, the commonality of this mentorship approach itself necessitates further investigation, especially regarding the social improvements and advances in college adjustment reported by these programs.

Finally, in terms of the research itself, studies contained an average of 27 participants (SD 16.34, range 7–59). These studies were usually conducted in one-on-one settings, either in entirety (six studies) or in part (two studies). Only one program, Connections, was studied entirely in the context of groups. Studies rarely described their settings, with no study taking place entirely in any one location. While few studies stated it, most studies could be presumed to be open trials, with only one program, STEPS, using an RCT approach. The remainder used either pre-post assessment measures (Connections, AMI, AMP, UNY) or these measures with interviews (CSMP, Horizons).

CONCLUSION AND CALL FOR RESEARCH

These programs stand as examples of empirically supported programs for college students with autism/ASD across two North American countries. However, it would seem that the vast majority of university-level programs which give service to students autism/ASD remain without empirical support. For example, CAN released "United States College Programs for Autistic Students" (McDermott et al., 2020), a document which reviews university autism-centered programs across the continental 48 United States. A total of 82 programs were described, including details about the operating university (city, usual length of program, etc.) and the university's affiliated autism-centered program, where applicable. We took a sample of 20 of these listed programs and searched for empirical evaluations using the following search engines: Academic Search Premier, Alternative Press Index, APA PsycArticles, APA PsycInfo, ERIC, and Google Scholar. No empirical support was found for programs reviewed, though some programs did have published material describing them (such as Texas A&M's Spectrum Living Learning Community; Hurley, 2020). While we do not dismiss the possibility of empirical support for reviewed programs (which may be in-press or in another database), this brief literature review suggests that most college autism services operate without empirical support. This may be understandable, given that the need for programming has far outpaced the field's ability to keep up in terms of identifying research-supported transition services.

However, some programs without direct empirical support may be more promising than others due to a connection with an already-supported program. For example, the TEAACH School Transition to Employment and Post-Secondary Education Program (T-STEP) is an extension and specialization of the well-known TEAACH method (see chapter 4). TEAACH itself is a program demonstrated to be effective at improving social skills, executive functioning, and maladaptive behavior rates in children and adolescents (Abshirini et al., 2020; Virues-Ortega et al., 2013). Based on well-established applied behavior analysis (ABA) principles, TEAACH can claim extensive empirical support for its services (TEAACH Autism Program, n.d.). T-STEP was founded as a specialization of this method in 2017, aiming to improve transition into both postsecondary education and employment. However, at the time of this writing, no published reports on the efficacy of T-STEP are available.

In summary, relatively few university-based autism support programs can draw on readily available empirical evidence. We hope to inspire additional research to validate these programs and to further investigate those which do have empirical support. We specifically call for investigation into under-researched methods of support, such as living learning communities (Hurley, 2020). The landscape of transition programs that exist, and the extant research base, suggest that supports typically involve some combination of skills training, peer mentoring, and experiential learning.

REFERENCES

Abshirini, M., Asgari, P., Heidari, A., & Naderi, F. (2021). The comparison of the effectiveness of training based on the theory of mind and the method of TEACCH on the executive functions of the children with an autism spectrum disorder in Bushehr City. *Jundishapur Journal of Chronic Disease Care, 10*(1): e103465.

Adreon, D., & Durocher, J. S. (2007). Evaluating the college transition needs of individuals with high-functioning autism spectrum disorders. *Intervention in School and Clinic, 42*(5), 271–279.

Alverson, C. Y., Lindstrom, L. E., & Hirano, K. A. (2019). High school to college: Transition experiences of young adults with autism. *Focus on Autism and Other Developmental Disabilities, 34*(1), 52–64.

Ames, M. E., McMorris, C. A., Alli, L. N., & Bebko, J. M. (2016). Overview and evaluation of a mentorship program for university students with ASD. *Focus on Autism and Other Developmental Disabilities, 31*(1), 27–36.

Buescher, A. V. S., Cidav, Z., Knapp, M., & Mandell, D. S. (2014). Costs of autism spectrum disorders in the United Kingdom and the United States. *JAMA Pediatrics, 168*(8), 721–728.

Capriola-Hall, N. N., Brewe, A. M., Golt, J., & White, S. W. (2021). Anxiety and depression reduction as distal outcomes of a college transition readiness program for adults with autism. *Journal of Autism and Developmental Disorders, 51*, 98–306.

Centre for Accessible Learning. (2020). Autism mentorship initiative. https://www.sfu.ca/students/accessible-learning/programs-and-services/autism-mentorship-program.html

Chancel, R., Miot, S., Dellapiazza, F., & Baghdadli, A. (2020). Group-based educational interventions in adolescents and young adults with ASD without ID: A systematic review focusing on the transition to adulthood. *European Child and Adolescent Psychiatry*, 1–21.

Children's Learning Projects. (2014). Autism Spectrum Disorders (ASD) Mentorship Program (AMP). https://bebko.apps01.yorku.ca/clp/?page_id=132

Cox, B. E., Nachman, B. R., Thompson, K., Dawson, S., Edelstein, J. A., & Breeden, C. (2020). An exploration of actionable insights regarding college students with autism: A review of the literature. *The Review of Higher Education*, *43*(4), 935–966.

Curtin University. (2020). *Autism and related conditions mentoring*. https://students.curtin.edu.au/experience/mentoring/autism-related-conditions/

Dipeolu, A. O., Storlie, C., & Johnson, C. (2014). Transition to college and students with high functioning autism spectrum disorder: Strategy considerations for school counselors. *Journal of School Counseling*, *12*(11), n11.

Gillespie-Lynch, K., Bublitz, D., Donachie, A., Wong, V., Brooks, P. J., & D'Onofrio, J. (2017, April). "For a long time our voices have been hushed": Using student perspectives to develop supports for neurodiverse college students. *Frontiers in Psychology*, *8*, 1–14.

Hamilton, J., Stevens, G., & Girdler, S. (2016) Becoming a mentor: The impact of training and the experience of mentoring university students on the autism spectrum. *PLOS One*, *11*(4):30153204.

Hillier, A., Goldstein, J., Murphy, D., Trietsch, R., Keeves, J., Mendes, E., & Queenan, A. (2018). Supporting university students with autism spectrum disorder. *Autism*, *22*(1), 20–28.

Hillier, A., Ryan, J., Buckingham, A., Schena, D., Queenan, A., Dottolo, A., & Abreu, M. (2020). Prospective college students with autism spectrum disorder: Parent perspectives. *Psychological Reports*, *122*(1), 88–107.

Hillier, A., Ryan, J., Donnelly, S. M., & Buckingham, A. (2019). Peer mentoring to prepare high school students with autism spectrum disorder for college. *Advances in Neurodevelopmental Disorders*, *3*(4), 411–422.

Hollander, E., Kolevzon, A., & Coyle, J. T. (Eds.). (2011). *Textbook of autism spectrum disorders*. American Psychiatric Publishing, Inc.

Hurley, G. (2020). Residence life accommodations for college students with autism spectrum disorders [Unpublished senior thesis]. Belmont University.

Maenner, M. J., Shaw, K. A., Baio, J., Washington, A., Patrick, M., DiRienzo, M., Christensen, D. L., Wiggins, L. D., Pettygrove, S., Andrews, J. G., Lopez, M., Hudson, A., Baroud, T., Schwenk, Y., White, T., Rosenberg, C. R., Lee, L.-C., Harrington, R. A., Huston, M., . . . Dietz, P. M. (2020). Prevalence of autism spectrum disorder among children aged 8 years—Autism and Developmental Disabilities Monitoring Network, 11 sites, United States, 2016. *MMWR Surveillance Summaries*, *69*(4), 1–12. https://doi.org/10.15585/mmwr.ss6904a1

Mazefsky, C. A., & White, S. W. (2014). Adults with autism. In F. R. Volkmar, S. Rogers, R. Paul, & K. A. Pelphrey (Eds.), *Handbook of autism and pervasive developmental disorders* (pp. 191–211). Wiley Press.

McDermott, N., Hartlage, A., Jackson, B., & Orlando, A. M. (2020). United States programs for college students. *College Autism Network*. https://collegeautismnetwork.org/wp-content/uploads/2020/10/Nachman-McDermott-2020-Autism-College-Programs-PPT-5.28.2020.pdf

McDonough, J. T., & Revell, G. (2010). Accessing employment supports in the adult system for transitioning youth with autism spectrum disorders. *Journal of Vocational Rehabilitation, 32*(2), 89–100.

McLeod, J. D., Meanwell, E., & Hawbaker, A. (2019). The experiences of college students on the autism spectrum: A comparison to their neurotypical peers. *Journal of Autism and Developmental Disorders, 49*(6), 2320–2336.

Roberts, N., & Birmingham, E. (2017). Mentoring university students with ASD: a mentee-centered approach. *Journal of Autism and Developmental Disorders, 47*(4), 1038–1050.

Roux, A. M., Shattuck, P. T., Cooper, B. P., Anderson, K. A., Wagner, M., & Narendorf, S. C. (2013). Postsecondary employment experiences among young adults with an autism spectrum disorder RH: Employment in young adults with autism. *Journal of the American Academy of Child and Adolescent Psychiatry, 52*(9), 931–939.

Shattuck, P. T., Narendorf, S. C., Cooper, B., Sterzing, P. R., Wagner, M., & Taylor, J. L. (2012). Postsecondary education and employment among youth with an autism spectrum disorder. *Pediatrics, 129*(6), 1042–1049.

Siew, C. T., Mazzucchelli, T. G., Rooney, R., & Girdler, S. (2017). A specialist peer mentoring program for university students on the autism spectrum: A pilot study. *PLoS ONE, 12*(7), 1–18.

Taylor, J. L., & Seltzer, M. M. (2011). Employment and post-secondary educational activities for young adults with autism spectrum disorders during transition to adulthood. *Journal of Autism and Developmental Disorders, 41*(5), 566–574.

Trevisan, D. A., Leach, S., Iarocci, G., & Birmingham, E. (2020). Evaluation of a peer mentorship program for autistic college students. *Autism in Adulthood, 3*(2), 187–194.

University of Massachusetts Lowell. (2018). Graduation rates. https://www.uml.edu/institutional-research/graduation-rates.aspx

U.S. Department of Health and Human Services. (2017). *Report to Congress: Young adults and transitioning youth with autism spectrum disorder.* https://www.hhs.gov/sites/default/files/2017AutismReport.pdf

Van Hees, V., Moyson, T., & Roeyers, H. (2015). Higher education experiences of students with autism spectrum disorder: Challenges, benefits and support needs. *Journal of Autism and Developmental Disorders, 45*(6), 1673–1688.

Virues-Ortega, J., Julio, F. M., & Pastor-Barriuso, R. (2013). The TEACCH program for children and adults with autism: A meta-analysis of intervention studies. *Clinical Psychology Review, 33*(8), 940–953.

Wei, X., Wagner, M., Hudson, L., Yu, J. W., & Javitz, H. (2016). The effect of transition planning participation and goal-setting on college enrollment among youth with autism spectrum disorders. *Remedial and Special Education, 37*(1), 3–14.

White, S. W., Elias, R., Capriola-Hall, N. N., Smith, I. C., Conner, C. M., Asselin, S. B., Howlin, P., Getzel, E. E., & Mazefsky, C. A. (2017). Development of a college transition and support program for students with autism spectrum disorder. *Journal of Autism and Developmental Disorders, 47*(10), 3072–3078.

White, S. W., Elias, R., Salinas, C. E., Capriola, N., Conner, C. M., Asselin, S. B., Miyazaki, Y., Mazefsky, C. A., Howlin, P., & Getzel, E. E. (2016). Students with autism spectrum disorder in college: Results from a preliminary mixed methods needs analysis. *Research in Developmental Disabilities, 56*, 29–40.

White, S. W., Ollendick, T. H., & Bray, B. C. (2011). College students on the autism spectrum: Prevalence and associated problems. *Autism, 15*(6), 683–701.

White, S. W., Smith, I. C., Miyazaki, Y., Conner, C. M., Elias, R., & Capriola-Hall, N. N. (2019). Improving transition to adulthood for students with autism: A randomized controlled trial of STEPS. *Journal of Clinical Child & Adolescent Psychology, 50*(2), 1–15.

6

Employment-
Focused Interventions

**CAROL SCHALL, STACI CARR, LAUREN AVELLONE,
AND PAUL WEHMAN ■**

KEY CONSIDERATIONS

- Competitive integrated employment provides benefits to individuals with ASD, including increased independence and socialization with peers without disabilities.
- Competitive integrated employment should be the first option for all individuals with ASD because of the benefits provided.
- Acquiring competitive integrated employment involves teaching the individual with ASD marketable skills *and* addressing the availability of needed supports and employer attitudes.
- There is a growing literature describing evidence-based and promising interventions that increase access for an individual with ASD to competitive integrated employment.
- Employment interventions requires an understanding of the strengths, interests, and preferences of an individual with ASD.
- Employers value their employees with ASD because of, not in spite of, some of the positive characteristics of ASD.
- The use of applied behavior analysis (ABA) may be useful for adults with ASD seeking or employed in competitive integrated employment.

RATIONALE FOR EMPLOYMENT INTERVENTION FOR ADULTS WITH ASD

It may seem odd to include a chapter regarding employment interventions in a book that focuses on psychological therapies for adults with ASD. After all, the focus of many therapeutic techniques is to ameliorate the impact of a disorder through a medical or psychological intervention. Many of the chapters in this book provide detailed reviews and case studies to demonstrate how a particular therapeutic technique, such as positive behavior support (see chapter 8) or dialectical behavior therapy (see chapter 12) can support a person with ASD in learning to deal with the challenges of disruptive behavior, depression, or neurosis.

This chapter, however, does not seek to discuss therapeutic techniques to improve the symptoms of a chronic psychiatric condition, or even teach the individual with ASD to adjust to the impact of the disorder. Instead, we think adults with ASD seeking employment are part of an ecological system that involves public policy, societal beliefs about disability, and the availability of supports at work. These are all issues that lie outside the scope of the person's individual skills and can either help or hinder their quest to gain competitive integrated employment (CIE; Wehman et al., 2019). Thus, interventions to increase CIE among adults with ASD must include both individual skill development and community connections. According to the United States Workforce Innovations Opportunity Act (WIOA; 2014), CIE is part- or full-time employment in a private, government, or public business where a person with a disability:

- is compensated at or above minimum wage,
- is paid the same rate as an employee without disabilities,
- is eligible for the same level of benefits provided to employees without disabilities,
- interacts with other persons without disabilities at the same level as other employees, and
- is eligible for promotions at the same level as other employees performing the same or similar work (29 U.S.C. §705, WIOA, 2014).

We know paid work is the defining activity of adulthood (Arnett, 2014; Wehman et al., 2019). Employment provides the adult without disabilities financial, physical, and psychological benefits (Modini et al., 2016). People with disabilities also report work as beneficial because it provides financial support, inclusion, socialization, and a source of identity (Akkerman et al., 2016; Heyman et al., 2016; Kocman & Weber, 2018; Saunders & Nedelec, 2014). Finally, there is evidence that employment is more beneficial for the young adult with ASD than remaining in high school. Specifically, Schall, Sima, Avellone, Wehman, McDonough, and Brown (2020) found that youth with ASD who participated in an intervention called Project Search plus ASD Supports (PS + ASD) and then gained employment demonstrated significantly lower support needs than an equally matched control group who remained in high school. Consequently, we consider CIE to be a therapeutic activity for the young adult with ASD. In fact, according to public policy and the state of our science, CIE should be the first option for every young adult with ASD graduating from high school or postsecondary education. Thus, before considering disability-only services in day support programs or sheltered work, *every* youth with ASD should be given every opportunity to learn the skills and behaviors needed in CIE while getting the necessary supports to increase their success (Schall et al., 2020; WIOA, 2014)

Unfortunately, this is not the current state of affairs for adults with ASD. Despite the many benefits associated with CIE for adults with ASD, the acquisition of employment remains elusive (Shattuck et al., 2011). Individuals with ASD face significantly greater challenges transitioning to adult life than do peers without disabilities and peers with other types of disabilities. Research indicates that many individuals with ASD experience poor outcomes after leaving high school, especially in the acquisition of CIE (Burke et al., 2019). Out of necessity, then, this chapter will focus on the ways for adults with ASD to access CIE for their own ongoing growth, development, and well-being. In particular, we focus on the individual characteristics of adults with ASD that may act as barriers to CIE and briefly discuss the evidence regarding the use of therapeutic strategies to address these. Then we turn our attention to the external factors that may play a significant role in the person with ASD acquiring and maintaining CIE, specifically the importance of business partnerships and interagency collaboration. Finally, we provide a selected review of evidence-based interventions for individuals with ASD who have high support needs and lower support needs. Each of these sections is followed by a case study illuminating these strategies.

INDIVIDUAL FACTORS AFFECTING EMPLOYMENT

The unique characteristics of ASD can profoundly influence employment success in positive and negative ways (Harmuth et al., 2018). Individuals with ASD may misread the emotion of others, fail to follow social norms, lack proper hygiene, or violate others' personal space (Hendricks, 2010; Ohl et al., 2017). Language and communication challenges can include improper tone, lack of eye contact, interrupting others, asking questions in an inappropriate way, relaying information inaccurately or incompletely, or misunderstanding instructions. These behaviors are not only off-putting to others but can also violate company policies about conduct and appearance, and they can often be grounds for termination even when the individual with ASD is performing job duties well. A recent survey of 59 businesses reported that their employees with ASD displayed quality of work and an overall work ethic that exceeded expected standards, but that one fifth of their employees with ASD struggled to interact with coworkers (Scott et al., 2017).

Maladaptive behaviors can also hinder employment success for individuals with ASD (Harmuth et al., 2018; Ohl et al., 2017). Display of physical or verbal aggression, tantrums, self-injurious behaviors, pica, or stereotypy can pose a liability to a company if the employee or others are injured or property is damaged as a result of problem behavior. Consequently, individuals with more challenging behavior typically end up in environments that are less integrated with the general community. For example, a study by Taylor and Seltzer (2011) found that individuals with ASD who exhibited maladaptive behaviors were less likely to gain CIE and more likely to be in segregated day activity centers (Taylor & Seltzer, 2011).

Challenges with executive functioning (EF) mean that individuals with ASD often have different learning needs than other employees (Bennett & Dukes, 2013; Hendricks, 2010; Lorenz et al., 2016; Ohl et al., 2017). Evidenced-based training techniques, specifically effective for individuals with ASD, are often necessary to help with overcoming impairments in working memory, problem solving, or attention. For example, an individual with ASD might need checklists created for job duties, visual schedules posted for routines, alarms or timers to cue work duration, or signs as reminders of workplace protocol. The inclusion of diagnosis-specific supports during employment training has been shown to be highly effective in prompting CIE outcomes. To illustrate, Wehman et al. (2019) reported a 73.4% employment rate for young adults who received ASD-specific supports.

Comorbid mental health disorders also negatively affect employment. Anxiety and depression can develop or be exacerbated by job demands or the social requirements which accompany a position. Employed adults with ASD interviewed by Hurlbutt and Chalmers (2004) reported sentiments of anxiety and exhaustion trying to navigate difficult social interactions while on the job. Individuals with ASD may also be personally affected by the environmental conditions within a job to an extent far greater than other employees. Sensitivity to sensory input is a symptom of ASD (Centers for Disease Control and Prevention, 2020) and, subsequently, jobs that are noisy, crowded, bright, or involve unregulated temperatures may be anxiety provoking to an individual with ASD. Many individuals with ASD use pharmacological interventions to lessen the symptoms of comorbid disorders. In a study of the health status of adults with ASD, Croen et al. (2015) found that adults with ASD had significantly increased rates of depression, anxiety, bipolar disorder, obsessive compulsive disorder, schizophrenia, and suicide attempts. While medications help reduce psychiatric symptoms, they also present side effects such as fatigue, mental cloudiness, nausea, and so forth that can negatively affect work attendance and performance.

These characteristics may seem daunting, yet, as we have noted, there are also strengths associated with ASD that predict success in the workplace. The presence of social communication impairments may be a barrier to some aspects of particular employment, yet it may also be an advantage to avoid social interaction while completing detailed repetitive tasks. In their 2014 journal article describing two case studies, Ham and colleagues described the strengths they observed in an employee with ASD who worked in a hospital pharmacy. Specifically, they noted that the young man (pseudonym, Darnell) had an excellent working memory and a strong focus on small details. They also noted his accuracy and neatness as a strength at work. These strengths are frequently recognized by employers, as they add value to their workplaces (McDonough et al., 2020; Solomon et al., 2020; Wright et al., 2020). While there is no doubt that the characteristics of ASD may require individuals to receive additional supports in employment, the external factors that influence employment are also relevant to this discussion, including the role businesses play in hiring people with ASD and the importance of collaboration between agencies supporting individuals with ASD.

EVIDENCED-BASED EMPLOYMENT INTERVENTIONS FOR ADULTS WITH ASD

Schall et al. (2020) identified four strongly recommended or recommended practices, and two emerging as recommended practices based on the strength of evidence in the research literature through a scoping review. Specifically, they noted that PS + ASD and supported employment (SE) are strongly recommended based upon the research literature. In particular, PS + ASD supports has demonstrated significantly better employment results in two randomized controlled trials (RCTs) for youth with significant support needs (Wehman et al., 2014, 2019). Likewise, SE is also strongly recommended. While there have been no RCTs for adults with ASD, there is a preponderance of high-quality research evidence from field-based prospective studies reporting very high employment outcomes for individuals with ASD across the spectrum of abilities and support needs (Schall et al., 2020). Two additional practices were identified as recommended based upon correlational analysis of large data sets. They were vocational rehabilitation (VR) services and high school transition services (Schall et al., 2020). Finally, there are a few research studies using prospective research methods that result in the emergence of two potential evidence based practices. These are customized employment (CE) and technology supports for work skills and schedules (Schall et al., 2020). Table 6-1 presents these practices with the quality of evidence provided. In the next sections, we present how these interventions are integrated into CIE supports for adults with ASD by describing the intervention and providing a case example.

MEETING THE EMPLOYMENT REQUIREMENTS OF ADULTS WITH HIGH SUPPORT NEEDS

PS + ASD

PS + ASD is a high school intervention that was specifically designed for individuals with significant support needs, while SE, high school transition services, and CE have all been successfully used for such individuals (Schall et al., 2020). Table 6-2 outlines the six elements that Wehman et al. (2019) described as essential to the success of the PS + ASD model. These elements compose much of

Table 6-1 RECOMMENDED INTERVENTIONS TO INCREASE CIE FOR ADULTS WITH ASD

Intervention	Studies	Level of Evidence	Population	Description
Project SEARCH + ASD Supports	• 3 RCTs	Highest	Youth/young adults; significant impact from ASD and comorbid disorders (ID and/or behavior challenges)	• Final year in HS • Immersed in business • 10-12 week unpaid internships learning work skills
Supported Employment	• 4 prospective quasi-experimental • 4 retrospective secondary data analysis	Very high	HS graduates; spectrum of abilities	• Individualized services for employment process (i.e., job search, development, training, and long-term support)
Vocational Rehabilitation Services	• 9 retrospective secondary data analysis	High	HS graduate with VR services; level of impact from ASD not specified	• State VR services (job placement, training, career counseling, diagnostic services, etc.)
High School Transition Services	• 2 retrospective secondary data analysis (national data sets)	High	Transition-aged students with ASD; level of impact from ASD not specified	• Career counseling • Employment experience in HS
Customized Employment	• 1 retrospective secondary data analysis (agency data)	Promising	Adults with ASD referred for CIE services; spectrum of abilities	• Discovery Process • Job created to meet employer needs/job seeker strengths
Technology for Skill-building/ Organizational Supports	• 1 prospective RCT (virtual reality interviewing) • 1 prospective RCT (personal digital assistant)	Promising	Adults with ASD seeking employment (study 1) Employed adults with ASD/ comorbid intellectual disability (study 2)	• Teach interview skills • Feedback via virtual reality • Visual task analyses, prompts, and navigation tools

SOURCE: Schall et al., 2020.
NOTE: High school (HS), intellectual disability (ID), randomized controlled trial (RCT), vocational rehabilitation (VR)

Table 6-2 SIX ELEMENTS OF PS + ASD SUPPORTING CIE

Element	Description	Key Components
Internships	Time limited, unpaid, educationally oriented work experiences in a real business setting.	• Repeated practice of work skills and professional behavior in real job settings • Shape skills to be more complex • Capitalize on the individual's strengths, interests, and preferences • Train co-workers/ supervisors about the social behavioral needs of intern
Systematic Instruction	Use of applied behavior analysis for skill development within workplace/ focus on development of social communication skills and successful work behaviors.	• Task analyses to teach work behaviors • Behavioral rehearsal of social communication skills • Prompting hierarchies • Generalization of skills • Functional behavior assessment for challenging behavior/ multi-component behavior intervention plans
Personalized Vocational Assessment	Participants try out various tasks and assess their success, desire to perform the task, and amount of support they require to learn the task.	• Match intern strengths, preferences, and interests to business needs • Customize internship to learn more about social behavioral needs of intern • Share information gained with collaborators/stakeholders • Assessments include tangential issues affecting employment (e.g., transportation, family support, personal independence)
Seamless Transition to Adult Services	Services provided by school, VR services organization, developmental disability agency, with strong family/ individual involvement.	• Multiple funding sources and concurrent service provision by multiple agencies (school, VR, developmental disability agency) • Avoids waiting lists by starting adult services before end of school services
Development of Résumé	Showcase skills in place of traditional interview.	• Video résumés show individuals completing real job tasks in a work environment • Working interviews; individuals performs job for a short period of time under the supervision of their employment support provider • Collection of recommendation letters from internship supervisors and mentors

(continued)

Table 6-2 Continued

Element	Description	Key Components
Focus on current employable skills in home community	Internships in real community businesses ensure that the person is learning marketable skills.	• Teach skills that are valued by the business and are completed by employees, *not* by volunteers • Intern learns real skills needed in the business • Teach skills that are marketable in the economy of the individual's community • Focus on meeting the business' needs while they help the intern learn skills • Encourage internship sites to consider hiring successful interns

SOURCE: Wehman et al., 2020.

the PS + ASD supports model. To date, this is the only packaged intervention with efficacy confirmed by two RCTs.

Supported Employment

SE is an individualized service during which a trained employment specialist assists a job seeker with a severe disability gain and maintain employment. For the purposes of this chapter, we do not consider supported employment to include group models, such as enclaves or work crews. Instead, we view SE as an individualized service designed to assist people with disabilities gain CIE. The main value of SE is to *employ then train*. This is a critical component of SE, as the assumption is that even those with significant impact from disabilities can both learn job skills and receive employment support to sustain their employment (Wehman et al., 2019). There has been very high-quality research documenting the efficacy of SE for individuals with ASD. Specifically, higher employment outcomes have been reported in both prospective quasi-experimental and retrospective data analysis of seven different teams of researchers in different countries (Brooke et al., 2018; Howlin et al., 2005; Lynas, 2014; McLaren et al., 2017; Schall et al., 2015; Wehman et al., 2012, 2016). This provides compelling evidence that SE is an evidence-based practice that results in higher CIE outcomes for adults with ASD.

Customized Employment

CE matches the unique strengths, interests, and support needs of the job candidate with the identified demands of the employer (Smith et al., 2015; Wehman et al.,

2018; WIOA, 2014). Rather than fitting the job seeker into an existing job, CE involves developing a job that did not previously exist to meet the business' needs and the job seeker's strengths (Brooke et al., 2018; Smith et al., 2015; Wehman et al., 2016, 2020). CE has been implemented with ASD supports as well, including (a) developing a work schedule with consistent structure, (b) teaching social communication skills and work expectations with applied behaviour analysis (ABA), (c) using visual supports to ensure consistent independent performance of work and social skills, and (d) implementing behavior supports (Wehman et al., 2012). CE provides a very suitable method for those with ASD and significant support needs. The highly individualized nature of the CIE outcome allows employment specialists to tailor the job to meet the needs of the business and the strengths, interests, and preferences of the employee.

CASE STUDY

Jamal is a 28-year-old man who was diagnosed with "classic autism" as a 6-year-old child. He displays challenging behavior, including flapping his hands and spinning in a circle. On occasion, he will yell, push on his chin, and bite his arm. He will also run from those around him. He is not able to read or write and has no mathematical skills. His verbal communication is also significantly impacted. Mostly, he speaks in one and two word phrases, such as "go home" and "eat." Jamal's employment specialist, Darius, used CE to negotiate a job for Jamal at the hospital's off-site sterilization department. The job required Jamal to move 2 meter tall by 1 meter wide (6.5 feet by 3 feet) rolling case carts into the sterilization unit and push buttons in a specific sequence to sterilize the instruments on the cart. While waiting for the unit to finish its sterilization routine, Jamal could pace, flap, and make noise. The employer also provided a quiet private space where he could take a break if he got too hot or became frustrated. Jamal earns $9.50 an hour (31% higher than minimum wage in his location), and works between 20 and 30 hours weekly. He is very reliable and hates to miss work.

Since Jamal has been working in central sterile, all of his co-workers have made errors when placing case carts in the sterilizing unit at one time or another—all, that is, except Jamal. Because of his attention to detail and his insistence that he complete repetitive tasks in precisely the same order every day, Jamal has never made an error when putting a case cart into the sterilization machine. Jamal is able to sign in and out of work with his employee badge, and he is also independent occupying his time while waiting for his parents. Darius is skilled in using ABA techniques to teach new skills and to analyze the function of Jamal's behavioral challenges if they arise or accelerate. Further, if needed, Darius is able to contact his supervisor and request additional support from a Board Certified Behavior Analyst to assist him. Without the availability of behavior analytic services, Jamal's success would be compromised by his episodic behavior challenges.

MEETING THE EMPLOYMENT REQUIREMENTS OF ADULTS WITH LOWER SUPPORT NEEDS

Adults with ASD and lower support needs also present unique challenges when acquiring and maintaining CIE. They have high verbal intelligence and strengths in academics, and they often excel in school and attend college. They may struggle when trying to obtain or maintain employment due to impairments in social skills, problem solving, and executive functioning. Unfortunately, adults with lower support needs often do not "meet requirements" for support from vocational rehabilitation services and are left to fend for themselves in an environment that may not understand these challenges or offer support or accommodations to make the job successful. In addition, many adults with lower support needs do not disclose to their employer that they have autism and require accommodations. This often leads to misunderstanding, missed deadlines, and termination. This does not have to be the case. Through targeted interventions, successful postsecondary education, and the support of vocational rehabilitation services, adults with ASD who have lower support needs can obtain competitive employment in jobs of their choosing that can lead to successful careers.

Postsecondary Education

Enrollment for this population is lower than that of many students with other disabilities (Newman et al. 2011; Roux et al. 2015; Shattuck et al. 2012). That said, recent research describing employment outcomes for postsecondary education (PSE) program participants is positive, with preliminary results representing high employment rates across disciplines (Moore & Schelling, 2015). Young adults with ASD can participate in PSE through traditional programs such as community college, vocational and career training, and 4-year universities. Time spent in PSE can offer instruction and practice in skills necessary for successful employment. Attending classes requires many skills that parallel employment, including self-determination, time management, and social skills, as well as managing stress anxiety in a fast-paced environment. A student seeking support from the disability services office can receive an array of supports and accommodations that can prove to be useful in the college setting and beyond. Thankfully, the availability of personal technology can be a way to address many of the challenges faced by adults with autism without making them stand out from their peers. Electronic organizers, alarms, timers, calendars, and other apps that can be downloaded to smart phones and computers are able to assist all individuals with (and without) disabilities to manage their time, assignments, routines. This addresses those EF tasks that are often the culprit of unsuccessful employment. In addition, it is important to consider the social aspect of PSE.

Cognitive Rehabilitation

Cognitive rehabilitation (CR) is a therapeutic approach designed to improve cognitive functioning for individuals who experience cognitive deficits. It includes a variety of evidence-based therapy methods that retrain or alleviate problems caused by impairment in attention, visual processing, language, memory, reasoning, problem solving, and executive functions. Cognitive rehabilitation includes interventions that are used to reinforce or reestablish previously learned patterns of behavior or to establish new compensatory mechanisms for cognitive processes. There has been extensive research to support the positive effect of CR in individuals with traumatic brain injury (TBI; Rumrill et al., 2016). More recently, researchers have begun to consider CR as a promising intervention for those with ASD. The desired outcome of cognitive rehabilitation is an improved quality of life including an increased ability to be actively engaged at home, work, and the community. Several therapies fall under the category of "cognitive rehabilitation" for adults with ASD, including the following promising practices: virtual reality training and social skills training.

Technology and the Use of Virtual Reality

The emerging technology of computerized instruction has led to an influx of treatment strategies and protocols internet-based and virtual reality-based treatment strategies and protocols that have demonstrated positive results in youth and adults with ASD (Smith et al., 2020; Walsh et al., 2017). Virtual reality provides an immersive experience into a simulated environment and stimulates different senses in the process. Adults with ASD, regardless of their support needs, often require systematic instruction that can be practiced frequently to build confidence and fluidity of the skill. Virtual reality provides a safe, controllable environment to practice these skills repeatedly. This application can target a variety of skills including specific job tasks, routines, communication, and social skills.

Vocational Rehabilitation Services

Vocational rehabilitation (VR) services for adults with ASD clearly results in successful employment (Sung et al., 2015). Research demonstrates that individuals with ASD often succeed in the workplace if transition and vocational rehabilitation services are tailored to meet their unique and individual needs (McDonough & Revell, 2010). Unfortunately, many individuals with lower support needs fail to meet the requirements to obtain these services, and thus are excluded from services. Of those who do receive services, many withdraw from the VR process because some traditional vocational rehabilitation practices are not only ineffective for people with ASD, but also actively distressing to them. Given the great variation in how ASD is experienced, VR providers must consider the unique interests, goals, and capabilities. The importance of a needs assessment in developing customized strategies to meet these unique needs is paramount. These assessments can lead to the design of engaging interventions, utilizing different processes and models to understand the social environment and job context. Some of the same strategies listed previously in PSE can be adapted to address the challenges faced on the job.

CASE STUDY

Amir is a 24-year-old man with a diagnosis of autism. He graduated from high school with a standard diploma while receiving support from his IEP team and special education. Amir attended a 4-year university to pursue a degree in history with a minor in art. While at the university, he received services from the student accessibility office to help with accommodations. Additionally, he and his mother contacted their local vocational rehabilitation office to seek support in finding employment while in college. He had some volunteer experience, but no paid employment. The case manager, Amir, and his mother explored his strengths and identified his support needs. A list of strengths emerged including a passion for history and historical events, attention to detail, and the ability to speak effectively about these topics. Through the help of his case manager, he was able to discuss tasks that he found difficult in high school, college, and potentially in employment. Through the support of an employment specialist, Amir learned self-advocacy and effective strategies and tools to maintain organization, and he developed more confidence. As a result, he joined an art club on campus and was able to secure hourly work at a local university-affiliated historical society, giving guided tours through a museum. Patrons found him to be so knowledgeable and professional that the museum staff asked him to increase his hours over the summers and guaranteed him a 30-hour per week position after graduation. Amir is very successful at work and has expanded his social network beyond the art club to include a group who does war reenactments. He finds great joy in both his work and social opportunities.

CONCLUSION

The purpose of this chapter was to describe the research evidence and discuss the implementation of employment interventions designed to increase adults' access to CIE. As we have noted, CIE may act as a protective factor from some of the ill effects that individuals with ASD face in adulthood when they are without daily structure. Specifically, we have found that adults with ASD who gain CIE continue to learn skills, are not isolated, and gain social interaction opportunities from working with their coworkers without disabilities. Future research should explore the benefits gained by adults with ASD in CIE to assess the degree to which it is a protective factor against isolation, plateauing of growth, depression, and anxiety disorders. Further, access to services such as ABA in the work place is not yet widespread. This is also something that should be addressed through public policy and funding. Nevertheless, people like Jamal and Amir have talents and gifts. They benefit from and provide benefit to their communities through their employment. It is beyond time for us as a society to take the message of inclusion to the workplace. We need these workers to enhance our own communities and workplaces.

REFERENCES

Akkerman, A., Janssen, C. G. C., Kef, S., & Meininger, H. P. (2016). Job satisfaction of people with intellectual disabilities in integrated and sheltered employment: An exploration of the literature. *Journal of Policy and Practice in Intellectual Disabilities, 13*(3), 205–216.

American Psychiatric Association. (2013). *Diagnostic and statistical manual of mental disorders* (5th ed.). https://doi.org/10.1176/appi.books.9780890425596

Arnett, J. J. (2014). *Emerging adulthood: The winding road from the late teens through the twenties.* Oxford University Press.

Bennett, K. D., & Dukes, C. (2013). Employment instruction for secondary students with autism spectrum disorder: A systematic review of the literature. *Education and Training in Autism and Developmental Disabilities, 48*(1), 67–75.

Brooke, V., Brooke, A. M., Schall, C., Wehman, P., McDonough, J., Thompson, K., & Smith, J. (2018). Employees with autism spectrum disorder achieving long-term employment success: A retrospective review of employment retention and intervention. *Research and Practice for Persons with Severe Disabilities, 43*(3), 181–193.

Burke, M. M., Waitz-Kudla, S. N., Rabideau, C., Taylor, J. L., & Hodapp, R. M. (2019) Pulling back the curtain: Issues in conducting an intervention study with transition-aged youth with autism spectrum disorders and their families. *Autism, 23*(2), 514–523.

Centers for Disease Control and Prevention. (2020). *Diagnostic criteria, Autism Spectrum Disorder (ASD).* https://www.cdc.gov/ncbddd/autism/hcp-dsm.html

Croen, L. A., Zerbo, O., Qian, Y., Massolo, M. L., Rich, S., Sidney, S., & Kripke, C. (2015). The health status of adults on the autism spectrum. *Autism: The International Journal of Research and Practice, 19*(7), 814–823.

Ham, W., McDonough, J., Molinelli, A., Schall, C., & Wehman, P. (2014). Employment supports for young adults with ASD: Two case studies. *Journal of Vocational Rehabilitation, 40*(2), 117–124.

Harmuth, E., Silletta, E., Bailey, A., Adams, T., Beck, C., & Barbic, S. P. (2018). Barriers and facilitators to employment for adults with autism: A scoping review. *Annals of International Occupational Therapy, 1*(1), 31–40.

Hendricks, D. (2010). Employment and adults with autism spectrum disorders: Challenges and strategies for success. *Journal of Vocational Rehabilitation, 32*(2), 125–134.

Howlin, P., Alcock, J., & Burkin, C. (2005). An 8 year follow-up of a specialist supported employment service for high-ability adults with autism or Asperger syndrome. *Autism, 9*(5), 533–549.

Hurlbutt, K., & Chalmers, L. (2004). Employment and adults with Asperger syndrome. *Focus on Autism and Other Developmental Disabilities, 19*(4), 215–222.

Heyman, M., Stokes, J. E., & Siperstein, G. N. (2016). Not all jobs are the same: Predictors of job quality for adults with intellectual disabilities. *Journal of Vocational Rehabilitation, 44*(3), 299–306.

Kocman, A., & Weber, G. (2018). Job satisfaction, quality of work life and work motivation in employees with intellectual disability: A systematic review. *Journal of Applied Research in Intellectual Disabilities, 31*, 1–22.

Lorenz, T., Frischling, C., Cuadros, R., & Heinitz, K. (2016). Autism and overcoming job barriers: Comparing job-related barriers and possible solutions in and outside of autism-specific employment. *PLOS ONE, 11*(1), Article e0147040.

Lynas, L. (2014). Project ABLE (Autism: building links to employment): A specialist employment services for young people and adults with autism spectrum condition. *Journal of Vocational Rehabilitation, 41*(1), 13–21.

McDonough, J., Ham, W., Brooke, A., Wehman, P., Wright, T., Godwin, J. C., Junod, P., & Hurst, R. (2020). Health care executive perceptions of hiring and retention practices of persons with disabilities: Results from executive focus groups. *Rehabilitation Counseling Bulletin, 64*(2), 75–85.

McDonough, J. T., & Revell, G. (2010). Accessing employment supports in the adult system for transitioning youth with autism spectrum disorders. *Journal of Vocational Rehabilitation, 32*(2), 89–100.

McLaren, J., Lichtenstein, J. D., Lynch D., Becker, D., & Drake, R. (2017). Individual placement and support for people with autism spectrum disorders: A pilot program. *Administration and Policy in Mental Health, 44*(3), 365–373.

Modini, M., Joyce, S., Mykletun, A., Christensen, H., Bryant, R. A., Mitchell, P. B., & Harvey, S. B. (2016). The mental health benefits of employment: Results of a systematic meta-review. *Australasian psychiatry: bulletin of Royal Australian and New Zealand College of Psychiatrists, 24*(4), 331–336.

Moore, E. J., & Schelling, A. (2015). Postsecondary inclusion for individuals with an intellectual disability and its effects on employment. *Journal of Intellectual Disabilities, 19*, 130–148.

Newman, L., Wagner, M., Knokey, A.-M., Marder, C., Nagle, K., Shaver, D., & Wei, X. (2011). *The post-high school outcomes of young adults with disabilities up to 8 years after high school: A report from the National Longitudinal Transition Study-2 (NLTS2)* (NCSER 2011–3005). SRI International. https://ies.ed.gov/ncser/pubs/20113005/pdf/20113005.pdf

Ohl, A., Grice Sheff, M., Small, S., Nguyen, J., Paskor, K., & Zanjirian, A. (2017). Predictors of employment status among adults with autism spectrum disorder. *Work, 56*(2), 345–355.

Roux, A. M., Shattuck, P. T., Rast, J. E., Rava, J. A., & Anderson, K. A. (2015). *National autism indicators report: Transition into young adulthood.* A. J. Drexel Autism Institute, Drexel University.

Rumrill, P., Elias, E., Hendricks, D. J., Jacobs, K., Leopold, A., Nardone, A., Sampson, E., Scherer, M., Stauffer, C, & McMahon, B. T. (2016). Promoting cognitive support technology use and employment success among postsecondary students with traumatic brain injuries. *Journal of Vocational Rehabilitation, 45*(1), 53–61.

Saunders, S. L., & Nedelec, B. (2014). What work means to people with work disability: A scoping review. *Journal of Occupational Rehabilitation, 24,* 100–110.

Schall, C., Sima, A. P., Avellone, L., Wehman, P., McDonough, J., & Brown, A. (2020). The effect of business internships model and employment on enhancing the independence of young adults with significant impact from autism. *Intellectual and Developmental Disabilities, 58*(4), 301–313.

Schall, C., Wehman, P., Avellone, L., & Taylor, J. P. (2020). Competitive integrated employment for youth and adults with autism: Findings from a scoping review. *Child and Adolescent Psychiatric Clinics of North America, 29*(2), 373–397.

Schall, C. M., Wehman, P., Brooke, V., Graham, C., McDonough, J., Brooke, A., Ham, W., Rounds, R., Lau, S., Allen, J. (2015). Employment interventions for individuals with ASD: The relative efficacy of supported employment with or without prior Project SEARCH training. *Journal of Autism and Developmental Disorders, 45,* 3990–4001.

Scott, M., Jacob, A., Hendrie, D., Parsons, R., Girdler, S., Falkmer, T., & Falkmer, M. (2017). Employers' perception of the costs and the benefits of hiring individuals with autism spectrum disorder in open employment in Australia. *PLOS ONE, 12*(5), Article e0177607.

Shattuck, P. T., Roux, A. M., Hudson, L. E., Taylor, J. L., Maenner, M. J., & Trani, J. F. (2012). Services for adults with an autism spectrum disorder. *Canadian Journal of Psychiatry. Revue Canadienne de psychiatrie, 57*(5), 284–291.

Shattuck, P. T., Wagner, M., Narendorf, S., Sterzing, P., & Hensley, M. (2011). Post high school service use among young adults with autism. *Archives of Pediatric and Adolescent Medicine, 165,* 141–146.

Smith, T. J., Dillahunt-Aspillaga, C., & Kenney, C. (2015). Integrating customized employment practices within the vocational rehabilitation system. *Journal of Vocational Rehabilitation, 42,* 201–208.

Smith, M. J., Pinto, R. J., Dewalt, L., Smith J. D., Sherwood, K., Miles, R., Taylor, J., & Hume, K. (2020). Using community-engaged methods to adapt virtual reality job-interview training for transition-age youth on the autism spectrum. *Research in Autism Spectrum Disorder, 71 Article # 101498.*

Solomon, C. (2020). Autism and employment: Implications for employers and adults with ASD. *Journal of Autism and Developmental Disorders, 50,* 4209–4217.

Sung, C., Sanchez, J., Kuo, H. J., Wang, C. C., & Leahy, M. J. (2015). Gender differences in vocational rehabilitation service predictors of successful competitive employment for transition-aged individuals with autism. *Journal of Autism and Developmental Disorders, 45,* 3204–3218.

Taylor, J. L. & Seltzer, M. (2011). Employment and post-secondary educational activities for young adults with autism spectrum disorders during the transition to adulthood. *Journal of Autism and Developmental Disorders, 41*(5), 566–574.

Walsh, E., Holloway, J., McCoy, A., & Lyndon, H. (2017). Technology-aided intervention for employment skills in adults with autism spectrum disorder: A systemic review. *Review Journal of Autism and Developmental Disorders, 4,* 12–25.

Wehman, P., Brooke, V., Brooke, A. M., Ham W., Schall, C., McDonough, J., Lau, S., Seward, H., & Avellone, L. (2016). Employment for adults with autism spectrum disorders: A retrospective review of a customized employment approach. *Research in Developmental Disabilities, 53–54*, 61–72.

Wehman, P., Iwanaga, K., Sima, A., McDonough, J., Chan, F., Brooke, A., Ham, W., Godwin, J., & Junod, P. (2020). Assessing attitudes of hospital staff toward working with co-workers with disabilities: A preliminary study. *Journal of Rehabilitation, 86*(4), 14–21.

Wehman, P., Lau, S., Mollinelli, A., Brooke, V., Thompson, K., Moore, C., & West, M. (2012). Supported employment for young adults with autism spectrum disorder: Preliminary data. *Research and Practice for Persons with Severe Disabilities, 27*(3), 160–169.

Wehman, P. H., Schall, C. M., McDonough, J., Kregel, J., Brooke, V., Molinelli, A., Ham, W., Graham, C. W., Riehle, J. E., Collins, H. T., & Thiss, W. (2014). Competitive employment for youth with Autism Spectrum Disorders: Early results from a randomized clinical trial. *Journal of Autism and Developmental Disorders, 44*, 487–500.

Wehman, P., Schall, C., McDonough, J., Sima, A., Brooke, A., Ham, W., Whittenburg, H., Brooke, V. Avellone, L, & Riehle, E. (2020). Competitive employment for transition-aged youth with significant impact from autism: A multi-site randomized clinical trial. *Journal of Autism and Developmental Disorders, 50*(6), 1882–1897.

Wehman, P., Taylor, J., Brooke, V., Avellone, L., Whittenburg, H., Ham, W., Molinelli B., A., & Carr, S. (2018). Toward competitive employment for persons with intellectual and developmental disabilities: What progress have we made and where do we need to go. *Research and Practice for Persons with Severe Disabilities, 43*(3), 131–144.

Workforce Innovation and Opportunity Act of 2014, Pub. L. No.113-128 128 Stat. 1425 (2014). https://www.govinfo.gov/content/pkg/PLAW-113publ128/pdf/PLAW-113publ128.pdf

Wright, T., Wehman, P., McDonough, J., Thomas, K., Ochrach, K., Thomas, K., Brooke, A., Ham, W., Godwin, J. C., & Junod, P. (2020). Charity-oriented versus human resource-oriented perspectives: Investigating staff understandings of employment practices for persons with disabilities. *Journal of Applied Rehabilitation Counseling, 51*(2), 146–167.

7

Social Skills Interventions

CYNTHIA I. D'AGOSTINO AND FRANCISCO M. MUSICH ■

KEY CONSIDERATIONS

- An adequate initial examination is important to conceptualize the case.
- Selection of social skills techniques or teaching and training programs will depend on the individual profile, needs, and hierarchy of priorities of each patient.
- Social skills interventions can be delivered via an individual or group approach and can include behavioral and cognitive techniques.
- Group social skills approaches can be effective for individuals who are interested in and motivated to improve and develop their social skills.
- It is important to take into account and to adapt interventions to the individual and cultural variables of each patient.

OVERVIEW

Communication, social interaction, and social skills are affected in autism spectrum disorders (ASD) from an early age and continue to be a challenging area for many individuals throughout their lives, regardless of their adaptive behavior or intellectual capabilities (Gaus, 2007, 2011; Howlin & Moss, 2012; Lord et al., 2020).

Transition into adulthood typically results in new challenges, contexts, and demands for social skills. For some adults, social requirements increase, as do the parameters within which social behaviors are observed, understood, and, sometimes, judged by others. For others, requirements decrease due to no longer being in mandated education but may result in social isolation. This increase in demands for the first group is often inversely proportional to the services and support available for both groups of patients.

It is important to consider that some individuals with comorbid intellectual disability will have a number of specific social skill challenges (Walsh et al., 2018; Wilkins & Matson, 2009), and others without intellectual disabilities will present more subtle impairments, but that does not mean that they will have less difficulty or distress (Spain & Blainey, 2015). Nonetheless, there are successful and well-adapted cases of social functioning of adults with ASD, but, for many, core difficulties in communication and social interaction persist in adulthood (Howlin & Moss, 2012; Laugeson & Ellingsen, 2014; Lord et al., 2020; White et al., 2010).

The Construct of Social Skills

The social skills construct lacks a universal general theoretical framework, both in assessment and training (Baker, 2003). Social skills can be defined as behaviors that are negatively or positively reinforced and the possibility of not performing behaviors that are punished or extinguished. It also implies behaviors in which a person can interpersonally express positive and negative feelings without the loss of social reinforcement (Caballo, 2002; Kelly, 2010). Social skills are context- and culture-dependent behaviors that emerge in early life, and many nonautistic individuals learn these skills more adeptly and generalize them more intuitively. This is not the case for individuals with ASD (Spain & Blainey, 2015; White et al., 2013).

Assessment of Social Performance

The first step in choosing and designing a treatment is a thorough clinical assessment (White et al., 2013). Substantial heterogeneity can be found in assessment instruments for social skills, social cognition, and autistic symptomatology for adults as well as children. This methodological heterogeneity in the assessment is also present in research and clinical literature and, to a degree, this is also what makes systematic reviews and generalization of research findings difficult (Spain & Blainey, 2015; White, 2010, 2013).

The assessment should incorporate a combination of different methods, including a robust and comprehensive evaluation of autistic symptomatology with standard and self-report measures, intellectual capabilities, cognitive functioning, social cognition, and social skills, including verbal and nonverbal communication skills (see Figure 7-1). Often, measurements are not only used in the assessment but also in evaluating progress and posttreatment outcomes. During the assessment, it is important to explore the presence of alexithymia, self-awareness (Frith & Happé, 1999; Happé, 2003; Williams, 2010; Williams & Happé, 2009), strengths and weaknesses, social motivation, presence of camouflaging, and coping resources. It is essential to know the history and trajectory of the individual's social context, their support networks, and previous positive or negative interaction experiences with peers that might have led to rejection, teasing or ostracism

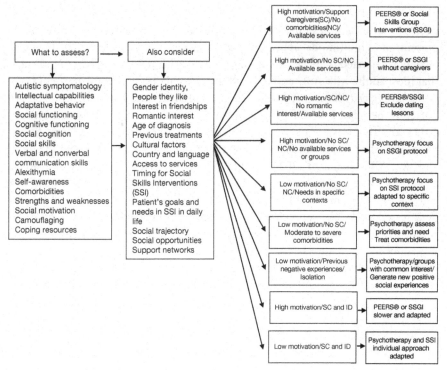

Figure 7-1 Assessment and Decision Making in Treatment Design
[A] Figure 7-1 is based on both clinical experience and research.
[B] Strategies and programs are suggestions, not research-informed mandates, as they do not take into account the full case conceptualization.

(White et al., 2010). Also, it is essential to consider gender identity, people with whom they enjoy spending their free time, and with whom they need or wish to expand their social life and skills, and their romantic or intimate interest if present. Furthermore, the age of ASD diagnosis and history of previous and present treatments is relevant, as this can provide clinicians with an understanding of whether social skills have been previously taught but not fully acquired, or if they need to be learned for the first time. This would also address performance or acquisition impairments (Bellini, 2008) and would be key in selection of the subsequent techniques.

Other key issues to assess include cultural factors, customs, and social codes in each individual's environment, geographical context, country, language; access to available specialized support services and general and mental health services; opportunities in each community; housing; access to university education and employment with and without support; and access to culture, sports, and leisure. These factors will help form an idea of the social context of the individual and the specific curricular needs in the design of the treatment option.

It is also crucial to assess physical and mental health comorbidities, in particular the co-occurrence of anxiety, which is multifaceted in ASD. It can be challenging to determine if the anxiety is primary or secondary to core impairments and might affect the treatment design (White et al., 2010). Anxiety should be addressed, if present, and a multimodal approach might be necessary (White et al., 2013). Social anxiety is reported to be present in many adults with ASD and research indicates that most adults with ASD and without intellectual disabilities are aware of their social struggles (Maddox & White, 2015). Moreover, social anxiety has been reported to be related to self-reported hostility in adults with ASD (White et al., 2012), and this feasibly plays a key role in case conceptualization. In addition, mood disorders and posttraumatic stress disorder (PTSD) are prevalent in adults with ASD (Rumball et al., 2020), and might affect social performance or even be caused by social events (Haruvi-Lamdan et al., 2020). Moreover, comorbidities can interfere and modulate outcomes in social skills interventions and should be assessed, addressed, and considered in the treatment design. Assessing if the timing for the intervention in social skills is the best or if other priorities are more urgent for the individual is necessary.

We believe that assessing and taking into account the patient's goals regarding their social skills treatment is relevant, regardless of the impression of the clinician or others in the patient's life. The rationale for this is that in our clinical experience, on average, patients tend to be more engaged in the treatment if they feel that they are working toward meaningful goals of their own. Frequently, addressing the patient's goal is a starting point in the treatment, and as this progresses, so do opportunities of including different goals. Also, goals might change as their confidence, knowledge, and skills increase during therapy.

Finally, although not always available, it is recommended to include reports from significant people in the adult's life, since they can provide very valuable and ecologically accurate information of our patient social performing.

Social Skills Interventions for Individuals With ASD: Techniques

Most research studies have focused on social skills interventions for children and adolescents, and to a lesser extent on people with intellectual disabilities (White et al., 2007), but not on adults with ASD without intellectual disabilities (Bishop-Fitzpatrick et al., 2013; Spain & Blainey, 2015).

Generally, manualized programs have in common the selection of a series of objectives, and these are usually limited in time and in number of sessions. Also, they provide didactic instructions, encourage behavioral rehearsals, role play, assignments, review, and feedback (Baker, 2003; Bellini et al., 2008; Gresham et al., 2001; Reichow et al., 2013; Spain & Blainey, 2015; White et al., 2007, 2010, 2012). Techniques used in teaching social skills can be multiple and can be combined in different ways in manualized programs or in individual interventions (Baker, 2003; Bellini et al., 2008; Winner & Crooke 2009). Some will be focused on performing specific behaviors, verbal and nonverbal, and other techniques will be focused on social cognition, social understanding, and perspective taking (White, 2012).

Table 7-1 STRATEGIES AND INTERVENTIONS FOR SOCIAL SKILLS TRAINING

Intervention Type	Techniques
Behavior and performance techniques	• Didactic instructions • Discrete trials • Chaining • Prompting • Modeling • Fading • Behavior rehearsals • Role plays • Video-modeling and video self-modeling • Practice assignments • Assignments review and feedback • Incidental teaching
Social cognition, perspective taking and hidden curriculum	• Social narratives • Social stories • Picture cognitive rehearsal • Comic strip conversations • Video analysis • Perspective taking exercises • Mind reading training • Social autopsy • Social problem solving • Self-awareness strategies • Hidden curriculum exercises

Various techniques are often reported in the literature (see Table 7-1), such as social narratives, social stories (Gray et al., 1993), and cognitive essays with drawings (Gray, 1994). Other techniques address social cognition, teaching of "the hidden curriculum" (Myles & Simpson, 2001), and perspective taking (Winner & Crooke, 2011). Similarly, techniques focused on the performance of specific behaviors are reported (White, 2012), including discrete rehearsal, direct and didactic instruction, modeling, chaining, fading, prompting, role play, and behavioral rehearsal (Baker, 2003; Bellini, 2008; Laugeson, 2010, 2017; Tincani & Bondy, 2015). For many individuals with ASD and moderate to severe intellectual disabilities, teaching will be mostly through behavioral techniques, discrete rehearsal, video modeling (Bellini, 2008; Tincani & Bondy, 2015; Walsh et. al., 2018), and adapting techniques for more able individuals with a slower pace and visual aids.

Evidence-Based Group Interventions Available for Adults With ASD

A recent systematic review of group social skills found that, while five studies showed preliminary evidence, interventions were effective for improving knowledge and understanding of social skills rather than for improving them, and they were very varied in content and objectives (Spain & Blainey, 2015). However, the samples were highly heterogeneous in size, and methodologies and were not always available in a manualized format or accessible for clinicians. Availability of these programs was reduced, and programs were not consistently available in a manual format.

Currently the most robust, available, and developed adult program for social skills in adults is the Program for the Education and Enrichment of Relationship Skills for Young Adults (PEERS-YA; Laugeson, 2017). This has the largest number of studies, participants, and replications. It also has the greatest accessibility in terms of manuals, format, training, and international availability. This program is adapted and extended from the original UCLA PEERS Program, a 14–16-week, parent-assisted social skills group intervention for adolescents with ASD (Laugeson & Frankel, 2010), maintaining the same format and the work methodology and supported by caregivers or social coaches. The program takes place over 16 weeks with simultaneous sessions of 1.5 hours, each involving a group of adults and a group of coaches who might be parents or other caregivers with two leaders for each group, and it is designed for individuals without intellectual disabilities. Sessions address conversational skills, electronic communication, how to choose friends, how to organize meetings and get-togethers, social etiquette for romantic dates, and conflict management among others. The teaching method comprises didactic and structured instruction, Socratic method, role play, perspective taking, behavioral rehearsals, modeling, assignments and reviews, and feedback in each session for 16 weeks. Both groups have their own leader but will work with the same objective and content. While adults receive didactic instructions and chances to role play and rehearse, caregivers (or coaches) will learn the step-by-step lesson and will gather ways of supporting the participant adult in the homework assignments and practice during each week. In order to benefit maximally from the PEERS-YA program, participants must be highly motivated to learn the proposed content, committed to the assigned tasks, attend all meetings, and have the support of a coach. An important novelty of this program are sessions related to romantic dates, which has not previously been addressed in other interventions and especially in group format. This is often left aside despite being highly required by some patients. However, it is important to take into account that clinicians will probably have to make adjustments to each country and culture regarding the romantic etiquette, since this can be a very culturally sensitive aspect. Those adjustments would be related to the specific content of the lessons, but not to the teaching methodology.

While the implementation of this specific program without caregivers or coaches is discouraged, the authors acknowledge that this may be the reality for many adults, and it can be unavoidable. In this instance, the authors recommend giving handouts of the sessions to caregivers or coaches, even if they do not attend the sessions, and involving them by giving them other additional resources and materials, such as books, apps, or websites to learn more about the program and how to support their adult during the training. In the case of individuals with intellectual disabilities, the authors recommend making the program longer and slower, simplifying lessons, and providing visual aids (Laugeson, 2017). Additionally, in the current context of increasing internet-based interactions and relationships, the intervention is being piloted via telehealth.

Individual Work of Social Skills and Techniques

For those individuals who might not benefit from group interventions for different reasons or if groups are not available for them, an individual approach and training is a treatment option. The initial assessment will be the same as the one proposed in the group section. The individual approach will include didactic instructions, role play, behavioral rehearsals, homework, practical assignments, perspective-taking exercises, and mixed techniques. These interventions can be well suited to the framework of individual psychotherapy and can also be coordinated in collaboration with different professionals, sometimes using manualized interventions as curriculum and intervention guides.

In this case, the clinician will deliver a tailor-made intervention, based on the needs and goals of the patient and the area of performance; sometimes this can be the work environment, social relationships, romantic relationships, or all the areas in general. Sometimes the clinician will work on teaching specific skills that apply to all areas, such as conversational skills, or in some other cases, specific abilities for a specific area, like handling disagreements with coworkers or inviting someone on a date. Just as in a social skills group intervention, it can be very useful to work with a social coach or caregiver, mentor, or friend who can troubleshoot in ecologically valid situations and help in implement real-world behavioral rehearsals, monitoring and giving feedback on the interactions of the consultant.

CASE STUDY

Sara is a 19-year-old woman studying design at local university with a recent diagnosis of ASD. She presented social struggles throughout her life and has no friends or social groups. She finds it very difficult to participate in social situations, to initiate and maintain conversations with others, and to handle disagreements and criticism. She appears socially awkward, rude, arrogant, and insensitive to others, which is the opposite reaction she wants to generate. Her parents reported the same and gave examples of how she tried to get closer to peers by being too clingy and not realizing when she was not welcome to a group or conversation.

She was motivated to learn social skills and all the lessons that were part of the PEERS-YA Program. She was an excellent candidate for group intervention, meeting all the inclusion criteria (she had no intellectual disabilities or comorbidities, she was socially motivated, and she could count on her mother to provide support alongside the intervention), yet there was no group available beginning any time soon for her.

It was decided that individual cognitive behavior therapy (CBT) and social skills training in two separate sessions a week in an individual format would be the best the treatment option. We followed the lessons from PEERS-YA almost in the same order they were presented in the manual: from conversational skills to complex social behaviors. Also, it was agreed that her mother would help her do her weekly assignments. The dating etiquette lessons from the PEERS-YA Program were omitted, as she was not interested in dating anyone romantically and focused on the lessons that involved finding sources of friends; conversational skills; entering, maintaining, and exiting conversations; electronic communication; appropriate use of humor; and handling rumors, gossip, and disagreements.

Strategies used in each session included didactic step-by-step instruction for each lesson, perspective-taking questions, one-on-one role play with her therapist, role play videos, practicing the assignments with the help of her mother in her natural settings, and reviewing the practice and feedback.

The highly structured method of each PEERS-YA sessions allowed her to go step by step in each behavior targeted, reviewing, practicing, and rehearsing her interactions. This gave her more security and self-efficacy. Previously, she would miss the key points of a specific social aspect and behavior involved and didn't realize exactly what went awry. With the intervention she could identify where she was failing and practice the step that she was missing or that was more difficult for her, noting which part of the skill needed to be corrected or improved. The individual approach worked for her, and sometimes she would take more than one session for each lesson if needed to ensure that the lesson was completely mastered before continuing with the following. PEERS-YA program might be useful also when working with an individual approach when group programs are not available.

CASE STUDY

Connan is a 24-year-old male with ASD and no intellectual disability. He received his diagnosis at the age of 5 and engaged in various treatments throughout his life. He had a longstanding history of social and communication impairments and lack of social motivation, and he had not been able to form significant bonds with peers. He attended university, where he obtained a degree in literature and education, and currently works as a teacher's aide at a school. His tasks are mainly helping teachers to prepare literature reading materials for adolescents in secondary school and to assist in administrative work. To perform his responsibilities, he needs to research and select books and short stories, prepare activities for students to solve, send them to the teachers, and work with them planning future assignments.

Connan sought therapy due to interpersonal problems at his workplace. During the initial assessment he reported procrastinating in his work and not knowing how to approach his coworkers, both personally and through electronic means. When probed by the clinician regarding his procrastination, he described concerns about failure in social work-related situations and worries about what his coworkers might think of him. There was an impression of anxiety interfering in his socialization. As he presented both social skills impairments and traits of social anxiety it was suggested to him to undergo social skills training and CBT for his anxiety symptoms. Connan agreed to it but explicitly informed the clinician that he did not intend to work toward expanding his social network and just wanted to "solve this issue at work." Taking into account the patient's goals, his lack of social motivation, and his co-occurring social anxiety, it was decided not to offer group interventions but to provide a tailor-made social skill training simultaneously with CBT.

The intervention was designed using didactic and structured instructions on how to use instant messaging services and write work emails and involved modeling and assisting Connan in writing, behavioral rehearsals, and role play with the clinician prior to sending any communication. There was no need to assist him in specific tasks such as selecting reading material or filling administrative forms. In addition, a modified CBT anxiety protocol was initiated. Modifications included offering more and longer sessions, fewer cognitive techniques, and more behavioral strategies. It was particularly helpful for him to reduce avoidance to note down what might go wrong, facing the feared situation, and fact checking if his initial thoughts indeed occurred. He reported fewer difficulties in facing social situations despite worrying he would confront anxiety-triggering situations. Nevertheless, Connan did not seem motivated to establish new relationships and was content with just being able to perform well at work.

In cases like Connan's it is important to thoroughly identify social skills impairments and co-occurring conditions such as anxiety or depression, since most of the times, these comorbidities can account for a percentage of the individual's social difficulties that superficially might strike as core ASD symptoms. Not addressing these adequately is usually associated with sub-clinical response to treatment and treatment dropout.

Underserved Populations

We believe that it is necessary for future lines of research and practice in social skills to include underseen populations, such as women and those with nonbinary gender identities and lesbian, gay, bisexual, transgender, queer and intersexed community (LBGTQI) individuals. These groups have been underrepresented in research and practice, and differential needs and supports in the social skills areas might not be fully addressed. It is essential that gender identity, diversity, and sexual orientation are respected and considered when designing practices (Hull et al., 2020; Strang et al., 2020), including social skills interventions, since this respect will increase engagement toward the treatment and will emotionally validate the individual's needs, rights, and goals.

It is important is to consider that women may present different social profiles than men (Carpenter et al., 2019; Happé & Frith, 2020; Halladay et. al, 2015;

Mandy & Lai 2017), with greater camouflaging strategies (Hull et al., 2017, 2019; Lai et al., 2021) and different social expectations for them across cultures. This will have an impact on the targeted skills in a specific curriculum and the technique selection. Also, women on the spectrum are more likely to have been exposed to physical, sexual, and psychological abuse (Haruvi-Lamdan et al., 2020), raising the issue of vulnerability of people with ASD in relationships (Bargiela et al., 2016). Preventing risks and promoting safety and healthy personal relationships should be a part of any social skills training for any adult on the spectrum of any biological sex and gender identity.

Future Directions

A promising area in social skills development is technology. Video modeling is already a well-documented evidence-based technique for teaching skills, but in some studies virtual reality and different apps and software for teaching social skills are being implemented and tested. It is important to consider the possibilities that this experimental and exploratory field can bring (Kandalaft et al., 2013). The use of technology and virtual reality can be well suited to the cognitive style of individuals with ASD (Parsons & Mitchell, 2002) and might be very promising combined with video modeling. Currently we still do not know the evidence of effectiveness of these interventions, but they will definitely provide new possibilities for accessing treatments that were not available before due to geographical distance or because of limited resources. This can be very beneficial and necessary for many communities in the future.

CONCLUSIONS

We still have a lot to do, research, and learn in order to better support adults with ASD generally. There is a limited, but encouraging, set of evidence-based programs and techniques in social skills program development whose aim will always be to increase the quality of the relationships and the quality of life of the patient.

When applying social skills interventions, clinicians should consider the following key points: performing a thorough assessment, selecting the goals and skills, deciding the best treatment option for the individual, and choosing the format that best suits the patient's needs at the moment of assessment. The following steps would be implementing, monitoring, and assessing the intervention and its outcomes. This process should be dynamic, since it might change over time, and it should take into account individual and cultural variables that are involved, keeping in mind aspects related to gender and diversity. It is important to remember that any social skills intervention will include training people with ASD but will also involve educating nonautistic people about ASD (Baker, 2003) and its full potential to contribute to a richer world.

When working with individuals with ASD, clinicians are usually trying to provide support to navigate successfully the world outside the spectrum. That other world, the autistic social world and point of view, with its plots and inner logic, is intriguing and fascinating for clinicians to explore and understand deeply its functioning and reveal its uniqueness in every treatment, individual, and therapeutic relationship. It will also be interesting to explore the communication, coping strategies, and the resources that arise from the interaction of individuals with ASD with each other. This knowledge could be invaluable and could be another important aspect of future interventions in social skills.

Those two social processing worlds are actually one we all share in practice, and the efforts to understand and to build bridges should be shared across research and clinical practice, advocates, stakeholders, autistic communities, and clinicians. The more bridges that are built, the more possibilities there will be for everyone to explore the infinite potential of human relationships.

REFERENCES

Baker, J. (2003) *Social skills training for children and adolescents with Asperger syndrome and social communication problems.* Autism Asperger Publishing Co.

Bargiela, S., Steward, R., & Mandy, W. (2016) The experiences of late-diagnosed women with autism spectrum conditions: An investigation of the female autism phenotype. *Journal of Autism Developmental Disorders, 46,* 3281–3294.

Bellini, Scott, and Jessica K. Peters. (2008) Social skills training for youth with autism spectrum disorders. *Child and Adolescent Psychiatric Clinics of North America, 17*(4), 857–873.

Bishop-Fitzpatrick, L., Minshew, N. J., & Eack, S. M. (2013). A systematic review of psychosocial interventions for adults with autism spectrum disorders. *Journal of Autism and Developmental Disorders, 43*(3), 687–694.

Caballo, V. E. (2002). *Manual de entrenamiento de las habilidades sociales.* Siglo XXI.

Carpenter, B., Happé, F., & Egerton, J. (Eds.). (2019). *Girls and autism: Educational, family and personal perspectives.* Routledge.

Frith, U., & Happé, F. (1999). Theory of mind and self-consciousness: What is it like to be autistic? *Mind & Language, 14,* 82–89.

Gaus, V. L. (2007). *Cognitive-behavioral therapy for adult Asperger syndrome.* Guilford Press.

Gaus, V. L. (2011) Adult Asperger syndrome and the utility of cognitive-behavioural therapy. *Journal of Contemporary Psychotherapy, 41,* 47–56.

Gray, C. (1994). *Comic strip conversations: Illustrated interactions that teach conversation skills to students with autism and related disorders.* Future Horizons.

Gray, C. A., & Garand, J. D. (1993). Social stories: Improving responses of students with autism with accurate social information. *Focus on Autistic Behaviour, 8*(1), 1–10.

Gresham, F. M., Sugai, G., & Horner, R. H. (2001). Interpreting outcomes of social skills training for students with high-incidence disabilities. *Exceptional Children, 67*(3), 331–344.

Halladay, A. K., Bishop, S., & Constantino, J. N. (2015). Sex and gender differences in autism spectrum disorder: Summarizing evidence gaps and identifying emerging areas of priority. *Molecular Autism, 6,* 36.

Happé F. (2003). Theory of mind and the self. *Annals of the New York Academy of Sciences, 1001*, 134–144.

Happé, F., & Frith, U. (2020). Annual research review: Looking back to look forward—changes in the concept of autism and implications for future research. *Journal of Child Psychology Psychiatry, 61*, 218–232.

Haruvi-Lamdan, N., Horesh, D., Zohar, S., Kraus, M., & Golan, O. (2020). Autism spectrum disorder and post-traumatic stress disorder: An unexplored co-occurrence of conditions. *Autism: The International Journal of Research and Practice, 24*(4), 884–898.

Howlin, P., & Moss, P. (2012). Adults with autism spectrum disorders. *Canadian Journal of psychiatry. Revue Canadienne de psychiatrie, 57*(5), 275–283.

Hull, L., Lai, M. C., Baron-Cohen, S., Allison, C., Smith, P., Petrides, K. V., & Mandy, W. (2019). Gender differences in self-reported camouflaging in autistic and non-autistic adults. *Autism, 24*(2), 352–363.

Hull, L., Mandy, W., & Petrides, K. V. (2017). Behavioural and cognitive sex/gender differences in autism spectrum condition and typically developing males and females. *Autism, 21*(6), 706–727.

Hull, L., Petrides, K. V., Allison, C., Smith, P., Baron-Cohen, S., Lai, M. C., & Mandy, W. (2017). "Putting on my best normal": Social camouflaging in adults with autism spectrum conditions. *Journal of Autism and Developmental Disorders, 47*(8), 2519–2534.

Kandalaft, M. R., Didehbani, N., Krawczyk, D. C. (2013). Virtual reality social cognition training for young adults with high-functioning autism. *Journal Autism Developmental Disorders, 43*, 34–44.

Kelly, R. A. (2010). *Entrenamiento de las habilidades sociales: Guía práctica para intervenciones/Jeffrey A. Kelly; [versión española Susana del Viso]*. Desclée de Brouwer, 1992.

Lai, M. C., Hull, L., Mandy, W., Chakrabarti, B., Nordahl, C. W., Lombardo, M. V., ... Livingston, L. A. (2021). Commentary: 'Camouflaging' in autistic people-reflection on Fombonne (2020). *Journal of Child Psychology and Psychiatry, 62*(8).

Lai, M. C., Lombardo, M. V., Auyeung, B., Chakrabarti, B., & Baron-Cohen, S. (2015). Sex/gender differences and autism: Setting the scene for future research. *Journal of the American Academy of Child & Adolescent Psychiatry, 54*(1), 11–24.

Laugeson, E. A. (2017). *PEERS® for young adults: Social skills training for adults with autism spectrum disorder and other social challenges*. Taylor & Francis.

Laugeson, E. A., & Frankel, F. (2010). *Social skills for teenagers with developmental and autism spectrum disorders: The PEERS Treatment Manual*. Routledge.

Laugeson, E. A., Frankel, F., Gantman, A., Dillon, A. R., & Mogil, C. (2012). Evidence-based social skills training for adolescents with autism spectrum disorders: The UCLA PEERS program. *Journal of Autism and Developmental Disorders, 42*(6), 1025–1036.

Laugeson, E. A., Gantman, A., Kapp, S. K., Orenski, K., & Ellingsen, R. (2015). A randomized controlled trial to improve social skills in young adults with autism spectrum disorder: The UCLA PEERS® program. *Journal of Autism and Developmental Disorders, 45*(12), 3978–3989.

Lord, C., McCauley, J. B., Pepa, L. A., Huerta, M., & Pickles, A. (2020). Work, living, and the pursuit of happiness: Vocational and psychosocial outcomes for young adults with autism. *Autism, 24*(7), 1691–1703.

Maddox, B. B., White, S. W. (2015) Comorbid social anxiety disorder in adults with autism spectrum disorder. *Journal of Autism Developmental Disorders*, a45, 3949–3960.

Mandy, W., & Lai, M.-C. (2017). Towards sex- and gender-informed autism research. *Autism, 21*(6), 643–645.

Myles, B. S., & Simpson, R. L. (2001). Understanding the hidden curriculum: An essential social skill for children and youth with Asperger syndrome. *Intervention in School and Clinic, 36*(5), 279–286.

Parsons, S., & Mitchell, P. (2002). The potential of virtual reality in social skills training for people with autistic spectrum disorders. *Journal of Intellectual Disability Research, 46*(5), 430–443.

Reichow, B., Steiner, A. M., & Volkmar, F. (2013). Cochrane review: Social skills groups for people aged 6 to 21 with autism spectrum disorders (ASD). *Evidence-Based Child Health, 8*(2), 266–315.

Rumball, F., Happé, F., & Grey, N. (2020). Experience of trauma and PTSD symptoms in autistic adults: Risk of PTSD development following DSM-5 and non-DSM-5 traumatic life events. *Autism Research, 13*(12), 2122–2132.Spain, D., & Blainey, S. H. (2015). Group social skills interventions for adults with high-functioning autism spectrum disorders: A systematic review. *Autism: The International Journal of Research and Practice, 19*(7), 874–886.

Spain, D., & Blainey, S. H. (2015). Group social skills interventions for adults with high-functioning autism spectrum disorders: A systematic review. *Autism, 19*(7), 874–886.

Strang, J. F., van der Miesen, A. I., Caplan, R., Hughes, C., daVanport, S., & Lai, M.-C. (2020). Both sex- and gender-related factors should be considered in autism research and clinical practice. *Autism, 24*(3), 539–543.

Tincani, M., & Bondy, A. (Eds.). (2015). *Autism spectrum disorders in adolescents and adults: Evidence-based and promising interventions*. Guilford Publications.

Walsh, E., Holloway, J., & Lydon, H. (2018) An evaluation of a social skills intervention for adults with autism spectrum disorder and intellectual disabilities preparing for employment in Ireland: A pilot study. *Journal of Autism and Developmental Disorders, 48*, 1727–1741.

Williams, D. (2010). Theory of own mind in autism: Evidence of a specific deficit in self-awareness? *Autism, 14*(5), 474–494.

Williams, D. M., Happé, F. (2009). What did I say? Versus what did I think? Attributing false beliefs to self amongst children with and without autism. *Journal of Autism Developmental Disorders, 39*, 865–873.

White, S. W., Keonig, K., & Scahill, L. (2006). Social skills development in children with autism spectrum disorders: A review of the intervention research. *Journal of Autism and Developmental Disorders, 37*(10), 1858–1868.

White, S. W., Koenig, K., & Scahill, L. (2010). Group social skills instruction for adolescents with high-functioning autism spectrum disorders. *Focus on Autism and Other Developmental Disabilities, 25*(4), 209–219.

White, S. W., Ollendick, T., Albano, A. M., Oswald, D., Johnson, C., Southam-Gerow, M. A., Kim, I., & Scahill, L. (2013). Randomized controlled trial: Multimodal anxiety and social skill intervention for adolescents with autism spectrum disorder. *Journal of Autism and Developmental Disorders, 43*(2), 382–394.

White, S. W., Kreiser, N. L., Pugliese, C., & Scarpa, A. (2012). Social anxiety mediates the effect of autism spectrum disorder characteristics on hostility in young adults. *Autism, 16*(5), 453–464.

White, S. W., Scarpa, A., Conner, C. M., Maddox, B. B., & Bonete, S. (2014). Evaluating change in social skills in high-functioning adults with autism spectrum disorder using a laboratory-based observational measure. *Focus on Autism and Other Developmental Disabilities, 30*(1), 3–12.

Wilkins, J., & Matson, J. L. (2009). A comparison of social skills profiles in intellectually disabled adults with and without ASD. *Behavior Modification, 33*(2), 143–155.

Winner, M. G., & Crooke, P. J. (2009). Social thinking: A training paradigm for professionals and treatment approach for individuals with social learning/social pragmatic challenges. *Perspectives on Language Learning and Education, 16*(2), 62–69.

Winner, M. G., & Crooke, P. J. (2011). Social communication strategies for adolescents with autism. *The ASHA Leader, 16*(1), 8–11.

8

Positive Behavioral Support

DARREN BOWRING AND SANDY TOOGOOD ■

KEY CONSIDERATIONS

- PBS is a framework model for designing person-centered, multicomponent interventions, based on a prior functional assessment.
- Functional assessment identifies motivative contexts and maintaining variables that account for the occurrence of challenging behavior (CB).
- PBS features data-informed decision making at assessment, intervention, and monitoring phases.
- PBS plans are a package of interventions that are constructional, nonaversive, effective, and least-restrictive and which involve stakeholder participation.
- The primary aim of PBS is to improve quality of life. Quality of life is both an intervention and outcome goal.
- Preliminary research indicates PBS is effective at reducing CB in individuals with ASD, but more robust research in larger samples is required to inform applied service development.

INTRODUCTION: CHALLENGING BEHAVIOR AND ASD

Challenging behavior (CB) is defined as

> Culturally abnormal behavior(s) of such an intensity, frequency or duration that the physical safety of the person or others is likely to be placed in serious jeopardy, or behavior which is likely to seriously limit use of, or result in the person being denied access to, ordinary community facilities (Emerson & Einfeld, 2011, p. 4).

CB includes, but is not restricted to, aggression, self-injury, property damage, and negative vocalizations. The term was adopted in the 1980s to focus attention on the challenges service providers faced in meeting people's support needs in the community rather than in institutional services, and to seek causal explanations within the social environment rather than the individual. The application of PBS to date has focused on populations with developmental disabilities, with research largely on intellectual disability populations, some of which include persons with an additional ASD diagnosis.

People with intellectual disabilities account for 1%–2% of the general population (British Psychological Society, 2011). Estimates vary, but it is thought that around 10% of people with intellectual disabilities will have an additional ASD diagnosis, rising to 50%–60% of people with severe or profound intellectual disabilities (Emerson & Baines, 2010). Approximately one third of people with an ASD diagnosis will also have intellectual disabilities (Emerson & Baines, 2010). ASD and ID are risk factors for CB that increase with severity of disability and presence of additional physical, sensory, or communication impairments (Bowring et al., 2017; Holden & Gitlesen, 2006; Jones et al., 2008; Lundqvist, 2013). Research in population samples suggests that approximately one in every five or six individuals with intellectual disabilities that are known to services will present with CB (Bowring et al., 2017; Jones et al. 2008; Lundqvist, 2013). A study by Hutchins and Prelock (2014) found the prevalence of CB in adults with both an intellectual disability and ASD diagnosis ranged from 35.8% to 63.4% with most studies finding that more than half of these individuals engaged in more than one CB. Studies in individuals with an ASD only diagnosis suggest 13%–30% of children engage in severe CB (Matson et al., 2008), with one in four presenting clinically challenging aggressive behavior (Hill et al., 2014).

AN OVERVIEW OF THE PBS APPROACH

Positive behavioral support (PBS) is a multicomponent framework for organizing, delivering, and evaluating the impact of interventions selected for an individual with developmental disorders whose behavior is complex and challenging (Carr et al., 1999; Horner, 2000; Kincaid et al., 2016; LaVigna & Willis, 2012). The principal aim in PBS is to enhance stakeholder quality of life (QoL). Stakeholders are persons whose behavior is challenging and those affected by the behavior such as parents, siblings, teachers, and care workers. Reducing CB represents one important way of enhancing stakeholder QoL, and enhancing QoL provides several important ways of reducing CB. Thus, QoL is both an intervention and an outcome. PBS is a person-centered approach in which behavior change procedures are determined on an individual basis following a period of functional and contextual assessment. Functional assessment identifies motivative contexts and maintaining variables that account for the occurrence of CB. Interventions are multicomponent modifications of behavior-environment interactions, indicated by assessment, such as environmental enrichment and supporting alternatives to CB. Intervention effects are carefully monitored and systematically evaluated using data.

ORIGINS OF PBS

PBS evolved in the 1980s from applied behavior analysis (ABA; Baer et al., 1968) amid concerns about nonfunctional analytic approaches involving the use of aversive stimuli such as aromatic ammonia (Tanner & Zeiler, 1975) and electric shock (Carr & Lovaas, 1983) to suppress severe problem behavior. ABA had developed as a field at a time of increasing public interest in civil rights and social justice. At the same time, work had begun in Scandinavia, leading eventually to the elaboration of the principles of normalization (Wolfensberger et al., 1972), which aimed to value people at risk of being devalued. Opinion divided sharply between empiricists and theorists. Pioneers of nonaversive approaches included Meyer and Evans (1989) and LaVigna and Donnellan (1986). Carr et al. (2002) described PBS as a synthesis of procedures from ABA, normalization theory, and the inclusive movement. Kincaid et al. (2016) present PBS as a dynamic and continually involving system that will come to include components as yet undiscovered.

The PBS Framework Approach

PBS is a framework for designing person-centered multicomponent interventions based on a prior functional assessment (Iwata et al., 1982; O'Neill et al., 2014). Intervention plans typically include a selection of social, behavioral, and educational procedures from ABA (Cooper et al., 2020) and evidence-based approaches from other related disciplines (such as occupational therapy, speech and language therapy, and clinical psychology) in ways that are internally coherent, consistent with assessment, and compatible with PBS core values. Intervention components are constructional (Goldiamond, 1974), nonaversive, effective, and the least restrictive available, with stakeholder participation a key component (Carr et al., 2002; Gore et al., 2013). PBS interventions pursue improvement at the individual, group, and systems levels, addressing, for example, issues such as service staff support, physical and mental health, and organizational structures.

PBS as a "Package" of Interventions

Addressing behavior change in natural settings requires multiple intervention procedures, and the combination of these into a "package" is what defines PBS (Smith, 2013).

The causal model of Hastings et al. (2013) suggests CB is maintained by biological and/or social consequences that includes the behavior of others. Maintaining processes can include stimulation, attention, tangible, and escape from demands (Carr, 1977). Pain reduction has recently been added to this list (Hastings et al., 2013). To understand CB, it is necessary to understand the circumstances that occur before and what happens after the behavior (Gore et al., 2013). People with developmental disorders have historically experienced impoverished social contact, low levels of engagement, and aversive interactions (Hastings et al., 2013). CB is often the most effective means of addressing these issues. In order to understand the maintaining processes, a functional behavioral assessment of the social and physical environment and context in which the CB occurs is needed (Miltenberger et al., 2019). This explains how the existing behavior helps the individual to manage or exert control over their environment, which informs the development of a more effective and person-centered intervention plan (Didden et al., 1997; Iwata et al., 1982; Miltenberger et al., 2019; O'Neill et al., 2014; Sprague & Horner, 1995). Research indicates that PBS interventions for CB have a greater chance of success if based on prior functional assessment (Carr et al., 1999; Hanley et al., 2003; Scott & Cooper, 2017).

Development of intervention plans in the PBS model is a collaborative endeavor with stakeholders to ensure good contextual fit (Albin et al., 1999; Monzale & Horner, 2020). While there is no set framework for the design of plans, they should be multielement and comprise some key components (LaVigna & Donnellan, 1986; McClean & Grey, 2012; Webber et al., 2011) including:

- Proactive strategies that are preventative, such as proactive management of physical and mental health; augmentative communication; strategies that modify the establishing operations that evoke CB (Michael, 1993); ABA-evidenced behavioral technology such as differential reinforcement of other behaviors (Vollmer & Iwata, 1992); strategies that promote person-centered QoL and give the individual choice, control, engagement; strategies that promote relationships; and community participation.
- Proactive strategies that are developmental, such as teaching new behaviors, promoting skills, teaching functionally equivalent behaviors, and teaching coping and tolerance skills.
- Secondary strategies, such as approaches to support the individual at early signs of distress, stimulus change, diversion to preferred activities, active listening, and a change of interactor or interactional style.
- Reactive strategies to reduce immediate risks and promote safety (LaVigna & Willis, 2012).
- Wider system approaches, such as staff/carer training and support for carers.

An emerging trend in PBS practice is an adaptation from the delivery of school-wide positive behavioral interventions and supports (PBIS) in the USA (Sugai & Horner, 2020), which describes a tiered level of support intensity. These are:

1. Universal support (preventative for everyone) which includes QoL interventions, clear procedures and routines, teaching prosocial behavior, promoting relationships, and reinforcing positive behavior.
2. Targeted support (additional, for those needing extra help in order to succeed), which includes targeted group interventions, social skills groups, brief functional assessments, and bespoke group support arrangements.
3. Intensive support (intervention for a few when behavior change is weak or not apparent), which would be based on a detailed functional assessment with individualized intervention plans.

A SUMMARY OF THE EMPIRICAL EVIDENCE FOR PBS

PBS has been used as a framework for intervention in services across the UK and in other countries (McClean & Grey, 2012). There is an emerging evidence base from meta-analytic reviews (Carr et al., 1999; LaVigna & Willis, 2012), and recent research studies with individuals with intellectual disabilities, including those with ASD (Allen et al., 2011; Hassiotis et al., 2009; McClean et al., 2007; McKenzie & Patterson, 2010), that PBS is effective at reducing levels of CB including aggression and self-injurious behavior. While initial results are encouraging, early research has been limited by methodological weaknesses (e.g., variations in definitions of CB, small sample sizes, lack of a control group, and assessment tools that have not been psychometrically evaluated or assessed for use in individuals with ASD; see McClintock et al., 2003) and a consistent failure to assess change in QoL and to explore the social validity impact of interventions (Carr et al., 2002; Kincaid et al., 2002; McClean et al., 2005). A meta-analysis of small randomized and quasi-randomized controlled trials (RCTs) concluded that behavioral interventions could be effective in helping people with ASD (Heyvaert et al., 2014), but that research designs with greater robustness in community settings were required.

In a study of four adults with ASD, McClean and Grey (2012) discovered substantial reductions in CBs following PBS intervention, along with improvement in mental health and QoL. Boettcher et al. (2003) used PBS to decrease CB in a child with ASD and her siblings, and the family experienced additional positive effects from this proactive intervention. A study by Lucyshyn et al. (2007) demonstrated that PBS led to a 75% reduction in CB for a child with ASD, and that the effects were maintained across a 7-year follow-up period. Associated outcomes included improved community engagement and social validity outcomes for parents. Bowring et al. (2017) considered individuals referred to a community-based PBS team, 53% of whom had ASD; they reported significant reductions in CB measured with the Behavior Problems Inventory—Short Form (BPI-S; Rojahn et al., 2012) with scores reducing from a mean of 37.74 (SD 30.54) at referral, to 12.12 (SD

12.24) at follow up, with a large effect size ($d = 0.84$). There was also significant improvement in QoL, health-related QoL and social validity impact such as reduced stress levels, greater knowledge on causes of CB, fewer injuries and damage to properties, improved relationships and greater access to joint community activities.

Despite these encouraging results, research into PBS as a framework model remains at the preliminary stage, and further studies have been advocated to inform theoretical understanding and applied service development (McClean et al., 2007; McKenzie, 2011). There is a need for further PBS studies, with larger samples, particularly in adult ASD populations, with more robust research designs, and with data examining QoL and social validity outcomes as well as CB. There has been a lack of robust RCT designs in ASD research (McGrew et al., 2016). One additional challenge for researchers is that PBS, as used in community service providers, is not a single treatment protocol, but a "package" of interventions (Stahmer et al., 2005). It is thus important that researchers have an agreement on the definition of PBS and evaluate the outcomes of PBS as a "package" in group studies (Smith, 2013), with ASD-specific samples.

CASE STUDY

Background

Michael was 19 years old and had a diagnosis of ASD and moderate intellectual disability. He had recently left school and transferred to an adult day service and respite provider. The local PBS practitioner received a referral due to Michael self-injuring in the form of punches to the right side of his face, occurring several times each day in all environments, resulting in an open wound just under his right eye.

The PBS practitioner met Michael and his parents at home. Parents reported a difficult transition for Michael from children to adult services with him struggling to adjust to the day service and different respite provider. They reported some self-injury during childhood in the form of wrist biting and head hitting, but nothing of the recent intensity. The PBS practitioner completed a BPI-S (Rojahn et al., 2012) and a QoL measure (based on Kincaid et al., 2002). The QoL scale assessed five domains: interpersonal relationships, self-determination, social inclusion, personal development, and emotional well-being. There has been a lack of measurement of QoL impact in PBS Studies (cf. LaVigna & Willis, 2012). Some studies, such as Hassiotis et al. (2011) and Allen et al. (2011) have focused on one QoL domain such as social inclusion, using the Guernsey Community Participation and Leisure Activities scale (Baker, 2000). Other small studies, such as McClean et al. (2007), have used tools such as Quality of Life Questionnaire (QoL-Q; Schalock et al., 1989).

The BPI-S identified the specific behaviors to target, alongside estimates of current frequency and severity. The QoL measure identified the lack of community presence and peer contact Michael had, as parents and services had reduced demands on him in recent months given the behavioral challenges. At the outset the PBS practitioner ensured there were data records in place to record instances of Michael hitting his face. Additionally, the PBS practitioner arranged investigations to rule out medical, dental, and psychiatric issues.

Functional Assessment

The PBS practitioner completed a detailed functional assessment in all the environments Michael accessed. The CB being assessed had been defined using BPI-S assessment. This involved:

- A review of previous professional reports such as Michael's ASD assessment, an educational psychology report; and recommendations from a speech and language therapy (SALT) assessment.
- Completion of motivational assessment "rating" scales (Durand & Crimmins, 1992) in all environments with key informants.
- Completion of a functional assessment interview (O'Neill et al., 2014) with key informants.
- Analysis of indirect antecedent behavior consequence (ABC) sheets with episodic severity data.
- Direct observations in all environments, particularly at times when CB had been more common, such as transitions.
- A visit to meet Michael's previous school and respite provider to collate information about previous supports and how the environments were set up to meet Michael's needs.
- A mediator analysis of staff support's understanding of Michael's preferred support arrangements and identification of training deficits.

The assessment concluded that Michael's underlying anxiety levels were higher due to the disruptive transition to adult services. The occupational therapist (OT) had completed a sensory profile assessment and identified that high levels of noise or visual stimulation (crowds) could serve as a setting event making a particular task (such as arriving at day services or playing bowling) more aversive. Results of the functional assessment concurred with this and concluded that the behavior of head hitting was maintained by negative reinforcement, as it led to immediate escape from aversive situations or termination of an aversive task (e.g., the bowling alley was very busy with a children's party, then Michael began head hitting, then he was taken home; arrived at day service and another service user was screaming, then Michael began head hitting, then Mum put him back in the car and drove around for a while until the situation had resolved).

PBS Plan and MDT Support

The PBS practitioner produced a short data-informed presentation on the above conclusions and presented this to Michael's multidisciplinary team (MDT).

The team involved the PBS practitioner, Michael's mother, his keyworker at day service, key worker at respite, SALT, OT and community nurse. The MDT all contributed to developing a multielement PBS plan based on this data. Everything included in the plan had good contextual fit: it could be delivered by the team in the environments where they supported Michael. The SALT worked with Michael to contribute to the plan. The SALT used pictorial and photo aids to support Michael to choose aspects of the plan, including activities to engage in, staff to support, and decoration for his day service room, such as the color of paint used on the walls. The SALT developed social stories to explain planning meetings and developed an easy-read version of the PBS plan that Michael could access. In this plan it listed:

Proactive Strategies

- The prime aim of the plan was to improve QoL. The plan listed approaches, people, and activities that were important to Michael and essential to promote his well-being who needed to be a regular part of his week. The plan prioritized giving Michael choice and control over his support arrangements and daytime program.
- The plan detailed communication strategies. The SALT supported Michael to choose his staff and activities in both environments. Visual planners (listing staff and activities) were made and placed at home and day service, with portable ones for everyone supporting Michael. SALT taught staff Makaton signs Michael used. Social stories were developed to support new initiatives and activities.
- The psychiatrist suggested low-arousal interventions to reduce stress around noise, complex language, crowds, proximity of others, changes to routines, and unfamiliar staff and transitions.
- A key aspect was predictable routines, sequences, and people. All providers began to collect Michael from home with a clear collection/transition plan.
- Timings for day service were changed for consistency to 11am–4pm; respite hours were changed to match this on weekends, to ensure predictable daily routines.
- A room at the day service was identified for Michael to begin and end his day, with lots of activities he enjoyed and visual aids present to communicate the structure and routine of the day. This replaced Michael arriving into the busy communal "day room" without a clear plan of his day.
- Michael's staff had photos taken and added to his visuals planner so he knew who would be supporting him each day.
- Staff who supported Michael were trained in ASD and low-arousal approaches by the local ASD Team.
- School staff delivered an additional training session (supported by parents) for day service and respite staff, sharing advice on Michael's likes and dislikes and support tips. Some school staff volunteered

to undertake shifts at day service and respite to coach and model approaches to staff.

- Skill teaching: day services introduced some educational approaches the school had suggested around ways Michael could communicate distress through signing.
- Differential reinforcement of alternative (DRA) behavior was introduced. This procedure involved reinforcing a behavior that served as a viable alternative for the problem behavior (Vollmer & Iwata, 1992). In this case Michael was taught the Makaton sign "worried" as an alternative to hitting his head. With each sign used, staff praised Michael and immediately communicated and fixed the issue. Once Michael had signed "happy," the activity continued and Michael was given a reinforcer in the form of a piece of candy. If Michael hit his head he was not praised or reinforced with candy.
- The sensory profile assessment led to Michael's day service room being adapted with blinds, new lights, less clutter, and clear walls, apart from visual planners. Regular sensory activities were introduced that Michael enjoyed.
- Michael would start and end the day in his room and access it at other times if finding some days difficult. Michael increasingly attended group activities from this safe space.
- As CB reduced, services began to reintroduce activities to key preferred places (bowling alley, activity park, and fishing) and to meet Michael's friends from school for joint activities.

Secondary Strategies

- Staff began to report knowing when Michael was becoming distressed as they became experienced in supporting him. They reported signs such as repeating key phrases, clearing his throat, and coughing as early indicators of distress.
- Staff were able to prompt Michael to sign what was wrong earlier (as he had been taught) and responded to these requests promptly, reinforcing these prosocial communication approaches.
- Michael's sister had produced some distraction activities, including Disney songs the staff were taught, which Michael enjoyed joining.
- The OT worked with Michael to develop coping skills. A range of replacement techniques were explored, not always successfully employed, but work continued on these.
- Support staff became skilled at working with Michael to change plans when he indicated, on some days, that he did not want to engage with certain activities.

Reactive Strategies

- If Michael started head hitting, staff and parents had agreed on low-arousal response strategies and would adapt activities to resolve the issue causing distress.

- Staff knew Makaton signs, which helped communicate with Michael and reassure him at these times.

Monitoring Phase

The PBS practitioner produced a clear graph detailing the frequency and severity of head hitting behavior. To the delight of Michael's MDT, this detailed a very quick downward reduction in severity, and after 8 weeks of PBS input Michael's wound had healed over. The MDT team continued to meet weekly to review progress, consider the data, review any incidents, and continue to develop the PBS plan collaboratively as a working document. These meetings, and the graphed data, were helpful to parents and staff, as they could see progress being made and they had support to review the times when things had not gone well. The PBS practitioner continued to complete direct observations to ensure implementation of the plan and support coaching and feedback to the team.

Outcomes

As things continued to improve the MDT meetings were extended to monthly. The team additionally focused on improvements in terms of QoL indicators given the behavioral improvements: Michael was meeting friends from school for activities, using the bus with support, visiting the cinema and going out for meals, increasingly joining in group activities at day services, and communicating verbally more. New targets and skills were discussed at MDT meetings to work on, based on work that SALT continued to do with Michael. Plans were made for Michael to begin vocational training.

After 12 months, the frequency of head hitting was such that the PBS practitioner was able to withdraw from the MDT, which continued with Michael's mother and keyworkers from respite and day services. The PBS practitioner could still attend by invitation if the team considered it helpful to discuss any issue.

CONCLUSIONS

ASD is a risk factor for CB that increases with the presence of additional cognitive, physical, sensory and communication impairments. PBS is a person-centered framework that targets improvement in stakeholder quality of life and the negative impacts of CB. In this chapter, we described PBS as a multicomponent "package" of interventions that are person centered, function based, evidence informed, and consistent with a set of values that emphasize empowerment and inclusion. Functional behavioral assessment is a crucial component of a PBS framework. PBS interventions typically enrich environments and help individuals to develop alternatives to CB. Our case study illustrated how, using a PBS approach, a small team was able to enhance the quality of a person's day-to-day life and reduce levels of self-injurious behavior. The PBS team was comprised of relevant stakeholders and the changes they made were both evidence based and evidence informed (i.e., data-based decision making). The evidence base for PBS is increasing. More studies are needed, however, with larger ASD populations and robust designs, including utilizing psychometrically evaluated tools for ASD populations, with measurement of QoL and social validity outcomes included. In the meantime, PBS offers an effective and ethically sound framework for addressing behavior and contexts that are complex and challenging.

REFERENCES

Albin, R. W., Lucyshyn J. M., Horner R. H., & Flannery K. B. (1999). Contextual fit for behavioural support plans: A model for "goodness of fit." In L. K. Koegel, R. L. Koegel, & G. Dunlap (Eds.), *Positive behavioural support: Including people with difficult behaviour in the community* (pp. 81–98). Paul Brookes Publishing.

Allen, D., Lowe, K., Baker, P., Dench, C., Hawkins, S., Jones, E., & James, W. (2011). Assessing the effectiveness of positive behavioural support: The P-CPO project. *International Journal of Positive Behavioural Support, 1,* 14–23.

Baer, D. M., Wolf, M. M., & Risley, T. R. (1968). Some current dimensions of applied behavior analysis. *Journal of Applied Behavior Analysis, 1,* 91–97.

Baker, P. A. (2000). Measurement of community participation and use of leisure by service users with intellectual disability: The Guernsey community participation and leisure assessment. *Journal of Applied Research in Intellectual Disabilities, 13,* 169–185.

Boettcher, M., Koegel, R. L., McNerney, E. K., & Kern Koegel, L. (2003). A family-centered prevention approach to PBS in a time of crisis. *Journal of Positive Behavior Interventions, 5*(1), 55–59.

Bowring, D. L., Totsika, V., Hastings, R. P., Toogood, S., & Griffiths, G. M. (2017). Challenging behaviours in adults with an intellectual disability: A total population study and exploration of risk indices. *British Journal of Clinical Psychology, 56,* 16–32.

British Psychological Society. (2011). *Commissioning clinical psychology services for adults with learning disabilities.* BPS.

Carr, E. G. (1977) The motivation of self-injurious behaviour: a review of some hypotheses. Psychological Bulletin, 84(4), 800-816.

Carr, E. G., Dunlap, G., Horner, R. H., Koegel, R. L., Turnbull, A. P., Sailor, W., Anderson, J. L., Albin, R. W., Koegel, L. K., & Fox, L., (2002). Positive behavior support: Evolution of an applied science. *Journal of Positive Behavior Interventions, 4,* 4–16.

Carr, E., Horner, R., Turnbull, A., Marquis, J., Magito-McLaughlin, D., McAtee, M., Smith, C., Anderson-Ryan, K., Ruef, M., & Doolabh, A. (1999). *Positive behavior support for people with developmental disabilities: A research synthesis.* American Association on Mental Retardation.

Carr, E. G., & Lovaas, O. I. (1983). Contingent electric shock as a treatment for severe behavior problems. In S. Axelrod & J. Apsche (Eds.), *The Effects of Punishment on Human Behavior* (pp. 221–245). New York, Academic Press.

Cooper, J. O., Heron, T. E., & Heward, W. L. (2020). *Applied behavior analysis* (3rd ed.). Pearson

Didden, R., Duker, P. C., & Korzilius, H. (1997). Meta-analytic study of treatment effectiveness for problem behaviours with individuals who have mental retardation. *American Journal on Mental Retardation, 101*(4), 387–399.

Durand, V. M., & Crimmins, D. B. (1992). *The Motivation Assessment scale (MAS) administration guide*. Monaco & Associates.

Emerson, E., & Baines, S. (2010). *The estimated prevalence of autism among adults with learning disabilities in England*. Improving Health and Lives: Learning Disabilities Observatory.

Emerson, E., & Einfeld, S. L. (2011). *Challenging behaviour* (3rd ed.). Cambridge University Press.

Goldiamond, I. (1974). Toward a constructional approach to social problems: Ethical and constitutional issues raised by applied behavior analysis. *Behaviorism, 2*(1),1–84.

Gore, N. J., McGill, P., Toogood, S., Allen, D., Hughes, J. C., & Baker, P. (2013). Definition and scope for positive behavioural support. *International Journal of Positive Behavioural Support, 3*(2), 4–23.

Hanley, G. P., Iwata, B. A., & McCord, B. E. (2003). Functional analysis of problem behavior: A review. *Journal of Applied Behavior Analysis, 36*, 147–185.

Hassiotis, A., Canagasabey, A., Robotham, D., Marston, L., Romeo, R., & King, M. (2011). Applied behaviour analysis and standard treatment in intellectual disability: 2-year outcomes. *British Journal of Psychiatry, 198*(6), 490–491.

Hassiotis, A., Robotham, D., Canagasabey, A., Romeo, R., Langridge, D., Blizard, R., Murad, S., & King, M. (2009). Randomized, single-blind, controlled trial of a specialist behavior therapy team for challenging behavior in adults with intellectual disabilities. *American Journal of Psychiatry, 166*, 1278–1285.

Hastings R. P., Allen D., Baker P., Gore N. J., Hughes J. C., McGill P., Noone, S. J., & Toogood, S. (2013). A conceptual framework for understanding why challenging behaviours occur in people with developmental disabilities. *International Journal of Positive Behavioural Support, 3*, 5–13.

Heyvaert, M., Saenen, L., Campbell, J. M., Maes, B., & Onghena, P. (2014). Efficacy of behavioral interventions for reducing problem behavior in persons with autism: An updated quantitative synthesis of single-subject research. *Research in Developmental Disabilities, 35*(10), 2463–2476.

Hill, A. P., Zuckerman, K. E., Hagen, A. D., Kriz, D. J., Duvall, S. W., Van Santen, J., Nigg, J., Fair, D., &Fombonne, E. (2014). Aggressive behavior problems in children with autism spectrum disorders: Prevalence and correlates in a large clinical sample. *Research in Autism Spectrum Disorders, 8*(9), 1121–1133.

Holden, B., & Gitlesen, J. P. (2006). A total population study of challenging behaviour in the county of Hedmark, Norway: Prevalence and risk markers. *Research in Developmental Disabilities, 27*, 456–465.

Horner, R. H. (2000). Positive behavior supports. *Focus on Autism and Other Developmental Disabilities, 15*, 97–105.

Hutchins, T. L., & Prelock, P. A. (2014). Using communication to reduce challenging behaviors in individuals with autism spectrum disorders and intellectual disability. *Child and Adolescent Psychiatric Clinics of North America, 23*(1), 41–55.

Iwata, B. A., Dorsey, M. F., Slifer, K. J., Bauman, K. E., & Richman, G. S. (1982). Toward a functional analysis of self-injury. *Analysis and Intervention in Developmental Disabilities, 2*, 3–20.

Jones S., Cooper S.-A., Smiley E., Allen L., Williamson A., & Morrison J. (2008). Prevalence of, and factors associated with, problem behaviors in adults with intellectual disabilities. *The Journal of Nervous and Mental Disease, 196*, 678–686.

Kincaid, D., Dunlap, G., Kern, L., Lane, K. L., Bambara, L. M., Brown, F., Fox, L., Knoster, T. P. (2016). Positive behavior support: A proposal for updating and refining the definition. *Journal of Positive Behavior Interventions, 18*(2), 69–73.

Kincaid, D., Knoster, T., Harrower, J. K., Shannon, P., & Bustamante, S. (2002). Measuring the impact of positive behaviour support. *Journal of Positive Behavior Interventions, 4*(2), 109–117.LaVigna, G. W., & Donnellan, A. M. (1986). *Alternatives to punishment: Solving behavior problems with non-aversive strategies.* Ardent Media.

LaVigna, G. W., & Willis, T. J. (2012). The efficacy of positive behavioural support with the most challenging behavior: The evidence and its implications, *Journal of Intellectual and Developmental Disability, 37*, 185–195.

Lucyshyn, J. M., Albin, R. W., Horner, R. H., Mann, J. C., Mann, J. A., & Wadsworth, G. (2007). Family implementation of positive behavior support for a child with autism: Longitudinal, single-case, experimental, and descriptive replication and extension. *Journal of Positive Behavior Interventions, 9*(3), 131–150.

Lundqvist, L. (2013). Prevalence and risk markers of behaviour problems among adults with intellectual disabilities. A total population study in Orebro County, Sweden. *Research in Developmental Disabilities, 34*, 1346–1356.

Matson, J. L., Wilkins, J., & Macken, J. (2008) The relationship of challenging behaviors to severity and symptoms of autism spectrum disorders. *Journal of Mental Health Research in Intellectual Disabilities, 2*(1), 29–44.

McClean, B., Dench, C., Grey, I. M., Shanahan, S., Fitzsimmons, E. M., Hendler, J., & Corrigan, M.(2005) Person focused training: A model for delivering positive behavioural supports to people with challenging behaviours. *Journal of Intellectual Disability Research, 49*(5), 340–352.

McClean, B., Grey, I. M., & McCracken, M. (2007). An evaluation of positive behavioural support for people with very severe challenging behaviours in community-based settings. *Journal of Intellectual Disabilities, 11*, 1–21.

McClean, B., & Ian Grey, I. M. (2012). A component analysis of positive behaviour support plans. *Journal of Intellectual & Developmental Disability, 37*(3), 221–231.

McClintock, K., Hall S., & Oliver C. (2003). Risk markers associated with challenging behaviours in people with developmental disabilities: A meta-analytic study. *Journal of Intellectual Disability Research, 47*, 405–416.

McGrew, J. H., Ruble, L. A., & Smith, I. M. (2016). Autism spectrum disorder and evidence-based practice in psychology. *Clinical Psychology: Science and Practice, 23*(3), 239–255.

McKenzie, K. (2011). Providing services in the United Kingdom to people with an intellectual disability who present behaviour which challenges: A review of the literature. *Research in Developmental Disabilities, 32*, 395–403.

McKenzie, K., & Patterson, M. (2010). The evaluation of an assertive outreach team: Implications for challenging behaviour. *British Journal of Learning Disabilities, 38*(4), 319–327.

Meyer, L. H., & Evans, I. M. (1989). *Nonaversive intervention for behavior problems: A manual for home and community*. PH Brookes.

Michael, J. (1993). Establishing operations. *The Behavior Analyst, 16*(2), 191–206.

Miltenberger, R. G., Valbuena, D., & Sanchez, S. (2019). Functional assessment of challenging behavior. *Current Developmental Disorders Reports, 6*, 202–208.

Monzale, M., & Horner, R. H. (2020). The impact of contextual fit enhancement protocol on behavior support plan fidelity and student behavior. *Behavioral Disorders, 46*(4), 267–278.

O'Neill, R. E., Albin, R. W., Horner, R. H., Storey, K., & Sprague, J. R. (2014). *Functional assessment and program development*. Nelson Education.

Rojahn, J., Rowe, E. W., Sharber, A. C., Hastings, R., Matson, J. L., Didden, R., Kroes, D. B. H., & Dumont, E. L. M. (2012). The Behaviour Problems Inventory—Short Form for individuals with intellectual disabilities: Part I: Development and provisional clinical reference data. *Journal of Intellectual Disability Research, 56*(5), 527–545.

Schalock, R. L., Keith, K. D., Hoffman, K., & Karan, O. C. (1989). Quality of life: Its measurement and use. *Mental Retardation, 27*, 25–31.

Scott, T. M., & Cooper, J. T. (2017). Functional behavior assessment and function-based intervention planning: Considering the simple logic of the process. *Beyond Behavior, 26*(3), 101–104.

Smith T. (2013). What is evidence-based behavior analysis? *The Behavior Analyst, 36*(1), 7–33.

Sprague, J. R., & Horner, R. H. (1995). Functional assessment and intervention in community settings. *Mental Retardation & Developmental Disabilities Research Reviews, 1*, 89–93.

Sugai, G., & Horner, R. H. (2020). Sustaining and scaling positive behavioral interventions and supports: Implementation drivers, outcomes, and considerations. *Exceptional Children, 86*(2), 120–136.

Stahmer, A. C., Collings, N. M., & Palinkas, L. A. (2005). Early intervention practices for children with autism: Descriptions from community providers. *Focus on Autism and Other Developmental Disabilities, 20*(2), 66–79.

Tanner, B. A., & Zeiler, M. (1975). Punishment of self-injurious behavior using aromatic ammonia as the aversive stimulus. *Journal of Applied Behavior Analysis, 8*(1), 53–57.

Webber, L., McVilly, K., Fester, T., & Chan, J. (2011). Factors influencing quality of behaviour support plans and the impact of plan quality on restrictive intervention use. *International Journal of Positive Behavioural Support, 1*(1), 24–31.

Wolfensberger, W. P., Nirje, B., Olshansky, S. Perske, R., & Roos, P. (1972). *The principle of normalization in human services*. Wolfensberger Collection. https://digitalcommons.unmc.edu/wolf_books/1

Vollmer, T. R., & Iwata, B. A. (1992). Differential reinforcement as treatment for behavior disorders: Procedural and functional variations. *Research in Developmental Disabilities, 13*, 393–417.

9

Cognitive Behavior Therapy

XIE YIN CHEW, ANN OZSIVADJIAN,
MATTHEW J. HOLLOCKS, AND ILIANA MAGIATI ■

KEY CONSIDERATIONS

- Neurocognitive differences and higher rates of vulnerability experiences in people with autistic increase their vulnerability to mental health difficulties.
- Cognitive Behavior Therapy (CBT) supports people to change their unhelpful thinking patterns and behaviors to more adaptive ways of thinking about, and responding to, distressing experiences and situations.
- The highly structured, logical, and here-and-now focus of CBT may make it a suitable and helpful approach for autistic adults with appropriate adaptations.
- Adaptations at every stage of CBT are important to support autism-related differences, needs, and preferences.
- Autistic clients may present with diverse and varied functioning in the social, communication, sensory, and neurocognitive domains with large differences between and within individuals; it is therefore important not to make assumptions about each client and to use adaptations flexibly and tailor them individually to each client.
- Many autistic adults have had substantial exposure to stressful, invalidating and/or threatening environments; therefore, it is important that clinicians utilize the CBT techniques while considering first whether the clients' thoughts and behaviors are in fact adaptive and should be accepted and encouraged, rather than being targeted for intervention.

Cognitive behavior therapy (CBT) is a goal-oriented, usually short-term therapy (on average 6–20 sessions) informed by cognitive and behavioral theories of human behavior and psychopathology. CBT is based on a few central ideas: (a) our *cognitions* or thoughts, *emotions* or feelings, and *behaviors* or responses are interlinked; (b) unhelpful thinking styles and responses toward distressing experiences contribute to the development and maintenance of mental health difficulties, and (c) distressing emotions can reinforce, and are in turn amplified by, the unhelpful thinking styles and behaviors in a vicious cycle, maintaining mental health difficulties (Westbrook et al., 2011).

At the cognitive level, CBT addresses unhelpful patterns of three levels of cognition: negative automatic thoughts (NATs), core beliefs, and dysfunctional assumptions (DAs; Beck, 2020; Westbrook et al., 2011). NATs are thoughts relating to specific situations that happen quickly and without effort (e.g., "They think I am weird" or "I can't do this"). Core beliefs represent a person's "deeper," absolute and overgeneralized ways of thinking (e.g., "I am unlovable," "Others will hurt me"). DAs are unrealistic attitudes or rules for living, often representing an unhelpful attempt for individuals to overcome their negative core beliefs (e.g., for someone with the core belief "I am unlovable," a relevant DA may be, "If I always please other people, then they will love me").

At the behavioral level, CBT aims to identify, understand, and replace unhelpful behaviors relating to withdrawal, avoidance, reassurance seeking or safety seeking, all of which reduce distress in the short-term, but perpetuate this in the longer-term (Salkovskis, 1991). CBT therefore aims to support people to become their own therapist by supporting them to develop their own knowledge, skills, and tools to change their unhelpful thinking patterns and behaviors (Fenn & Byrne, 2013). While CBT incorporates early life events in understanding the origin of the difficulties, these early events are not necessarily processed during treatment; instead, the focus of CBT is on evaluating and developing alternative, more balanced thoughts and responses in the present.

THE EVIDENCE BASE FOR CBT IN NON-AUTISTIC ADULTS

CBT has a well-established evidence base (David et al., 2018). It is often recommended as a first-line psychological intervention for many mental health conditions, including anxiety disorders, depression and bipolar disorder, obsessive compulsive disorder (OCD), and posttraumatic stress disorder (PTSD; National Institute for Health and Care Excellence [NICE], 2011). CBT is at least as effective as, or more effective than, other interventions (e.g., psychodynamic therapy, interpersonal therapy) and more effective than waitlist or nonspecific controls (Butler et al., 2006; Cuijpers et al., 2013; Hofmann et al., 2012).

MAIN CBT STRATEGIES AND TECHNIQUES

CBT can be delivered through face-to-face individual or group sessions, and also through guided self-help approaches or computerized/online delivery (Cuijpers et al., 2019). Commonly used CBT strategies include psychoeducation;

collaborative formulation; behavior-focused strategies, such as behavioral activation, relaxation training, and graded exposure/behavioral experiments; and cognitively focused strategies, such as cognitive restructuring, problem-solving, and behavioral experiments (Beck, 2020).

CBT FOR AUTISTIC ADULTS

Mental health difficulties are considerably more prevalent in autistic people compared to the general population (Hollocks et al., 2019; Lai et al., 2019). Various neurocognitive differences have been proposed to account for these higher prevalence rates, including alexithymia (difficulties identifying and describing one's own and others' emotions; Bird & Cook, 2013); emotional regulation (Cai et al., 2018); information processing and thinking styles, such as intolerance of uncertainty (IU; Boulter et al., 2014); cognitive inflexibility (i.e., Ozsivadjian et al., 2020); and negative processing biases (e.g., Hollocks et al., 2016). Autistic people are also known to experience high rates of victimization, social isolation, and discrimination, which also contribute to more mental health difficulties (Gaus, 2011a; Griffiths et al., 2019; South & Rodgers, 2017). Such experiences can, and often do, lead to the development of negative beliefs and assumptions, such as "I am weird" or "incompetent," "others are not to be trusted," or "if I keep away from people, I won't get hurt"). In stressful events, these beliefs are activated, and autistic people often experience distressing emotions which may then be further perpetuated by unhelpful thinking and behavioral patterns. CBT therefore has the potential to be helpful to autistic people and co-occurring mental health difficulties.

However, some reservations in relation to offering CBT to autistic people have been expressed by professionals (see Maddox et al., 2019, 2020). For example, there were initial concerns that core autism-related characteristics could potentially limit the suitability, acceptability, or effectiveness of CBT, such as in relation to the therapeutic alliance and engagement (Anderson & Morris, 2006) and in identifying, evaluating, and/or shifting their feelings and thoughts (Gaus, 2011a, 2011b; Spain, 2019). Yet the highly structured, logical, and here-and-now focus of CBT may align well with the needs and preferences of autistic adults and could lend itself to being a suitable and helpful approach for them with appropriate adaptations (Spain & Happé, 2020).

THE EVIDENCE BASE FOR CBT FOR AUTISM PEOPLE

Empirical research on the application of CBT with autistic people has largely been conducted in children and adolescents, but there is a growing number of studies in adult populations (see Weston et al., 2016). Two systematic reviews on the effectiveness of CBT for autistic adults (Benevides et al., 2020; Spain, 2019) looked at 15 studies (a combination of four randomized controlled trials [RCTs], other intervention studies, and case studies) involving a total of 301 autistic adults. The majority focused primarily on co-occurring mood and anxiety difficulties (including social anxiety and OCD). Overall, CBT, whether delivered individually or in groups, was effective for improving self- and clinician-rated mood and anxiety and can be considered an emerging evidence-based approach for autistic adults (Benevides et al., 2020; Spain, 2019). To our knowledge, no meta-analysis of CBT for autistic adults has been conducted to date. However, studies to date have primarily excluded autistic adults with an intellectual disability and routinely excluded more complex mental health conditions, such as psychosis, bipolar disorder, suicidality, and substance misuse (Spain, 2019), which limits conclusions about the effectiveness of CBT for autistic adults with intellectual disabilities and/ or more complex mental health difficulties.

ADAPTATIONS/MODIFICATIONS TO CBT FOR AUTISTIC ADULTS

Based on the existing empirical literature, we outline in the sections that follow recommended adaptations for different stages of the CBT process (for more details, see Anderson & Morris, 2006; Blainey, 2019; Kerns et al., 2016, Maddox et al., 2020; NICE, 2012; Russell et al., 2019; Spain & Happé, 2020); these are illustrative rather than exhaustive and will need to be individually considered for different clients, as not all adaptations will suit or be needed with all autistic adults.

Engagement, Rapport, and Therapist Communication

Therapists may need to spend more time learning how each of their autistic clients communicates in order to form a strong therapeutic relationship. For example, eye contact or conveying emotion through facial expressions may be uncomfortable or difficult for some autistic adults. It is also important to discuss the client's interests and insights into their own neurodiverse differences as a way to build rapport. Some clients may need additional time to process verbal information and concepts and to formulate a response. Clinicians will need to be patient and comfortable with possible silences and slower pacing. Asking closed questions may be helpful, if the open/Socratic method of questioning does not elicit sufficient information. Language use may need to be more specific, concrete, and direct with some clients (i.e., the use of metaphors, ambiguity, and hypothetical situations may need to be reduced or explained more explicitly), but not with others who make excellent use of metaphor, and therefore any adaptations will need to be individually tailored and used flexibly.

CBT Assessment

The first few CBT sessions, when assessment usually takes place, may be stressful or confusing for some autistic clients. Providing information in advance about what to expect is helpful. Clinicians may need to conduct assessment over several sessions to build rapport and to gain a clear understanding of the presenting issues, including how autism-related experiences potentially contributed to the clients' current difficulties, the clients' own understanding and experience of their autism, and their unique profile of strengths, interests, and associated needs and difficulties. Therefore, therapists must have a good understanding of autism and its heterogeneity. As clients may have idiosyncratic ways of describing thoughts and emotions, it may be helpful to operationalize and use the clients' own terminology. Significant others could be invited, with the client's permission, for support and to contribute additional information and perspectives to the assessment.

CBT assessment often includes the completion of standardized rating scales in addition to clinical interviews and observations. When these are used, it is important to help autistic clients clarify the scale's items as needed. Ratings scales may be used as a starting point, with follow-up or clarifying questions asked to try to tease out autism-related from other experiences (see Chew et al., 2020, for clarifying OCD and social anxiety scale items). Clinicians should be pragmatic when interpreting ratings from existing screening measures, as their validity has not yet been established for autistic people.

Practical Adaptations to CBT Delivery

Practical adaptations to minimize demands, meet autism-related needs, or reduce unnecessary stress/anxiety may also be necessary. It will be important at the outset to set clear and shared expectations about therapy with the clients and significant others regarding the number, frequency and duration of sessions offered. An agenda can collaboratively be agreed upon, and regular appointments with a similar structure for each session can be provided. In terms of sensory sensitivities, it will be helpful to ask about and accommodate these in-session and at waiting areas (e.g., using the same clinic room, reducing crowding, dimming the lights, etc.). Clinicians will also need to be flexible with session duration: shorter sessions could be offered to some clients, while longer/additional time, for example to process information and for inclusion of regular breaks, may be needed for others.

Goal Setting

Goals for CBT should be functional, respectful, and relevant for autistic adults and should address co-occurring emotional or behavioral difficulties, so as to improve well-being, independence, and/or quality of life. Based on the client's presenting difficulties and autism-informed formulation, shared specific, realistic, and measurable goals need to be set collaboratively and explicitly. However, executive functioning (EF) difficulties may make goal setting more difficult for some clients. So clinicians may need to spend more time than usual developing therapy goals and providing suggestions and help with generating alternatives. Additionally, some clients may not be as motivated or may experience anxiety/concerns about change. In this case, it may be helpful to discuss the "pros and cons" of certain changes/goals in relation to their presenting difficulties and life, to help them with decision-making.

CBT Formulation

The collaborative CBT formulation would need to be specifically adapted to integrate autism-related neurocognitive and psychosocial vulnerabilities and life events in the conceptualization of the development and maintenance of mental health problems (see Blainey, 2019, for anxiety; Gaus, 2011a for developmental autism-informed CBT model of anxiety/depression; see also Spain & Happé, 2020). The therapist should periodically review the formulation with the client to ensure they have a continuing shared understanding. Additionally, it will be important to highlight the client's strengths, skills, resilience, and protective factors in the formulation. It may be helpful to discuss with the client the possibility of sharing the formulation with significant others so that they also understand the therapy rationale, particularly if significant others respond to the client's distress in unhelpful ways.

CBT Intervention Strategies or Techniques

GENERAL

Throughout the intervention, therapists may need to use more visual aids/tools (e.g., written session agenda, worksheets, thought bubbles) to support communication and understanding. Incorporating their client's interests into sessions may also increase engagement (e.g., using apps with a client who is tech-savvy; using different art expressions with an artistic client; incorporating examples from Harry Potter for the client who is passionate about this). As some autistic people may benefit from additional support, it may be helpful to involve other providers, family, friends, or carers when helpful and agreed to by the client, while bearing in mind that for other clients such involvement may not be needed or may even negatively impact their self-determination and independence.

PSYCHOEDUCATION

Emotional literacy is a necessary, important foundation for the rest of the CBT work. Thus, it is important to spend more time (perhaps a few sessions) on psychoeducation about autism, emotions, and socialization to the CBT model for the clients who may have difficulties with interoception or identifying emotions, in order to strengthen skills in emotional awareness, particularly in supporting the individual to identify and label their emotions (e.g., the physical and behavioral cues) and developing a joint language for these concepts. Therapists may need to explore flexible and creative approaches to explain concepts, for example using drawings, images, or computers.

Cognitive Restructuring

Neurocognitive differences may make it difficult for some clients to engage in cognitive strategies. Some clients may feel they are being "persuaded" to change their thinking and may be uncomfortable with this. If clients find it difficult to evaluate/challenge negative thinking, therapists can try alternative strategies such as redirecting attentional focus, mindfulness, problem solving, and validation of negative cognitions that may indeed be realistic as well as negative (Blainey, 2019). It may also be helpful to place more emphasis on behavioral change, rather than targeting cognitions, and using the behavioral change as the starting point for cognitive work. Adding greater structure and making cognitive concepts more concrete may also be important—for example, providing worksheets listing helpful and unhelpful thoughts. Additionally, allowing multiple-choice options (e.g., a list of common unhelpful thoughts from which to choose) to reduce the pressure to generate novel solutions may be helpful. It is crucial to understand that many autistic adults have had substantial exposure to stressful and/or invalidating environments and therefore their thoughts about themselves, others, or the world may have served an adaptive function. It is important that therapists do not invalidate their clients' lived-in experiences through cognitive restructuring, but rather explore what experiences may have led to these thoughts being developed in the first place as well as ways in which clients can think about themselves and others that are more balanced and helpful to them.

Behavioral Strategies

Because many autistic individuals prefer routine and certainty, changes during CBT may trigger anxiety or concern. New behaviors also require planning and flexibility, which may be challenging for some clients. Explaining clearly the rationale and aims of behavioral work may make this aspect of therapy more personally meaningful for the client. Therapists should take a graded approach to introducing changes in behavior, breaking these down into smaller, more manageable chunks. It is important also to scaffold and support behavior change in CBT through, for example, modeling and role playing new skills and behaviors during sessions and as much as possible in real-world settings. Encouraging clients to make coping cards, or having phone or app reminders to cue the use of coping strategies or to track mood, may also reduce additional cognitive demands. Additionally, teaching skills and coping strategies to augment CBT if indicated, such as emotion regulation, problem solving, organizational skills, assertiveness, and managing uncertainty may be helpful on an individualized basis for some clients.

As with cognitive restructuring, many behaviors adopted by autistic people are not safety or avoidance behaviors, but rather appropriate, helpful, and needed accommodations to their differences and needs. For this reason, the therapist must work together with the client to identify which behaviors are essential and helpful for the client's well-being and which are unhelpful. For example, wearing noise-canceling headphones to manage sensory needs, or declining some social invitations, are in all likelihood appropriate accommodations to overwhelming sensory and social environments to prevent burnout and to respect individual preferences and choices. Other behaviors, however, may be unhelpful and will maintain the client's low mood or anxiety; for example, declining an invitation from a much loved close friend to go for a walk in the forest, previously the client's favorite activity, may be avoidance behavior stemming from low mood, and thus an appropriate behavior to target in behavioral work.

HOMEWORK

Initially, clinicians may need to be somewhat more direct and offer suggestions for homework, encouraging the client to pick, rather than generate, ideas while setting attainable homework goals. They need to discuss clearly with the clients about the "who," "what," "where," "when," and "how" of homework, as well as possible obstacles to completion and solutions. Clinicians may also support some clients' cognitive/EF needs by creating written instructions, routines, reminders, and checklists if and as needed. Additionally, when clients agree, trusted others can support activity schedules or behavioral experiments between sessions.

MANAGING ENDINGS

To reduce potential anxiety, clinicians should be explicit about the number of sessions to be offered and discuss/plan endings in advance. As in traditional CBT, it is important to review progress and develop a relapse prevention "blueprint." When indicated, a cohesive handover with other services that will continue supporting the client is helpful. As autism is a lifelong condition with high rates of recurrence of anxiety and mood difficulties, clinicians should be mindful that some clients may need to start and resume CBT several times and that this is not in any way an indication of failure of the clinician, client, or intervention.

CASE STUDY

Brief Background and Reason for CBT Referral

Jo is a 28-year-old woman with a diagnosis of autism since early childhood and a history of expressive language difficulties. She was referred to a clinical psychologist after a brief period of hospitalization due to depression. She also frequently became panicky in social situations and everyday situations, such as engaging in a hobby or cooking a meal, where there was a risk of perceived failure.

Brief Relevant History

Jo had attended a number of schools, including a mainstream school followed by a special educational need school for her secondary education. One particularly difficult period for her was being held back a year in her mid-teens to catch up academically, which made her feel, in her words, "stupid." She also had memories of people at home and school becoming irritated with her for not understanding or keeping up. After school, she became a primary school teaching assistant and at the time of the referral she was working as a part-time nursery assistant in a job she had held for some months. She had few friends. Jo enjoyed creative activities in her spare time, although at the time of referral these had tailed off to nonexistent due to her anxieties about failing. In terms of her autism-related differences, Jo became easily overwhelmed in loud places or in groups of more than a few people.

Goals in CBT

Jo's goals were to be less anxious in social situations, to be able to deal with her feelings better, and to be able to talk to people more easily. She specifically wanted to resume cooking meals for her family and roommate and to be able to talk to strangers to ask questions when she was out in the community. Therefore, specific goals included "Research and cook two meals per week for my family," "Begin and complete a creative activity," and "Ask at least one question of a sales assistant when I am in a shop." She was encouraged to write her thoughts/reflections and also rate her anxiety before and after each activity.

CBT Formulation

Social situations such as transactions in a shop, or large family gatherings, frequently triggered NATs such as "I never know what to say" and "People will think I'm stupid." Everyday activities such as cooking or artistic pursuits triggered thoughts such as "I can't do this, what's wrong with me" and "I'm useless." Dysfunctional assumptions included "It's better to reject people, before they reject you" and "I have to do things perfectly, otherwise I will have failed," while her core beliefs were "I'm useless" and "People don't like me." Autism-related experiences and/or differences contributing to these cognitions included experiences of being socially rejected and teased at school and feeling "stupid" for having to repeat a year of school when she was 13 years old.

CBT Work

CBT followed a fairly standardized approach, developing a collaborative formulation and identifying key thoughts and beliefs, while taking into account language difficulties and reduced cognitive flexibility, which Jo accepted was a feature that affected her interactions with people. For example, she found it very difficult to accept when people around her asked her questions about her choices, perceiving this as criticism. Jo and her therapist set weekly behavioral experiments, to test out alternative explanations and develop distress tolerance skills. For example, Jo set herself a task of cooking more family meals, both to test out whether she would fail at the task of following a recipe, and also to learn to tolerate the distress this activity caused her, as well as to accept others' compliments of her cooking, which she found excruciating and usually rejected.

In terms of adaptations to "traditional" CBT, the sessions were carefully paced, allowing time for language processing difficulties. Jo was also encouraged to keep a notebook and bring it with her to each session, to record key points and strategies discussed. Jo's parents were also intermittently involved. For example, while it was all-too-easy for adults around her to talk over her and finish her sentences for her, given her expressive language difficulties, her parents were enabled to give Jo time to speak and to encourage others in her family to do so.

During the therapeutic process, we evaluated and challenged negative thoughts and assumptions, identifying the inertia caused by thoughts such as "there's no point trying this, as I will fail" and also breaking negative cycles caused by thoughts such as "I may as well reject them, because they'll end up rejecting me." Collectively, these new learning experiences were also used to construct a new narrative and identity, encouraging Jo to accept that she is no longer the teenager who felt stupid for being held back a year, but now an independent adult, who requires support for some of her needs, but who is also competent and able to overcome many difficulties, as well as a warm and engaging person. A key part of this new narrative was the inclusion of her neurodiverse characteristics as strengths and differences, rather than deficits. As an example, reduced flexibility may on one hand present some social challenges for Jo, but may also contribute to higher determination to complete a task, once Jo had started it.

After 12 sessions, Jo's mood had improved on formal self-report screening measures and also qualitative observations from herself and her parents. She remained socially anxious, but she was able to cook meals for herself and her family several times per week, resume some of her art pursuits, and approach people she didn't know with more confidence. Her subjective units of anxiety distress reduced from 8/10 at the beginning to 4/10 toward the end of therapy. She also hoped and planned how she would continue to build on these skills going forwards.

CONCLUSION

CBT is a highly structured, practical, and present-focused approach that is relevant and suitable for autistic adults with co-occurring mood and anxiety difficulties. The general consensus in the emerging evidence base and clinical practice is that individualized adaptations are recommended with autistic adults for different stages of the CBT process. Further research into the effectiveness of such adaptations, as well as into the effectiveness of CBT for other co-occurring mental health conditions other than depressive and anxiety-related difficulties, is needed.

REFERENCES

Anderson, S., & Morris, J. (2006). Cognitive behaviour therapy for people with Asperger syndrome. *Behavioural and Cognitive Psychotherapy, 34*(3), 293–303.

Beck, J. S. (2020). *Cognitive behavior therapy: Basics and beyond* (3rd ed.). Guilford Press.

Benevides, T. W., Shore, S. M., Andresen, M.-L., Caplan, R., Cook, B., Gassner, D. L., Erves, J. M., Hazlewood, T. M., King, M. C., Morgan, L., Murphy, L. E., Purkis, Y., Rankowski, B., Rutledge, S. M., Welch, S. P., & Wittig, K. (2020). Interventions to address health outcomes among autistic adults: A systematic review. *Autism, 24*(6), 1345–1359.

Bird, G., & Cook, R. (2013). Mixed emotions: The contribution of alexithymia to the emotional symptoms of autism. *Translational Psychiatry, 3*(7), e285–e285.

Blainey, S. (2019). General anxiety. In E. Chaplin, D. Spain, & C. McCarthy (Eds.). *A clinician's guide to mental health conditions in adults with autism spectrum disorders: Assessment and interventions* (pp. 97–110). Jessica Kingsley Publishers.

Boulter, C., Freeston, M., South, M., & Rodgers, J. (2014). Intolerance of uncertainty as a framework for understanding anxiety in children and adolescents with autism spectrum disorders. *Journal of Autism and Developmental Disorders, 44*(6), 1391–1402.

Butler, A. C., Chapman, J. E., Forman, E. M., & Beck, A. T. (2006). The empirical status of cognitive-behavioral therapy: A review of meta-analyses. *Clinical Psychology Review, 26*(1), 17–31.

Cai, R. Y., Richdale, A. L., Uljarević, M., Dissanayake, C., & Samson, A. C. (2018). Emotion regulation in autism spectrum disorder: Where we are and where we need to go. *Autism Research, 11*(7), 962–978.

Chew, X. Y., Leong, D.-J., Khor, K. M., Tan, G. M. Y., Wei, K.-C., & Magiati, I. (2021). Clarifying self-report measures of social anxiety and obsessive-compulsive disorder to improve reporting for autistic adults. *Autism in Adulthood, 3*(2), 129–146.

Cuijpers, P., Berking, M., Andersson, G., Quigley, L., Kleiboer, A., & Dobson, K. S. (2013). A meta-analysis of cognitive-behavioural therapy for adult depression, alone and in comparison with other treatments. *The Canadian Journal of Psychiatry, 58*(7), 376–385.

Cuijpers, P., Noma, H., Karyotaki, E., Cipriani, A., & Furukawa, T. A. (2019). Effectiveness and acceptability of cognitive behavior therapy delivery formats in adults with depression: A network meta-analysis. *JAMA Psychiatry, 76*(7), 700–707. https://doi.org/10.1001/jamapsychiatry.2019.0268

David, D., Cristea, I., & Hofmann, S. G. (2018). Why cognitive behavioral therapy is the current gold standard of psychotherapy. *Frontiers in Psychiatry, 9*(4).

Fenn, K., & Byrne, M. (2013). The key principles of cognitive behavioural therapy. *InnovAiT, 6*(9), 579–585.

Gaus, V. L. (2011a). Adult Asperger syndrome and the utility of cognitive-behavioral therapy. *Journal of Contemporary Psychotherapy, 41*(1), 47–56.

Gaus, V. L. (2011b). Cognitive behavioural therapy for adults with autism spectrum disorder. *Advances in Mental Health and Intellectual Disabilities, 5*(5), 15–25.

Griffiths, S., Allison, C., Kenny, R., Holt, R., Smith, P., & Baron-Cohen, S. (2019). The Vulnerability Experiences Quotient (VEQ): A study of vulnerability, mental health and life satisfaction in autistic adults. *Autism Research, 12*(10), 1516–1528.

Hofmann, S. G., Asnaani, A., Vonk, I. J., Sawyer, A. T., & Fang, A. (2012). The efficacy of cognitive behavioral therapy: A review of meta-analyses. *Cognitive Therapy and Research, 36*(5), 427–440.

Hollocks, M. J., Lerh, J. W., Magiati, I., Meiser-Stedman, R., & Brugha, T. S. (2019). Anxiety and depression in adults with autism spectrum disorder: A systematic review and meta-analysis. *Psychological Medicine, 49*(4), 559–572.

Hollocks, M. J., Pickles, A., Howlin, P., & Simonoff, E. (2016). Dual cognitive and biological correlates of anxiety in autism spectrum disorders. *Journal of Autism and Developmental Disorders, 46*(10), 3295–3307.

Kerns, C. M., Roux, A. M., Connell, J. E., & Shattuck, P. T. (2016). Adapting cognitive behavioral techniques to address anxiety and depression in cognitively able emerging adults on the autism spectrum. *Cognitive and Behavioral Practice, 23*(3), 329–340.

Lai, M.-C., Kassee, C., Besney, R., Bonato, S., Hull, L., Mandy, W., Szatmari, P., & Ameis, S. H. (2019). Prevalence of co-occurring mental health diagnoses in the autism population: A systematic review and meta-analysis. *The Lancet Psychiatry, 6*(10), 819–829.

Maddox, B. B., Crabbe, S., Beidas, R. S., Brookman-Frazee, L., Cannuscio, C. C., Miller, J. S., Nicolaidis, C., & Mandell, D. S. (2020). "I wouldn't know where to start": Perspectives from clinicians, agency leaders, and autistic adults on improving community mental health services for autistic adults. *Autism, 24*(4), 919–930.

Maddox, B. B., Crabbe, S. R., Fishman, J. M., Beidas, R. S., Brookman-Frazee, L., Miller, J. S., Nicolaidis, C., & Mandell, D. S. (2019). Factors influencing the use of cognitive–behavioral therapy with autistic adults: A survey of community mental health clinicians. *Journal of Autism and Developmental Disorders, 49*(11), 4421–4428.

National Institute for Health and Care Excellence. (2011). *Common mental health disorders: Identification and pathways to care* (Clinical Guideline No. 123 [CG123]). Retrieved December 1, 2020, from http://www.nice.org.uk/guidance/cg123

National Institute for Health and Care Excellence. (2012). *Autism spectrum disorder in adults: diagnosis and management* (Clinical Guideline No. 142 [CG142]). Retrieved December 1, 2020, from http://www.nice.org.uk/guidance/cg142

Ozsivadjian, A., Hollocks, M. J., Magiati, I., Happé, F., Baird, G., & Absoud, M. (2021). Is cognitive inflexibility a missing link? The role of cognitive inflexibility, alexithymia and intolerance of uncertainty in externalising and internalising behaviours in young people with autism spectrum disorder. *Journal of Child Psychology and Psychiatry, 62*(6), 715–724.

Russell, A., Jassi, A., & Johnston, K. (2019). *OCD and autism: A clinician's guide to adapting CBT*. Jessica Kingsley Publishers.

Salkovskis, P. M. (1991). The importance of behaviour in the maintenance of anxiety and panic: A cognitive account. *Behavioural Psychotherapy, 19*(1), 6–19.

South, M., & Rodgers, J. (2017). Sensory, emotional and cognitive contributions to anxiety in autism spectrum disorders. *Frontiers in Human Neuroscience, 11*(20).

Spain, D. (2019). Cognitive behaviour therapy. In E. Chaplin, D. Spain, & C. McCarthy (Eds.). *A clinician's guide to mental health conditions in adults with autism spectrum disorders: Assessment and interventions* (pp. 290–307). Jessica Kingsley Publishers.

Spain, D., & Happé, F. (2020). How to optimise cognitive behaviour therapy (CBT) for people with autism spectrum disorders (ASD): A Delphi study. *Journal of Rational-Emotive & Cognitive-Behavior Therapy, 38*(2), 184–208.

Westbrook, D., Kennerley, H., & Kirk, J. (2011). *An introduction to cognitive behaviour therapy: Skills and applications* (2nd ed.). SAGE Publications.

Weston, L., Hodgekins, J., & Langdon, P. E. (2016). Effectiveness of cognitive behavioural therapy with people who have autistic spectrum disorders: A systematic review and meta-analysis. *Clinical Psychology Review, 49*, 41–54.

10

Mindfulness-Based Interventions

KELLY B. BECK ■

KEY CONSIDERATIONS

- Research supports the efficacy of mindfulness-based interventions (MBIs) improving co-occurring mental health symptoms and quality of life in samples of adults with autism spectrum disorders (ASD).
- Emotion regulation (ER) is a likely mechanism of change in mindfulness-based interventions for adults with ASD.
- Clinicians with personal meditation practices are more adept at adjusting mindfulness-based interventions for adults with ASD.
- Most mindfulness-based intervention literature adapts programs for use with adults with ASD, particularly meditation length, session structure, and simplified language.
- New evidence suggests that mindfulness-based interventions may be appropriate for adults with ASD without modification.
- Future research must address accessible mindfulness training and implementation supports for providers interested in using mindfulness-based interventions for adults with ASD.

Mindfulness is an experience of present-moment awareness that is cultivated through meditation practices. Mindfulness has rapidly emerged as an evidence-based treatment for various physical, emotional, and behavioral conditions (Gotink et al., 2015). Mindfulness-based interventions (MBIs) may be ideally suited to support adults with autism spectrum disorder (ASD), as they do not require a high degree of insight or awareness, are experiential and repetitive in nature, and can be tailored to a wide range of functioning. There is evidence supporting the feasibility, acceptability, and efficacy of MBIs for improving co-occurring psychiatric symptoms and quality of life in samples of adults with ASD (Beck, Greco, et al., 2020; Cachia et al., 2016; Hartley et al., 2019; Kiep et al., 2014; Spek et al., 2010, 2013; White et al., 2018). Adults with ASD experiencing impaired emotion regulation (ER) may respond well to MBIs. Clinically elevated ER impairment is four times more common in ASD than age-equivalent peers, and it frequently underlies suicidality, hospitalization, and mood disorders (Conner et al., 2020). ER is a mechanism of change in MBIs (Gu et al., 2015) and there is emerging evidence that MBIs improve ER in ASD samples (Beck, Conner, et al., 2020; Conner & White, 2018; Conner et al., 2019). Individuals with ASD have unique cognitive needs that influence mindfulness delivery, such as difficulty with abstract language, attention span, and internal awareness (Beck, Conner, White, & Mazefsky, 2020). As such, this chapter aims to provide a resource to current and future clinicians serving adults with ASD. Mindfulness, mindfulness meditation, and MBIs are introduced and then followed by a summary of empirical evidence supporting MBIs in samples of adults with ASD. Common clinical delivery challenges and strategies are provided through a case study exemplar for clinicians interested in using MBIs with adults with ASD.

WHAT IS MINDFULNESS?

Current applications of mindfulness have roots in centuries-old teachings from Guatama Buddha that have been modernized to fit into secular healthcare (Hwang & Singh, 2016). In the scientific community, mindfulness is operationally defined as "the awareness that emerges through paying attention on purpose, in the present moment, and nonjudgmentally to the unfolding of experience moment by moment" (Kabat-Zinn, 2006). Hwang & Singh provide a comprehensive and thorough contextual history of mindfulness in their chapter reviewing MBIs for individuals with intellectual disability (Hwang & Singh, 2016).

Nonjudgmental awareness can be described as a cognitive and emotional distancing from an observed experience, in an impartial or neutral state (Gunaratana, 2015). For instance, one would notice pain as "hot" or "sharp" rather than labeling it as "undesirable" or "unbearable." Nonjudgmental awareness has been widely misunderstood in the proliferation of mindfulness, often cited simply as "acceptance." The English word acceptance implies consent or approval, leading many to believe that practicing mindfulness means approving all experiences. A more appropriate description is impartial *acknowledgment* of experiences without labeling or judgment. This distinction is particularly relevant for use in ASD given the tendency for literal language and concrete thinking.

MINDFULNESS MEDITATION

Mindfulness can be cultivated through meditation practice, which consists of concentration exercises that train the mind to focus (Gunaratana, 2015). There are many different meditation practice traditions, all with different religious and philosophical roots (Gunaratana, 2015). Most contemporary MBIs used in healthcare settings use practices from Vipassana meditation, also synonymous with "insight meditation" or "mindfulness meditation." These meditations are concentration practices that focus on direct, present-moment experiences and are commonly packaged together in MBIs without the original religious or philosophical teachings (Crane et al., 2016). Common practices include awareness of breathing or sitting meditation, walking meditation, body scans, and mindful movement. Vipassana meditations are taught in sequence, beginning with meditations focused on physical sensations (body scans, breathing) to build awareness and then progressing to thought and emotion identification. This sequence allows individuals with limited insight or awareness (often adults with ASD) to build concentration skills and awareness before attempting to work with thoughts or emotions. Walking and movement meditations are easily tailored for individuals with ASD and are often useful for individuals who engage in repetitive movement behaviors. The Vipassana awareness of breathing meditation can be substantially simplified for co-occurring ASD and intellectual disability. Thus, Vipassana meditations are uniquely applicable to individuals with ASD and guidance is easily simplified without modifying the core practice.

MINDFULNESS-BASED INTERVENTIONS

Jon Kabat-Zinn introduced the first MBI, mindfulness-based stress reduction (MBSR), in 1979 for individuals with severe chronic pain conditions who were not responding to medical and pharmaceutical intervention (Kabat-Zinn, 2006; Kabat-Zinn et al., 1985). MBIs then gained traction as researchers explored the use of mindfulness with other chronic health conditions, demonstrating efficacy of improved stress, depression, anxiety, and quality of life (Gotink et al., 2015). Mindfulness has since exploded in popular Western culture as an exciting and innovative mind-body treatment to improve a variety of conditions with biopsychosocial impairments (Hwang & Singh, 2016).

MBSR is a standardized, experiential group of 12–30 of individuals who complete eight weekly 2.5-hour sessions, one 7.5 full-day silent meditation retreat, and learn Vipassana meditations. MBSR is considered evidence-based for chronic pain and has demonstrated large effects in stress reduction, reducing anxiety and depression, and improving quality of life in samples of individuals with chronic illness (e.g., cancer, cardiovascular disease) and mental health disorders (e.g., anxiety; Gotink et al., 2015).

Nearly all MBIs have been developed and adapted from MBSR, and most of the MBIs that do not cite MBSR as a foundational model utilize the Vipassana meditations taught in MBSR (Crane et al., 2016). Mindfulness-based cognitive therapy (MBCT) combines MBSR and cognitive behavioral therapy (CBT) to treat individuals with recurrent major depressive disorder (Segal et al., 2002). Acceptance and commitment therapy (ACT) and dialectical behavior therapy (DBT) incorporate attitudes of mindfulness and nonjudgment but do not utilize formal meditation practices (Baer, 2003; Cheisa & Malinowski, 2011). Chapters 11 and 12 review emotion-focused therapies (including ACT) and DBT for ASD respectively.

MINDFULNESS TRAINING AND CLINICAL DELIVERY

Despite the growing efficacy, MBIs pose significant dissemination and implementation challenges. MBI delivery and training is underresearched, and formal MBI training pathways that do exist are expensive, take several years to complete, and often involve multiple intensive trainings (7–10 days), 10-day silent meditation retreats, and regular supervision. These training programs emphasize that experiential learning and establishing a personal meditation practice are far superior to didactic learning (McCown et al., 2011). While mindfulness training modalities (experiential vs. didactic) have not been empirically tested, research has found that clinicians with formal training and personal meditation practice deliver MBIs with more skill, ultimately impacting clinical outcomes (Ruijgrok-Lupton et al., 2018). However, it is not feasible, practical, or sustainable for all clinicians to complete formal mindfulness trainings. This is a challenge that researchers and clinicians must collaboratively address as the field moves from research efficacy to widespread community implementation. At a minimum, clinicians planning to use MBIs should establish a personal meditation practice, either independently or through the support of a formal course such as MBSR.

MINDFULNESS-BASED INTERVENTIONS FOR ADULTS WITH ASD

While MBI research for adults with ASD is still relatively new, MBIs have demonstrated comparable outcomes to other psychotherapy treatments, such as CBT, for adults with ASD (Hartley et al., 2019; Sizoo & Kiuper, 2017). The MBIs that have been developed and tested in adult ASD samples are reviewed in the following sections.

Mindfulness-Based Therapy—Autism Spectrum (MBT-AS)

Mindfulness-based therapy—autism spectrum, or MBT-AS, has the most empirical support for adults with ASD, with demonstrated efficacy in improving co-occurring anxiety and depression symptoms. Spek and colleagues developed this group MBI by adapting MBSR into a 9-week intervention with 2.5-hour sessions (Spek et al., 2010, 2013). MBT-AS is a more structured version of MBSR with an added didactic session, additional time for processing speed impairments, and simplified language (e.g., the removal of metaphors). Pilot testing of MBT-AS established feasibility, satisfaction, and statistically significant improvement in depressive symptoms at posttreatment (Spek et al., 2010). MBT-AS was then tested in a randomized controlled trial (RCT; n = 50) and demonstrated efficacy in reducing depression, anxiety, rumination symptoms, and improving well-being (Kiep et al., 2014; Spek et al., 2013).

Subsequently, Sizoo and Kiuper slightly modified MBT-AS into 13 weekly 90-minute group sessions with shortened meditation practices (2017). This version of MBT-AS was compared to CBT in an RCT (n = 59). Both MBT-AS and CBT demonstrated significant, large effect changes in depression, anxiety, and rumination (Sizoo & Kiuper, 2017). This suggests that MBT-AS may be equivalent to CBT in addressing co-occurring mental health symptoms among adults with ASD. One might consider MBT-AS over CBT with adults who have difficulty identifying thoughts, understanding abstract language, limited verbal comprehension and expression, or who did not respond to previous CBT treatment.

Mindfulness-Based Stress Reduction

Prior to 2020, all published MBIs for adults with ASD were adapted specifically for ASD diagnostic characteristics. While the results were promising, this limits widespread dissemination and implementation in a population that already experiences huge service gaps. Beck and colleagues tested the feasibility, acceptability, and need for modification of traditional (i.e., nonadapted) MBSR (Beck, Greco, et al., 2020). This small pilot found that MBSR was appropriate for adults with ASD without intellectual disabilities (Beck, Greco, et al., 2020). All participants (n = 12) completed the 7.5-hour silent meditation retreat day and reported high satisfaction with the group. Feasibility, acceptability, participant satisfaction benchmarks were met, and the sample reported preliminary large effect size changes in positive outlook, quality of life, and mindfulness. While no modifications were needed, the group leader made small clinical adjustments and participants required supports (e.g., public transportation) outside of group sessions.

Braden and colleagues conducted an RCT comparing MBSR to a stress reduction control group with a sample of adults with ASD (n = 28; Pagni et al., 2020). MBSR was minimally adapted from 2.5- to 2-hour sessions and the full-day retreat was eliminated, but the content was consistent with the standardized curriculum and it was taught by a certified MBSR teacher. Participants in the MBSR group reported significant reduction in self-reported depressive symptoms and corresponding neural changes in the middle cingulate cortex and higher order cognitive brain regions were detected (Pagni et al., 2020).

Other Mindfulness-Based Interventions

Conner & White designed the first brief MBI for adults with ASD. This brief MBI consisted of six, 1-hour individual therapy sessions to target emotion dysregulation in a sample of adults with ASD (n = 9). This intervention was based on MBCT, with modifications made to the intervention delivery (individualized), shortened sessions (from 2.5 hours to 50 minutes), shortened meditation practices (from 1 hour to 20 minutes), simplified language, and psychoeducation on depression was replaced with emotion regulation content (Conner & White, 2018). The study demonstrated feasibility (100% retention), adequate fidelity, and acceptable treatment satisfaction. Most participants reported reliable change in impulse control, access to emotion regulation strategies, or emotional acceptance (Conner & White, 2018)

Gaigg and colleagues conducted an RCT that compared two self-guided online interventions, traditional CBT and brief MBCT, in a sample of adults with ASD (n = 54; 2020). A readily available online MBCT program endorsed by the National Health Service in the United Kingdom was used; thus, it was not designed specifically for ASD. Participants completed 4 modules over 4 weeks and received automated email reminders, notifications, and invitations to new material and mindfulness practices. Many participants experienced clinically significant improvements in anxiety symptoms in the MBCT (66.7%) and CBT (57.1%) groups, with no significant differences between groups. There were slightly more individuals who did not complete the CBT program compared to the MBCT group.

The emotion awareness and skills enhancement (EASE) program is an MBI developed and tested for adolescents and young adults (ages 12–21) with ASD and ER impairment (Conner et al., 2019). EASE is a 16-week individual MBI that incorporates cognitive strategies taught in MBCT but utilizes Vipassana meditation practices drawn from MBSR. The open pilot established feasibility, satisfaction, and preliminary efficacy, with large effect size changes in reduced functional impairment, less maladaptive emotion regulation strategies, and improved depression in an adolescent sample (n = 20). It is currently being tested in an ongoing RCT.

EASE is currently being adapted for individuals with co-occurring ASD and intellectual disabilities up to age 25, in a team-based approach for caregivers and participants (EASE-Teams). EASE-Teams uses Vipassana breathing and walking meditations that have been significantly shortened (30 seconds long) and simplified for adults with limited verbal ability. Meditations are taught and repeated throughout sessions and clinicians work with families to incorporate mindfulness into already established daily routines.

Summary of the Evidence

The current state of science suggests that there is potential to improve outcomes for adults with ASD through MBIs. Most of the research utilizes group MBIs with group sizes ranging from 7 to 12 individuals. Efficacy has been established for improving co-occurring depressive symptoms and quality of life in group MBIs, with changes detected through self-report and neurophysiological assessment.

More recent literature demonstrated preliminary feasibility and acceptability using individual MBIs to improve ER among young adults with ASD. To date, two studies have evaluated MBI programs that were not designed or modified specifically for ASD (Beck, Greco, et al., 2020; Gaigg et al., 2020); both studies found that the MBIs were appropriate for ASD and demonstrated preliminary efficacy in improved mental health and quality of life. Despite this promising evidence, MBI research is limited to feasibility and efficacy with pilot, quasi-experimental, and a few RCT designs (Hartley et al., 2019).

MBIs can be a good alternative to more traditional psychotherapy, such as CBT, especially for clients who have a history of limited improvement in treatment. MBIs can be individually tailored to ASD-specific characteristics, communication ability, and intellectual functioning (White et al., 2018). Clinicians might consider MBIs for clients who present with limited insight, impaired ER, or significant rumination or perseveration. The experiential meditation training in MBIs can be helpful for clients who have difficulty with "talk therapy." Adults with ASD who have limited verbal skills or co-occurring intellectual disability are able to actively participate in modified Vipassana meditation practices. MBIs have been used extensively in samples of adolescents with intellectual disability (Hwang & Singh, 2016), providing opportunity for MBIs to be used with the large population of adults with co-occurring ASD and intellectual disability. Finally, MBIs can be implemented in different environments in order to foster generalization of skills.

Clinical Strategies for MBI Delivery

Adults with ASD have unique cognitive and social needs that can impact MBI delivery (Beck, Conner, et al., 2020). Social challenges, such as limited social reciprocity and difficulty with group interactions, can make group-based MBIs challenging for clinicians. Limitations in attention span, abstract language, and awareness can also impact meditations and intervention delivery (Beck, Conner, et al., 2020). In nearly all of the evidence summarized previously, research labs utilized teams with extensive ASD experience *and* mindfulness experts. This level of dual expertise is unlikely to occur in most community-based service settings. Thus, considerations and suggestions for clinicians utilizing MBIs with adults with ASD are detailed in what follows and in Table 10-1.

Mindfulness Meditations for Adults With ASD

Meditations are a core component of MBIs and allow for in-vivo, experiential practice to approach challenges and problems in new ways. Meditation guidance is greatly enhanced by having familiarity with the meditations to make necessary adjustments to meditation scripts moment by moment. For clinicians just starting with MBIs, until comfortable it is much better to play a meditation recording and practice *with* the client than to read from a printed meditation script.

Table 10-1 Suggested Adjustments for Utilizing MBIs With Adults With ASD

ASD Characteristic	Challenge	Practical Solution or Technique	Exemplar Language
Slow processing speed	Meditation instruction can be too fast; group processing makes it difficult to follow or share	Provide substantial empty space (long pauses) and slow the speed in meditations.	
		Provide specific and repetitive directions in meditation guidance.	"Now, bringing the attention to the [breathing; left arm; chest]."
		Lead the group in a brief exercise to allow time to process.	
Concrete thinking	Meditation language	Eliminate metaphors and provide specific and repetitive meditation guidance.	"Bringing the attention to sensations of air entering the nose and exiting the nose."
Difficulty with unstructured conversations	MBI group processing; listening and speaking in dyads was difficult and uncomfortable	Provide concrete mindfulness inquiry discussion questions on paper.	"Please point to one sensation you noticed in your body."
		Explicitly time and direct discussions.	"When the bell rings, it's your partner's turn to share."
Limited social reciprocity & perseveration	Perseverating on past or excessive story-telling during group	Re-establish story-telling guidelines at beginning of each session.	"I may stop stories so all can participate, and we can talk about things that are happening right now."
		Stop participant with prompt and lead impromptu breathing meditation and inquiry.	"I see we're getting stuck on the past. Let's pause and breathe together."
Spatial awareness	Difficulty maintaining one's space during meditations	Re-establish "rules" before each session.	"We are going to stay on our mat while we complete this practice."
		Direct placement of yoga mats in room.	Consider placing individual with spatial difficulties near clinician.

(continued)

Table 10-1 Continued

ASD Characteristic	Challenge	Practical Solution or Technique	Exemplar Language
Sensory sensitivity	Difficulty with sensory sensitivity during meditations (e.g., background noise)	Normalizing with psychoeducation on sensory sensitivity in ASD. Meditation suggestions to anchor attention to neutral area during heightened sensitivity.	"Let's find an area of your body that is neutral. How about the bottom of your feet?"
Attention span	Looking at phone during meditation; obvious inattention; visible impatience with the meditation	Lengthen meditation (>5 minutes) to allow thoughts to settle. Maintain enough silence in meditation but add extra guidance on bringing attention back to breathing. Acknowledge boredom and inattention during inquiry. Incorporate movement meditations into session.	"Noticing that the attention wandered, and gently bringing the attention back to the breathing." "Nice job noticing boredom. Where did you feel that in your body?"
Limited internal awareness	Not able to identify physical sensations, thoughts, or emotions	Model noticing basic physical sensations. Suggest something observed during inquiry. Incorporate external object and fade use as client builds awareness (e.g., stuffed animal)	"I noticed my breathing in my chest. What did you notice?" "I noticed you were scratching your arm. Did you notice itchiness?" "Feeling sensations of [Fluffy] rising and falling on your chest."

Mindful inquiry, a brief discussion on meditation practice, occurs following a meditation. The general process includes asking, "what did you notice in that practice?" and a brief discussion. This discussion is intended to stay present-focused on physical sensations, thoughts, or emotions noticed during the meditation practice. It is common for clients with ASD to be unsure or not have any sensations to notice during the meditation. Other clients may become overly analytical about the meditation process, engage in story telling, or try to understand the "why" behind a thought or emotion. A common mistake for clinicians new to mindfulness is to ask too many follow-up questions or to try to help the client understand the "why." Instead, clinicians can model responses (e.g., "I noticed my breathing in my nose") and encourage more meditations (e.g., "I see you're stuck; Let's breathe together"). Engaging in thought challenging, problem solving, discussions about past experiences, or explicit relaxation would be counter to the theoretical framework of mindfulness (Crane, Kuyken, et al., 2012; Crane, Brewer, et al., 2016).

Common MBI Challenges of Adults With ASD

Group MBIs have more social interaction in comparison to individual MBI sessions and have the potential to be more cost-effective. However, group MBIs are also more challenging given social impairments that are characteristic of ASD. Over-correction for disruptive behaviors can be counterproductive to the foundations of mindfulness. Instead of traditional prompting, reward systems, or behavior training, it is recommended that clinicians use kind, repetitive reminders throughout the sessions. Clinicians can also use brief meditation practices to interrupt unwanted group behavior and reorient the group to present-moment experiential learning. Challenges and techniques for MBI group management are detailed in Table 10-1.

Other limitations common in ASD, such as perseveration, spatial awareness, sensory sensitivity, attention span, and limited internal awareness, are likely to emerge when utilizing MBIs with adults with ASD. Many of these limitations can be addressed with minimal adjustments to the meditation practice, discussion, or session structure without formal adaptation (Table 10-1).

CASE STUDY

This case study presents information regarding a single MBSR group that consisted of 12 adults with ASD (Full Scale IQ>70; Beck, Greco, et al., 2020). ASD-specific mindfulness techniques utilized with two clients, Deborah and Freddy, are presented in detail. Deborah is an adult Caucasian female diagnosed with ASD and co-occurring attention deficit/hyperactivity disorder (ADHD). Deborah described ER challenges that led to difficulty maintaining employment, social relationships, and engaging in activities of daily living (i.e., grocery shopping). Freddy, an adult

Caucasian male diagnosed with ASD and co-occurring generalized anxiety disorder, joined the MBSR group to improve "stress" and challenges maintaining employment due to "freezing" when stressed. Both clients participated in an MBSR group that followed the standard curriculum and attended all sessions (Beck, Greco, et al., 2020; Santorelli et al., 2017; Santorelli, 2001). Additional detail on the procedures, methods, and analyses have been previously published (Beck, Greco, et al., 2020).

Deborah had difficulty with limited social reciprocity and perseveration during group interactions, and she would often escalate while describing her past negative experience. She had limited awareness and difficulty noticing her escalation and perseveration in the moment. This behavior impacted group dynamics because other participants were frustrated that she would frequently break the "rules." The clinician managed this by stopping her mid-story and providing the group with the instruction, "I see you are stuck. Let's all bring our attention to the breathing in *this* moment." Deborah would occasionally get frustrated with the interruption, but the instruction allowed her to practice meditation in the moment of dysregulation and perseveration. As the group progressed, she was able to notice her dysregulation in the moment without instructor prompting and reported to generalize this skill in her daily life.

Freddy had difficulty with problem solving, organization of time, processing speed, and ER, all of which impacted his group participation and required additional supports. He needed to be encouraged to leave his house and come to group at the start of each session (often 45 minutes late), as he would often freeze in fear of being late and disrupting the group. Freddy benefited from text message reminders (2x a week) to attend. During groups, Freddy needed extra time to organize his thoughts for group discussions and meditations. Vipassana meditations can be easily simplified to remove metaphors, and the clinician added substantially longer pauses and more silence into the meditations. During discussions, the clinician led brief 30-second breathing practices when it was Freddy's turn to talk so that he could gather his thoughts and share. His ability to gather his thoughts and quickly share improved as the group progressed.

Deborah and Freddy both indicated very high satisfaction with the MBSR program and reported substantial changes in quality of life, positive outlook, mindfulness, and anxiety. During exit interviews, Deborah described improved ER as the greatest benefit of the MBSR group, which impacted her social relationships and daily functioning:

> It helped me communicate my needs and disappointments and things of that nature before things get to be too bad. . . . The last couple meltdowns I still had them, but I was able to explain myself and calm myself down. . . . Like say the store is crowded and I can't go in, I used to force myself no matter what and now I think to myself do I really need to do this right now.

Freddy cited benefits that positively impacted daily functioning and employment:

Having quicker reaction time on tough situations. The getting that thinking process started. That is a big help because there were days where I just freeze all day because I didn't know what to do. I'm infinitely more productive. . . . I used to not have gotten to work until 3 and instead I have gotten to work at 1.

CONCLUSION

MBIs are promising evidence-based treatment options for adults with ASD, with demonstrated changes in co-occurring depression, rumination, anxiety, ER, and quality of life (Hartley et al., 2019). Much of the evidence supporting MBIs for adults with ASD utilize group formats. Common adaptations include simplified language, structural changes to sessions, and shortening meditation practices. The experiential focus of MBIs allow for individual tailoring to communication skills and cognitive functioning, and there is new research exploring the use of MBIs for individuals with co-occurring ASD and intellectual disabilities. Recent research suggests that some adults with ASD may be able to participate in MBIs without adaptation (Beck, Greco, et al., 2020; Gaigg et al., 2020). This has potential to increase service options for adults with ASD, as some may be able to participate in readily available community-based MBIs.

Widespread dissemination and implementation of MBIs for ASD will require thoughtful implementation strategies and training programs. MBI training pathways are arduous and are not traditionally incorporated into graduate school curriculums. Clinicians can begin by engaging in a personal mindfulness meditation practice on their own or enrolling in a community-based mindfulness course (e.g., MBSR). ASD characteristics can influence MBI delivery but small adjustments can be made without changing the meditation. Future research should systematically explore the clinical delivery and training needs while balancing scientific rigor and real-life context in order to test the effectiveness and implementation of MBIs into community-based settings for adults with ASD.

Funding Acknowledgment: This work was supported by the National Center For Advancing Translational Sciences of the National Institutes of Health under Award Number KL2TR001856 (Author: KB). The content is solely the responsibility of the author and does not necessarily represent the official views of the National Institutes of Health.

REFERENCES

Baer, R. (2003). Mindfulness training as a clinical intervention: A conceptual and empirical review. *Clinical Psychology: Science and Practice, 10*(2), 125–143.

Beck, K. B., Conner, C. M., White, S. W., & Mazefsky, C. A. (2020). Mindfulness "Here and Now": Strategies for Helping Adolescents With Autism. *Journal of the American Academy of Child & Adolescent Psychiatry, 59*(10), 1125–1127.

Beck, K. B., Conner, C. M., Breitenfeldt, K. E., Northrup, J., White, S. W., & Mazefsky, C. A. (2020). Assessment and treatment of emotion regulation impairment in autism spectrum disorder across the life span: Current state of the science and future directions. *Child and Adolescent Psychiatric Clinics, 29*(3), 527–542.

Beck, K. B., Greco, C. M., Terhorst, L. A., Skidmore, E. R., Kulzer, J. L., & McCue, M. P. (2020). Mindfulness-based stress reduction for adults with autism spectrum disorder: Feasibility and estimated effects. *Mindfulness, 11*, 1286–1297.

Cachia, R. L., Anderson, A., & Moore, D. W. (2016). Mindfulness in Individuals with Autism Spectrum Disorder: A Systematic Review and Narrative Analysis. *Review Journal of Autism and Developmental Disorders, 3*(2), 165–178.

Chiesa, A., & Malinowski, P. (2011). Mindfulness-based approaches: Are they all the same? *Journal of Clinical Psychology, 67*(4), 404–424.

Conner, C. M., Golt, J., Righi, G., Shaffer, R., Siegel, M., & Mazefsky, C. A. (2020). A Comparative Study of Suicidality and Its Association with Emotion Regulation Impairment in Large ASD and US Census-Matched Samples. *Journal of Autism and Developmental Disorders, 50*(10), 3545–3560.

Conner, C. M., & White, S. W. (2018). Brief report: Feasibility and preliminary efficacy of individual mindfulness therapy for adults with autism spectrum disorder. *Journal of Autism and Developmental Disorders, 48*(1), 290–300.

Conner, C. M., White, S. W., Beck, K. B., Golt, J., Smith, I. C., & Mazefsky, C. A. (2019). Improving emotion regulation ability in autism: The Emotional Awareness and Skills Enhancement (EASE) program. *Autism, 23*(5), 1273–1287.

Crane, R. S., Brewer, J., Felman, C., Kabat-Zinn, J., Santorelli, S., Williams, J. M. G., Kuyken, W. (2016). What defines mindfulness-based programs: The warp and the weft. *Psychological Medicine, 47*, 990–999.

Crane, R. S., Kuyken, Q., Williams, M. G., Hastings, R. P., Cooper, L., & Fennell, M. J. (2012). Competence in teaching mindfulness-based courses: Concepts, development and assessment. *Mindfulness, 3*, 76–84.

Gaigg, S. B., Flaxman, P. E., McLaven, G., Shah, R., Bowler, D. M., Meyer, B., Roestorf, A., Haenschel, C., Rodgers, J., & South, M. (2020). Self-guided mindfulness and cognitive behavioural practices reduce anxiety in autistic adults: A pilot 8-month waitlist-controlled trial of widely available online tools. *Autism, 24*(4), 867–883.

Gotink, R., Chu, P., Busschback, J., Benson, H., Fricchione, G., & Hunink, M. (2015). Standardised mindfulness-based interventions in healthcare: An overview of systematic reviews and meta-analyses of RCTs. *PLOSONE, 10*(4), 1–17.

Gu, J., Strauss, C., Bond, R., & Cavanagh, K. (2015). How do mindfulness-based cognitive therapy and mindfulness-based stress reduction improve mental health and wellbeing? A systematic review and meta-analysis of meditation studies. *Clinical Psychology Review, 37*, 1–12.

Gunaratana, H. (2015). *Mindfulness in plain English.* Wisdom Publications.

Hartley, M., Dorstyn, D., & Due, M. (2019). Mindfulness for children and adults with autism spectrum disorder and their caregivers: A meta-analysis. *Journal for Autism and Developmental Disabilities, 49*, 4306–4319.

Hartmann, K., Urbano, M. R., Raffaele, C. T., Kreiser, N. L., Williams, T. V., Qualls, L. R., & Elkins, D. E. (2019). Outcomes of an emotion regulation intervention group in young adults with autism spectrum disorder. *Bulletin of the Menninger Clinic, 83*(3), 259–277.

Hwang, Y., & Singh, N. N. (2016). Mindfulness. In N. N. Singh (Ed.), *Handbook of evidence-based practices in intellectual and developmental disabilities* (pp. 311–346). Springer Nature.

Kabat-Zinn, J. (2006). Mindfulness-based interventions in context: Past, present, & future. *Clinical Psychology Science and Practice, 10*(2), 144–156.

Kabat-Zinn, J., Lipworth, L., & Burney, R. (1985). The clinician use of mindfulness meditation for the self-regulation of chronic pain. *Journal of Behavioral Medicine, 8*(2), 163–189.

Kiep, M., Spek, A. A., & Hoeben, L. (2014). Mindfulness-based therapy in adults with an autism spectrum disorder: Do treatment effects last? *Mindfulness, 6*(3), 637–644.

McCown, D., Reibel, D., & Micozzi, M. S. (2011). *Teaching mindfulness: A practical guide for clinicians and educators*. Springer.

Pagni, B. A., Walsh, M. J., Foldes, E., Sebren, A., Dixon, M. V., Guerithault, H., Braden, B. B. (2020). The neural correlates of mindfulness-induced depression reduction in adults with autism spectrum disorder: A pilot study. *Journal of Neuroscience Research, 98*(6), 1150–1161.

Ruijgrok-Lupton, P. E., Crane, R. S., & Dorjee, D. (2018). Impact of mindfulness-based teacher training on MBSR participant well-being outcomes and course satisfaction. *Mindfulness, 9*(1),117–128.

Santorelli, S. (2001). *Mindfulness-based stress reduction (MBSR): Standards of practice*. Center for Mindfulness in Medicine, Health Care & Society.

Santorelli, S. F., Meleo-Meyer, F., Koerbel, L., & Kabat-Zinn, J. (2017). *Mindfulness-Based Stress Reduction (MBSR) Authorized Curriculum Guide©*. Center of Mindfulness in Medicine, Health Care, & Society.

Segal, V., Williams, J. M. G., Teasdale, J. D. (2002). *Mindfulness-based cognitive therapy for depression*. Guilford Press.

Sizoo, B. B., & Kuiper, E. (2017). Cognitive behavioural therapy and mindfulness based stress reduction may be equally effective in reducing anxiety and depression in adults with autism spectrum disorders. *Research in Developmental Disabilities, 64*, 47–55.

Spek, A. A., van Ham, N. C., & van Lieshout, H. (2010). Effectiviteit van Mindfulness Based Stress Reduction bij volwassenen met een autismespectrumstoornis. *Wetenschappelijk Tijdschrift Autisme, 9*(3), 82–88.

Spek, A. A., van Ham, N. C., Nyklicek, I. (2013). Mindfulness-based therapy in adults with autism spectrum disorder: A randomized controlled trial. *Research in Developmental Disabilities, 34*, 246–253.

White, S. W., Simmons, G. L., Gotham, K. O., Conner, C. M., Smith, I. C., Beck, K. B., & Mazefsky, C. A. (2018). Psychosocial treatments targeting anxiety and depression in adolescents and adults on the autism spectrum: Review of the research and recommended future directions. *Current Psychiatry Reports, 20*(82), 1–10.

11

Emotion-Focused Therapies

ANNA ROBINSON AND CAITLIN M. CONNER ■

KEY CONSIDERATIONS

- Autistic adults often experience emotional difficulties and may have differences in their abilities to recognize their own emotions, express and regulate their emotions, and recognize others' emotions.
- Autistic adults are more likely to have co-occurring psychiatric conditions such as anxiety and depression.
- Emotion-focused therapy, a humanistic therapy approach, has been adapted to help adults on the autism spectrum who struggle with emotions and past traumatic experiences.
- Several studies have also targeted emotion regulation impairment in autism using mindfulness-based and cognitive behavioral approaches
- Future research in this area should examine which treatment works best for whom on the spectrum, how or whether to adapt interventions for those on the autism spectrum who do not have intellectual disability, and how to make interventions adaptable to those on the autism spectrum with an intellectual disability.

OVERVIEW OF EMOTION-FOCUSED THERAPIES

Differences in emotional expression and regulation have been present since the earliest descriptions of autism (Kanner, 1943). Autistic individuals display differences in emotional development across the lifespan (see Conner et al., in press, for review).

To date, research has shown differences or impairments in several domains of emotion processing in autistic individuals. Studies of autistic adults indicate that impairments in emotion awareness, including the inability to notice, describe, and distinguish among one's own emotions, is present in nearly half of adults sampled

(Berthoz & Hill, 2005). While some research indicates that autistic individuals are able to recognize others' emotional expressions, the ability to distinguish more subtle, complex, and dynamic emotional expressions is thought to be impaired in at least some autistic adults (Eack et al., 2015; Rigby et al., 2018). Differences in emotion expression, such as flattened, atypical, exaggerated, and incongruent expressions, have been reported in studies of autistic individuals (Costa et al., 2017; Trevisan et al., 2018). Lastly, studies of emotion regulation (ER), the ability to modify one's own emotions, in autistic individuals have indicated early and frequent difficulties, such as overly relying on maladaptive strategies like suppression and avoidance and difficulties managing strong, very reactive emotional responses (Mazefsky & White, 2014).

Given that differences or difficulties in emotion-related areas may present in a sizable number of autistic individuals, it is likely that emotional difficulties may lead to other downstream adverse effects. For example, ties between emotional impairments and social abilities are likely, as impairments in the abilities to label, demonstrate, and respond optimally to emotions can dampen social connections. For example, facial expressions of autistic adults were found to appear more "unnatural" when judged by neurotypical peers (Faso et al., 2014). A meta-analysis of research in autism found that impaired emotion recognition was associated with poorer social functioning (Trevisan & Birmingham, 2016). In a study comparing quantity of social interactions in autistic and non-autistic adults, impairments in emotional awareness, but not autistic symptom severity, were associated with fewer social interactions (Gerber et al., 2019).

Co-occurring psychiatric conditions are highly prevalent throughout the lifespan in autism, with analyses of a multi-site sample of autistic youth demonstrating that a majority of autistic 8-year-olds have at least one co-occurring psychiatric condition (Soke et al., 2018). Adult prevalence rates of anxiety or depressive disorders range widely, from 20%–80% (Rosen et al., 2018). Impairments in ER have been shown to be associated with co-occurring psychopathology and suicidality (Conner et al., 2020; Mazefsky & White, 2014) as well as use of inpatient psychiatric services, crisis services, and psychotropic medication (Conner et al., 2021).

Thus, treatment of emotional difficulties is vitally important for autistic adults. This chapter will focus on interventions that directly target emotional difficulties, such as emotion-focused therapy, dialectical behavior therapy (DBT), and cognitive behavior therapy (CBT) for ER. We will close our chapter with a discussion of future directions.

INTERVENTIONS

Despite evidence that emotional difficulties contribute to social impairments in autism, there are no widespread interventions available to ameliorate emotion-focused issues. Furthermore, extant treatment research regarding emotion awareness, expression, and recognition has largely focused on autistic children and adolescents. Most of the research utilizes computer-based programs for training recognition and expression of facial emotion expressions (see Berggren et al., 2018, for review; Wieckowski et al., 2020). One of the few studies that has focused on autistic adults used a computer program called Mind Reading to teach adults emotion recognition of complex facial emotion expressions; while results across several groups of adults indicated increased recognition, generalizability outside of the computer program was questionable (Golan & Baron-Cohen, 2006).

Similarly, little research to date has examined interventions directly targeting ER, and most of this research has occurred with autistic children and adolescents (see Beck, Conner, et al., 2020, for a review). The emotion awareness and skills enhancement (EASE) program was developed to improve ER impairment in autistic adolescents and adults through teaching emotional awareness with mindfulness-based techniques. An initial open trial found improvements in ER, as well as decreases in depression, anxiety, and irritability symptoms (Conner et al., 2019). However, this trial (n = 20) of EASE did not include adults, and a larger, randomized controlled trial (RCT) including adults is still underway (Conner et al., 2019).

Conner and White (2018) adapted mindfulness-based cognitive therapy into an individual therapy targeting ER impairment. The six-session therapy focused on teaching mindfulness meditation techniques, discussion of ER strategies considered traditionally "adaptive" and "maladaptive," and practice of adaptive ER strategies. Nine young autistic adults (age 18–25) completed the intervention and self-reported improvement in ER strategies as well as decreased negative affect (Conner & White, 2018).

Emotion-related outcomes have likewise been recorded in interventions targeting other areas. The majority of extant psychosocial intervention research in autism has focused on treatment of co-occurring anxiety disorders in children and adolescents using CBT (Weston et al., 2016). In CBT-focused research, studies have typically used programs either developed or adapted specifically for autistic individuals. The largest RCT of CBT for anxiety treatment in autistic youth to date compared traditional CBT to a CBT adapted specifically for autism, and found that a traditional format was effective for some youth on the spectrum (Wood et al., 2020). To date, fewer studies have used CBT with adults on the spectrum. A systematic review of CBT and mindfulness studies involving autistic adults found only six studies and, of those, only two were RCTs comparing CBT or mindfulness to a waitlist or comparison treatment condition (Spain et al., 2015). One study compared CBT versus an anxiety management approach for autistic adults and obsessive compulsive disorder (OCD), with nearly half of the CBT group considered treatment responders, more than twice than that of the anxiety management condition (Russell et al., 2013). CBT studies concerning autistic adults have also targeted social anxiety, agoraphobia, posttraumatic stress disorder (PTSD), depression, self-harming behaviors, and substance use disorders (Helverschou et al., 2019; Spain et al., 2015).

More research has investigated mindfulness-based interventions with autistic adults, including mindfulness-based stress reduction (MBSR), a group-based approach that increased emotion awareness, life satisfaction, and trait mindfulness

(Beck, Greco, et al., 2020); a study of acceptance and commitment therapy (ACT) that decreased stress (Pahnke et al., 2019); and a study that investigated the efficacy of online self-help programs (one CBT and one mindfulness-focused) for autistic adults with co-occurring anxiety (Gaigg et al., 2020). Results suggest that, for at least some autistic adults, such online programs could be a cost-effective and accessible means to treatment when in-person psychotherapy is unavailable or not obtainable.

Emotion-focused therapy (EFT) is a humanistic-experiential psychotherapy that combines relational principles from the person-centered approach (Rogers, 1951) with more directive evocative interventions from Gestalt and other experiential therapies (Greenberg et al., 1993). Within EFT, the therapeutic relationship is seen as a key curative element that integrates active approaches of psychodrama (Moreno & Moreno, 1959), process-guiding methods from Gestalt therapy (Perls et al., 1951), and experiential therapy, such as Gendlin's focusing (1981). There is increasing evidence of the effectiveness of EFT for treating depression (Goldman et al., 2006), generalized anxiety disorder (Timulak et al., 2017), and social anxiety disorder (Shahar et al., 2017).

Emotion-focused therapy for autism spectrum (EFT-AS; Robinson & Elliott, 2017) is an integrative group psychotherapy approach grounded in humanistic values and EFT theory and practice, and it also uses video-assisted interpersonal process recall (IPR; Kagan, 1984) as a process-guiding method making experiential and self-other relational processing more accessible and concrete. EFT is process-marker driven, working with an empathic relationship using markers to guide interventions for different types of problems that arise in session. EFT-AS follows a three-step model consisting of two kinds of alternating sessions: a group therapy session and a video-assisted IPR session. The therapist analyses each therapy session to select three short clips; these edited clips contain the task markers and are played in the following IPR session. The therapist is guided by IPR selection principles, for example, looking for moments of interpersonal ruptures between clients, clients engaged in dialogue of painful experiences, or an absence of emotion dialogue. In all sessions, the therapist offers empathic attunement with client emotions, helping clients by focusing their attention inwards on bodily feelings. Emotion processing is further supported by the therapist guiding clients through a range of therapeutic tasks in directed awareness and emotion stimulation using imagery and psychodramatic enactments, interpersonal exchanges, and video IPR.

In EFT, working with primary and secondary emotions are key concepts. The primary emotion is the first emotion a person feels when they react to a situation, and these are usually adaptive emotional responses. Secondary emotions come afterward and often mask or hide the primary emotion (i.e., anger hiding the primary hurt emotion). In EFT, the therapist works with the secondary emotion to help the client locate the primary, hidden emotion. This primary emotion is either adaptive or maladaptive, and the maladaptive emotion is what we call core pain. The core pain has an unmet need embedded in it (i.e., if I feel fear then I need to feel safe). In EFT, the therapist empathically follows the client and helps them reach their core pain, and the unmet need emerges from this state.

The aim of EFT is to change a maladaptive emotion with an adaptive emotion following six key principles. The first is developing awareness of emotions—being able to access them and be in touch with their internal emotional experiences. This is followed by the second principle, which is having clients express their emotions, mostly with enactment tasks, using chair dialogues. The use of imaginary chair dialogues such as two-chair dialogue for conflict split, two-chair dialogue for self-interruption, or empty chair dialogue for unfinished business (Elliott et al., 2004), heightens awareness and evokes more adaptive emotions. The third focuses on ER, helping clients to regulate their emotions so they do not become too overwhelmed and can thereby process their emotions. Following this, the fourth principle involves helping clients to gain insight and understanding of their own emotions by reflecting upon their emotional experience, where they are engaged in creating new narratives. In EFT, positive outcomes involve the final two key principles in which emotion transformation occurs. The first of these is changing emotion with emotion, with the client replacing one emotion by experiencing a more powerful emotion. The sixth key principle is the corrective emotional experience, which involves changing the maladaptive emotion (core painful emotion) with another more adaptive emotion, but within the interpersonal relationship. In individual therapy this is with the therapist; as EFT-AS is a group therapy this can be with the therapist, but often the therapist facilitates interpersonal opportunities with other group members. To date, positive preliminary findings for EFT-AS have been reported (Robinson & Elliott, 2016), as well as a number of case conceptualizations from clinical data of clients working through specific presenting problems. These include misempathy (Robinson & Elliott, 2017) leading to compassion for self and self-soothing; accessing trauma-related experiences with healing from evoked affective empathy and compassion responses from other (Robinson, 2018) and relational rupture and repair (Robinson, 2020).

CASE STUDY

The following presents a case example of working with trauma-related experiences (for the case conceptualization model, see Robinson, 2018) following an emotional-deepening model (Pascual-Leone & Greenberg, 2007). The case of Martin (with Carla and Matt), demonstrates working with trauma-related experiences using the deepening model as a guide (see Figure 11-1). Martin, a 39-year-old male diagnosed with Asperger syndrome in adulthood, was unemployed at the time and living with his mother and brother at their family home. Martin dropped out of college toward the end of his first year and came to therapy seeking support for social isolation, depression, and anxiety related to repetitive, intrusive, destructive thoughts. In the first phase of therapy (see Figure 11-1, phase 1), clients tend to start with a global undifferentiated emotion. Frequently, clients are out of touch with their inner emotions, stating "I don't feel my emotions." The therapist's goal is to help the client to specify or differentiate what kind of feeling they have, with

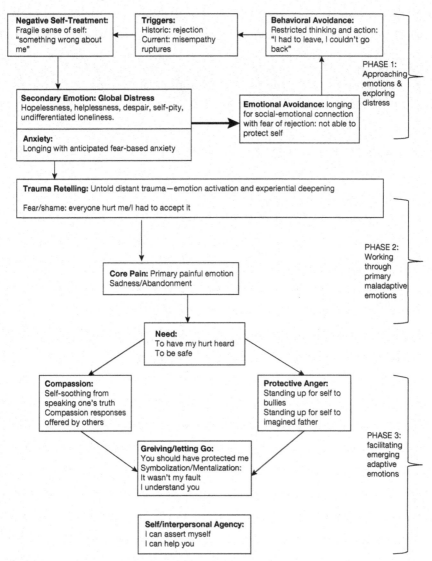

Figure 11-1 Emotion-Focused Therapy Case Conceptualization of Trauma-Related Experiences
See Robinson, 2018.

tasks that help clients turn their attention inwards, so they can experience these emotions, label them, and articulate them.

In EFT-AS, emotional misunderstanding has been identified as an emotion marker because this often presents in therapy as misempathy ruptures between group members or dialogue of these repeated occurrences outside of the therapy sessions, as part of the client's narrative history. Therefore, misempathy is seen as a trigger and defined as a lack of synchronized empathic attunement to the other's felt sense or expressed feelings (Robinson & Elliott, 2017). Therapists are looking for emotion markers to identify and change negative interaction cycles. Martin talks about how he has experienced misempathy ruptures in different situations:

> MARTIN: I got pulled upstairs by the supervisor I worked with for doing something wrong, they did say I'd been confrontational and aggressive when I was trying to be assertive.

These negative interpersonal experiences are often followed by restricted thinking, such as a stuck cognitive loop, that the person feels powerless to change, resulting in behavioral avoidance:

> MARTIN: I ended up having to leave; I ended up having to leave there, I couldn't go on.

The client engages in negative self-treatment dialogue. These negative self-judgments manifest as a fragile sense of self, often as a consequence of concrete experiences of habitual failed interpersonal encounters (Robinson, 2018) and reinforce a lack of self-agency within these exchanges:

> MARTIN: They talk about conversations that I don't know about and you feel guilty about not knowing about them. . . . I can't have conversations.

Feared triggers and the emotional pain they bring are accompanied with a longing desire to connect, but a lack of understanding of how to socially and emotionally read typically developing others generates an apprehensive anxiety:

> MARTIN: I went to University to find friends, to get more of a social life, but it didn't happen. I was stuck in my room, I couldn't do anything to get it.

In EFT-AS, IPR is used as a process guide to support clients in accessing the emotional pain contained within their stories. Martin entered therapy with a low level of emotion regulation. He was upregulated, with flat affect and limited nonverbal emotional expressions, and his discourse possessed limited emotional experiences. This missing emotional response to self was evident in his narration of his own stories, but also in IPR reflection to self:

> MARTIN: I look like a statue; I don't really use gestures or look at people when I'm talking.

The therapist uses tasks to help the client deepen their emotional experience, by using edited clips of video for IPR to evoke emotional responses to self and engaging in chair enactments. The therapist is listening for an emotion compass or the painful experiences recalled in the client's story. In EFT, *reprocessing tasks* help clients with trauma retelling, through systematic evocative unfolding and in creating meaning bridges through trauma retelling and emotion connection to sense making (Paivio & Pascual-Leone, 2010). Experiences of extreme and chronic rejection and peer victimization (Maiano et al., 2016) form part of their unprocessed trauma-related experiences, which often manifest as a fragile sense of self (Robinson, 2018).

> MARTIN: I felt that there was something not right about me. Something wrong. I just didn't think there was anything to do and that there was no point in trying anymore, so I became more isolated and stuck in my flat on my own.

This unfolding moves to a slightly deeper emotion response, typically a secondary reactive emotion that is an emotion which is a reaction to another emotion that came before it. This is often the symptom that the client brings to therapy, whether they are depressed, anxious, or experiencing post-trauma difficulties. In the deepening process we work with the primary maladaptive emotion; the client will often be stuck in these emotions, so the therapist helps the client work with this. The client often experiences the feeling of helplessness or a sense of despair:

> MARTIN: I did feel like it was too late like I said, I do feel like it's too late in some ways.
> THERAPIST: Too late. . . .
> MARTIN: For recovery. I'll never be normal. . . . . I'll never have a relationship, I'll always be alone.

Toward the middle phase of therapy (see Figure 11-1, phase 2) the therapist helps the client work through primary maladaptive emotions to access and give voice to these trauma experiences:

> MARTIN: I was horrendously upset by bullying when I was a child. . . . Even teachers called me the names.

The therapist uses IPR as a process guide to evocative unfolding of recalled trauma, which can lead to tapping into feelings associated with the memory and to accessing the adaptive emotion that counters feelings of hopelessness, helplessness, and fear. Martin initially connects with his anger at the violation by others who bullied him:

> MARTIN: I could viciously attack them all. . . . I didn't. I feel like doing that now.

In a heightened state of arousal by accessing his distant trauma memories, Martin initially becomes underregulated, feeling the anger in the here and now. EFT-AS unfolds memories to access emotional experiences in order to transform these with a more adaptive emotion:

THERAPIST: There is strength in your voice. It sounds, a strong anger.

MARTIN: I am angry with all those people who called me the name as if that was ok, as if I accepted it. I didn't.

The final phase of therapy is *emotional transformation* (see Figure 11-1, phase 3). The client achieves this through engagement in enactment tasks. One of the most helpful is empty chair enactments, which can help the client access the adaptive emotion and express it:

MARTIN: I feel like going out and doing violence to those people who harmed me.

THERAPIST: If you could tell those people who called you those names what would you say? [Therapist brings up an empty chair] Let's put them in that chair. What would you say to them?

MARTIN: It wasn't ok. It wasn't ok to call me that name. That wasn't my name.

THERAPIST: It wasn't my name. [Points at empty chair.]

[Therapist helps Martin put each person who harmed him in the chair.]

This deepening process continues until the underlying painful memory is accessed:

MARTIN: My dad thought it was because of the way I react. I was just able to express the way I felt at home, and my dad thought that that was how I reacted, but I didn't react I was just trying to express how it hurts.

The therapist helps the client to identify what in the primary maladaptive emotion is their core pain; that is, what hurts the most. This core pain is at the deepest level, that thing that feels most painful. It is often a sense of feeling "broken," "abandoned," or "unlovable." The therapist offers empathy while being alongside the clients as they experience their core pain. The therapist asks the client, What does this sense of being "abandoned," what does this part of you need? When the client is able to articulate this, such as "to be protected," they engage in an imagined chair enactment of *speaking one's truth*:

THERAPIST: If you could speak to your Dad, if he was here sitting in that chair, what would you like to say to him?

MARTIN: I'd just ask him why didn't you stand up for me? . . . [Lowers head.]

THERAPIST: [Lowers tone of voice and points to empty chair.] Tell him.

MARTIN: Why did you not defend me when I was getting called all these names? You sided with all the people who used to call me it.

THERAPIST: You didn't defend me. Tell him. . . . [Points to empty chair.]

MARTIN: Why didn't you care about the way you made me feel?

THERAPIST: I felt . . .

MARTIN: Sad . . . yeah . . . sad.

As the client begins to access the core pain and the unmet needs that they point to, the therapist will then ask the client "what will meet that unmet need?" In EFT, the thing that will meet that need is a different emotion. If this is the client feeling vulnerable, it would be protective anger, that is, anger that protects; or if feeling a sense of abandonment, it would be compassion, or connecting sadness (sadness that connects). In therapy, the client then bridges from a primary maladaptive emotion to an adaptive emotion through the unmet need associated with the core pain. These adaptive emotions from the unmet need are particularly useful for meeting the unmet need of different core pain, such as protective anger for trauma, by helping the client access a part of them that protects and supports the part that is feeling hurt. In EFT-AS, the aim is to help the client access self-compassion to transform the stuck primary maladaptive emotion. Emotion transformation occurs by replacing one emotion by experiencing a more powerful emotion, which is most effective within an interpersonal relationship. Self-compassion and self-soothing is often difficult to achieve, but in EFT-AS, other group members can offer compassion to soothe:

> CARLA: I feel as if I want to give Martin a hug. . . . It's a protective feeling, it's a protective feeling that I've got. [Pause.] I want to protect.
> THERAPIST: Where are the emotions coming from?
> CARLA: I want to give Martin a hug. [Carla looks toward Martin, who holds her gaze; they hold each other's warm gaze.]

The final stage of task resolution is meaning creation, and this facilitates acceptance with self-agency and marks the ending of therapy. Reduced cognitive (but not affective) empathy has been reported in autistic adults (Holt et al., 2018). Therefore, creation of cognitive empathic understanding supports the new changing narrative, which is best achieved within interpersonal understanding and involves grieving and letting go:

> THERAPIST: And how do you feel about your Dad just now?
> MARTIN: It's still sad that he got it wrong. . . . I wasn't diagnosed then and that's why he didn't understand me.

SUMMARY

While co-occurring psychiatric conditions are common in autistic adults, research into treatments is still emerging. Several evidence-based treatments such as CBT and DBT for neurotypical populations have shown some efficacy in improving emotion-related outcomes for autistic adults (Hartmann et al., 2019; Spain et al., 2017). Less research has examined approaches that directly target emotional concerns, such as EFT, emotion recognition training, and therapies to improve ER impairment. Far more research that recruits larger samples to determine individual factors influencing treatment outcomes is needed to better understand and recommend effective treatments for autistic adults who present with emotion-related concerns.

Effective treatments for autistic adults must also be accessible. While the evidence base suggests that the treatments discussed in this chapter have clinical benefit for individuals on the autism spectrum, oftentimes general mental health providers are hesitant to treat autistic individuals (White et al., 2020). Given the difficulties of locating a mental health professional with autism expertise, it offers hope that autistic adults could see symptom improvement from a general provider. However, research that has tracked autistic adults through Medicare records (U.S. government-provided healthcare for individuals with disabilities or low-income individuals) has found that autistic adults are more likely to receive psychotropic medications than therapy for depression or anxiety when compared to their non-autistic peers (Maddox et al., 2018). Overall, mental health professionals who serve neurotypical adults may require access to training materials to serve adults on the spectrum, or even just the knowledge that their standard treatments for emotional difficulties may prove effective for autistic adults with little to moderate adaptation.

REFERENCES

Beck, K. B., Conner, C. M., Breitenfeldt, K. E., Northrup, J. B., White, S. W., & Mazefsky, C. A. (2020). Assessment and Treatment of Emotion Regulation Impairment in Autism Spectrum Disorder Across the Lifespan. *Child and Adolescent Psychiatric Clinics of North America*, *29*(3), 527–542.

Beck, K. B., Greco, C. M., Terhorst, L. A., Skidmore, E. R., Kulzer, J. L., & McCue, M. P. (2020). Mindfulness-based stress reduction for adults with autism spectrum disorder: Feasibility and estimated effects. *Mindfulness*, *11*(5), 1286–1297.

Berggren, S., Fletcher-Watson, S., Milenkovic, N., Marschik, P. B., Bölte, S., & Jonsson, U. (2018). Emotion recognition training in autism spectrum disorder: A systematic review of challenges related to generalizability. *Developmental Neurorehabilitation*, *21*(3), 141–154.

Berthoz, S., & Hill, E. L. (2005). The validity of using self-reports to assess emotion regulation abilities in adults with autism spectrum disorder. *European Psychiatry*, *20*, 291–298.

Conner, C. M., Golt, J., Righi, G., Shaffer, R., Siegel, M., & Mazefsky, C. A. (2020). A comparative study of suicidality and its association with emotion regulation impairment in large ASD and US census-matched samples. *Journal of Autism and Developmental Disorders*, *50*(10), 3545–3560.

Conner, C. M., Golt, J., Shaffer, R. C., Righi, G., Siegel, M., & Mazefsky, C. A. (2021). Emotion dysregulation is substantially elevated in autism compared to the general population: Impact on psychiatric services. *Autism Research*, *14*, 169–181.

Conner, C. M., & White, S. W. (2018). Brief report: Feasibility and preliminary efficacy of individual mindfulness therapy for adults with autism spectrum disorder. *Journal of Autism and Developmental Disorders, 48*(1), 390–400.

Conner, C. M., White, S. W., Beck, K. B., Golt, J., Smith, I. C., & Mazefsky, C. A. (2019). Improving emotion regulation ability in autism: The emotional awareness and skills enhancement (EASE) program. *Autism, 23*(5), 1273–1287.

Conner, C. M., Wieckowski, A. T., Day, T. N., & Mazefsky, C. A. (in press). Emotion development in autism. In A. Samson, E. Walle, & D. Dukes (Eds.), *Emotion development*. Oxford University Press.

Costa, A. P., Steffgen, G., & Samson, A. C. (2017). Expressive incoherence and alexithymia in autism spectrum disorder. *Journal of Autism and Developmental Disorders, 47*(6), 1–14.

Eack, S. M., Mazefsky, C. A., & Minshew, N. J. (2015). Misinterpretation of facial expressions of emotion in verbal adults with autism spectrum disorder. *Autism, 19*(3), 308–315.

Faso, D. J., Sasson, N. J., & Pinkham, A. E. (2014). Evaluating posed and evoked facial expressions of emotion from adults with autism spectrum disorder. *Journal of Autism and Developmental Disorders, 45*(1), 75–89.

Elliott, R., Watson, J. C., Goldman, R. N., & Greenberg, L. S. (2004). *Learning emotion-focused therapy: The process-experiential approach to change.* Washington,DC: APA.

Gaigg, S. B., Flaxman, P. E., McLaven, G., Shah, R., Bowler, D. M., Meyer, B., Roestorf, A., Haenschel, C., Rodgers, J., & South, M. (2020). Self-guided mindfulness and cognitive behavioural practices reduce anxiety in autistic adults: A pilot 8-month waitlist-controlled trial of widely available online tools. *Autism* Advance online publication. doi:10.1177/1362361320909184

Gendlin, E. T. (1981). *Focusing* (2nd ed.). Bantam Books.

Gerber, A. H., Girard, J. M., Scott, S. B., & Lerner, M. D. (2019). Alexithymia—not autism—is associated with frequency of social interactions in adults. *Behaviour Research and Therapy, 123*, 1–11.

Golan, O., & Baron-Cohen, S. (2006). Systemizing empathy: Teaching adults with Asperger syndrome or high-functioning autism to recognize complex emotions using interactive multimedia. *Development and Psychopathology, 18*(2), 591–617.

Goldman, R. N., Greenberg, L. S., & Angus, L. (2006). The effects of adding emotion-focused interventions to the client-centered relationship conditions in the treatment of depression. *Psychotherapy Research, 16*, 536–546.

Greenberg, L., Rice, L., & Elliott, R. (1993). *Facilitating emotional change: The moment by moment process.* Guilford.

Hartmann, K., Urbano, M. R., Raffaele, C. T., Kreiser, N. L., Williams, T. V., Qualls, L. R., & Elkins, D. E. (2019). Outcomes of an emotion regulation intervention group in young adults with autism spectrum disorder. *Bulletin of the Menninger Clinic, 83*(3), 259–277.

Helverschou, S. B., Brunvold, A. R., & Arnevik, E. A. (2019). Treating patients with co-occurring autism spectrum disorder and substance use disorder: A clinical explorative study. *Substance Abuse: Research and Treatment, 13*. Advance online publication. doi:10.1177/1178221819843291

Holt, R., Upadhyay, J., Smith, P., Allison, C., Baron-Cohen, S., & Chakrabarti, B. (2018). The Cambridge sympathy test: Self-reported sympathy and distress in autism. *PLOS ONE, 13*(7), e0198273.

Kagan, N. (1984). Interpersonal process recall: Basic methods and recent research. In D. Larson (Ed.), *Teaching psychological skills* (pp. 229–244). Brooks Cole.

Kanner, L. (1943). Autistic disturbances of affective contact. *Nervous Child, 2,* 217–250.

Maddox, B. B., Kang-Yi, C. D., Brodkin, E. S., & Mandell, D. S. (2018). Treatment utilization by adults with autism and co-occurring anxiety or depression. *Research in Autism Spectrum Disorders, 51,* 32–37.

Maiano, C., Normand, C. L., Salvas, M. C., Moullec, G., & Aime, A. (2016). Prevalence of school bullying among youth with autism spectrum disorders: A systematic review and meta-analysis. *Autism Research, 9*(6), 601–615.

Mazefsky, C. A., & White, S. W. (2014). Emotion regulation. *Child and Adolescent Psychiatric Clinics of North America, 23*(1), 15–24.

Moreno, J. L., & Moreno, Z. T. (1959). *Foundations of psychotherapy.* Beacon House.

Pahnke, J., Hirvikoski, T., Bjureberg, J., Bölte, S., Jokinen, J., Bohman, B., & Lundgren, T. (2019). Acceptance and commitment therapy for autistic adults: An open pilot study in a psychiatric outpatient context. *Journal of Contextual Behavioral Science, 13,* 34–41.

Paivio, S. C., & Pascual-Leone, A. (2010). *Emotion-focused therapy for complex trauma: An integrative approach.* American Psychiatric Association.

Pascual-Leone, A., & Greenberg, L. S. (2007). Emotional processing in experiential therapy: Why "the only way out is through." *Journal of Consulting and Clinical Psychology, 75,* 875–887.

Perls, F. S., Hefferline, R. E., & Goodman, P. (1951). *Gestalt therapy: Excitement and growth in the human personality.* Dell.

Rigby, S. N., Stoesz, B. M., & Jakobson, L. S. (2018). Empathy and face processing in adults with and without autism spectrum disorder. *Autism Research, 11*(6), 942–955.

Robinson, A. (2018). Emotion-focused therapy for autism spectrum disorder: A case conceptualization model for trauma-related experiences. *Journal of Contemporary Psychotherapy, 48,* 133–1433.

Robinson, A. (2020). Enhancing empathy in emotion-focused group therapy for adolescents with autism spectrum disorder: A case conceptualization model for interpersonal rupture and repair. *Journal of Contemporary Psychotherapy, 50,* 133–142.

Robinson, A., & Elliott, R. (2016). Brief Report: An Observational Measure of Empathy for Autism Spectrum: A Preliminary Study of the Development and Reliability of the Client Emotional Processing Scale. *Journal of Autism and Developmental Disorders, 46,* 2240–2250.

Robinson, A., & Elliott, R. (2017). Emotion-focused therapy for clients with autistic process. *Person-Centered and Experiential Psychotherapies, 16*(3), 215–235.

Rogers, C. (1951). *Client-centered therapy: Its current practice, implications and theory.* Constable.

Rosen, T. E., Mazefsky, C. A., Vasa, R. A., & Lerner, M. D. (2018). Co-occurring psychiatric conditions in autism spectrum disorder. *International Review of Psychiatry, 30*(1), 40–61.

Russell, A. J., Jassi, A., Fullana, M. A., Mack, H., Johnston, K., Heyman, I., Murphy, D. G., Mataix-Cols, D. (2013). Cognitive behavior therapy for comorbid obsessive-compulsive disorder in high-functioning autism spectrum disorders: A randomized controlled trial. *Depression and Anxiety, 30*(8), 697–708.

Shahar, B., Bar-Kalifa, E., & Alon, E. (2017). Emotion-focused therapy for social anxiety disorder. *Journal of Consulting and Clinical Psychology, 85*(3), 238–249.

Soke, G. N., Maenner, M. J., Christensen, D., Kurzius-Spencer, M., & Schieve, L. A. (2018). Prevalence of co-occurring medical and behavioral conditions/symptoms among 4- and 8-year-old children with autism spectrum disorder in selected areas of the United States in 2010. *Journal of Autism and Developmental Disorders, 48*, 2663–2676.

Spain, D., Blainey, S. H., & Vaillancourt, K. (2017). Group cognitive behaviour therapy (CBT) for social interaction anxiety in adults with autism spectrum disorders (ASD). *Research in Autism Spectrum Disorders, 41*, 20–30.

Spain, D., Sin, J., Chalder, T., Murphy, D., & Happé, F. (2015). Cognitive behaviour therapy for adults with autism spectrum disorders and psychiatric co-morbidity: A review. *Research in Autism Spectrum Disorders, 9*, 151–162.

Timulak, L., McElvaney, J., Keogh, D., Martin, E., Clare, P., Chepukova, E., & Greenberg, L. (2017). Emotion-focused therapy for generalized anxiety disorder: An exploratory study. *Psychotherapy, 54*(4), 361–366.

Trevisan, D. A., & Birmingham, E. (2016). Are emotion recognition abilities related to everyday social functioning in ASD? A meta-analysis. *Research in Autism Spectrum Disorders, 32*, 24–42.

Trevisan, D. A., Hoskyn, M., & Birmingham, E. (2018). Facial expression production in autism: A meta-analysis. *Autism Research, 11*(12), 1586–1601. doi:10.1002/aur.2037

Weston, L., Hodgekins, J., & Langdon, P. E. (2016). Effectiveness of cognitive behavioural therapy with people who have autistic spectrum disorders: A systematic review and meta-analysis. *Clinical Psychology Review, 49*, 41–54.

White, S. W., Conner, C. M., Beck, K. B., & Mazefsky, C. A. (2021). Clinical update: The implementation of evidence-based emotion regulation treatment for clients with autism. *Evidence-Based Practice in Child and Adolescent Mental Health, 6*(1), 1–10.

Wieckowski, A. T., Flynn, L. T., Richey, J. A., Gracanin, D., & White, S. W. (2020). Measuring change in facial emotion recognition in individuals with autism spectrum disorder: A systematic review. *Autism, 24*(7), 1607–1628.

Wood, J. J., Kendall, P. C., Wood, K. S., Kerns, C. M., Seltzer, M., Small, B. J., Lewin, A. B., Storch, E. A. (2020). Cognitive behavioral treatments for anxiety in children with autism spectrum disorder: A randomized clinical trial. *JAMA Psychiatry, 77*(5), 473–484.

12

Dialectical Behavior Therapy

LORNA TAYLOR, ERMIONE NEOPHYTOU,
AND KATE JOHNSTON ■

KEY CONSIDERATIONS

- Therapeutic telephone/text contact between sessions may be required when supporting emotional monitoring.
- The therapeutic relationship provides an opportunity for social learning.
- The development of emotion regulation skills can depend on the skill of the therapist in modeling and naming emotions as they occur in session and between session.
- A client's potentially reduced emotional expression should be considered by the therapist and considered when exploring wider emotional and social difficulties.
- It is important not to overlook everyday functional impairments that may trigger emotional and relational difficulties.

AN OVERVIEW OF DIALECTICAL BEHAVIOR THERAPY

Dialectical behavior therapy (DBT) is a cognitive behavioral approach that was developed by Marsha Linehan (Linehan, 1993) as a comprehensive treatment to address emotional regulation (ER) difficulties experienced by chronically suicidal women with a diagnosis of borderline personality disorder (BPD). The evidence base for DBT has grown rapidly and it is now recommended as a first-line treatment for those with a diagnosis of BPD (e.g., National Institute for Health and Care Excellence guidelines in the UK). A meta-analysis has shown the approach to be effective at reducing suicidal and self-harm behaviors in adults with a diagnosis of BPD (Kliem et al., 2010), and DBT has increasingly been applied to other populations where underlying emotion dysregulation is a key maintaining factor in difficulties, such as substance misuse (Linehan et al., 1999), attention deficit/hyperactivity disorder (ADHD) (Nasri et al., 2020), and eating disorders (Rosenfeld et al., 2007; Sampl et al., 2010). DBT has also been extended into older (Lynch et al., 2003) and younger populations, specifically adolescents (Rathus & Miller, 2002).

The increasing application of DBT to various psychopathologies and across different settings points to its comprehensive nature and approach, incorporating cognitive, behavioral and third wave psychological approaches. While focusing on addressing core ER difficulties and problematic resulting behaviors, the approach also allows a careful integration of a biosocial formulation. Linehan's biosocial model posits that difficulties arise following a transaction between an individual's vulnerabilities and environmental influences. She outlined that individuals with BPD experience heightened emotional sensitivity, difficulties regulating emotional responses, and a slow return to baseline following emotional arousal. This ER pattern leads to dysfunctional responding during challenging situations. Difficulties emerge when this occurs in an invalidating developmental context, characterized by a lack of understanding of the individual's emotional experiences. This leads the individual to fail to develop effective ER. Patterns of oscillation between emotional inhibition and extreme lability emerge.

Dialectics is a method of philosophical reasoning which states that two opposing statements can be true at the same time. The primary dialectic in DBT consists of simultaneous acceptance of things "as they are" and of the individual's need to implement changes to their responding and behaviors to "build a life worth living" (Linehan, 1993). This acceptance-change dialectic sets DBT apart from cognitive behavioral therapy (CBT), which focuses on precipitating change, which can be considered invalidating to an individual who experiences a high level of constant emotional distress. In therapy, the dialectic translates to the balance of focus on increasing emotional awareness, acceptance, and understanding while also focusing on behavioral change and careful management of contingencies. The approach is typically a 12-month intensive therapy that includes four "modes": weekly individual therapy, weekly skills groups, telephone coaching, and weekly therapist consult.

Individual therapy sessions focus on developing a formulation of presenting difficulties and a hierarchy of therapeutic goals. There is a focus on the client recording emotions and problematic behaviors between sessions on a "diary card." This is then collaboratively reviewed in session to enable prioritization of any risk behaviors or difficulties that have arisen. Within individual sessions, behavioral chain analysis is then employed to explore risk behaviors. This involves a moment-by-moment break down and understanding of thoughts, actions, and emotions that occurred prior to and following any incident of risk. While initially led by the clinician, over time the client learns to complete this task with increasing independence. As therapy progresses and skills are learned, solution analyses (a process of identifying appropriate points to introduce appropriate adaptive skills) are completed as a way of introducing new, adaptive ways of managing difficult situations.

Skills groups consist of didactic teaching of four skills modules: mindfulness, emotion regulation, distress tolerance, and interpersonal effectiveness. These skills are referred to in individual therapy sessions. Mindfulness is considered a core skill in DBT, often introduced as the first module and subsequently incorporated into other modules. Research suggests that mindfulness skills are an essential determinant of treatment success.

DBT uses phone coaching to provide in-the-moment support with the goal of coaching clients to implement DBT skills to effectively cope with difficult situations that arise in their everyday life. The calls are typically brief and will often follow a set protocol (e.g., where a client calls and expresses suicidal behavior).

DBT consult is a weekly meeting attended by clinicians delivering the intervention. Clinicians bring dilemmas or difficulties arising in their individual work, including their own reactions or emotions to this. The DBT consultation is essential to help therapists monitor their fidelity to the treatment, develop their skills, and sustain their motivation to work with high-risk, challenging clients.

DBT WITH AUTISTIC INDIVIDUALS

Working Therapeutically With Risk

Self-reported suicidal ideation and attempts are relatively prevalent in autistic individuals; up to two thirds report experiencing suicidal ideation and one third report at least one suicide attempt (Hedley & Uljarevic 2018; Segers & Rawana, 2014). Research also highlights increased rates of wider risk behavior across the lifespan of autistic individuals, including aggression and self-injurious behavior (Lacavalier et al., 2006). Despite widely documented risks, at present there is no evidence-based treatment available to address risk behavior for this group.

Emotion Regulation as a Treatment Target

The rationale for the utilization of a DBT approach with autistic individuals lies within the recognition of difficulties with ER and the evident adverse and debilitating impact that this has (Mazefsky et al., 2013). ER is a complex process involving neurobiology, cognition, behavior, and emotion (Thompson, 2011) that allows an individual to monitor and modify emotional arousal and reactivity to engage in adaptive behavior. Unsurprisingly, compared to the general population, autistic individuals are four times more likely to have clinically significant difficulties with ER (England-Mason, 2020). A growing body of research suggests that this impairment manifests in a range of behavioral and mental health problems, including aggression and self-injury (Charlton et al., 2020; Damiano et al., 2014; Mazefsky & White, 2014; White et al., 2014).

Although existing psychosocial interventions for autistic individuals have traditionally focused on diagnosis-specific interventions (e.g., CBT for anxiety), there is increasing support for considering ER as a treatment target (Beck et al., 2020; Cai et al., 2018; England Mason 2020; White et al., 2020;). Recent mindfulness-based treatments and CBT approaches that teach effective ER to autistic children and/or their parents have demonstrated feasibility and improvements in ER skills with associated potential reductions in wider features associated with autism (Conner et al., 2019; Reyes et al., 2019; Thomson et al., 2015).

White et al. (2020) suggest that remediation of ER problems is an element in many psychological intervention models and highlight that it is the cornerstone of several approaches, perhaps most notably DBT (Linehan, 1993; Rathus & Miller, 2014). Hartmann and colleagues (2012) outline a theoretical argument for the use of DBT given recent models positing underlying emotion dysregulation as a core feature of autism (Mazefsky et al., 2013), high rates of self-harm and suicidality, and difficulties with social skills/relationships. To date, only one study has used DBT with autistic individuals (Hartmann et al., 2019). The study examined the effectiveness of a 12-week ER group intervention for autistic adults. Findings indicated significant improvements in social communication and interaction, social awareness, and social cognition. While the findings require replication, the results are encouraging regarding group approaches to ER in autism and potential benefits for social interaction.

Considering Co-Morbidities

DBT has been successfully adapted for people with neurodevelopmental differences (Ingamells & Morrissey, 2014; McNair et al., 2017) and there is emerging evidence regarding its use for individuals with ADHD (Nasri et al., 2017) and intellectual disability (Sakdalan et al., 2010). Although separate conditions, ADHD, autism, and intellectual disability co-occur and have impairments in common. Stevens, Peng, and Barnard-Brak (2016) reported that ADHD co-occurred in 59% of autistic individuals and research suggests that almost half of autistic individuals have diagnosed intellectual disability (Postorino et al., 2016). The high rates of co-occurrence and emerging evidence base for DBT in wider neurodevelopmental difficulties further point to its potential application for autistic people.

Rationale for Aspects of DBT

There are a number of aspects of DBT treatment that are compatible with adaptations recommended for psychological interventions for autistic individuals (Cooper et al., 2018; Walters et al., 2016), namely the long-term nature of the therapy, focus on mindfulness, behavior management, provision of support to generalize skills, and the importance of the therapeutic relationships and social learning opportunities.

As outlined previously, mindfulness is a key aspect of DBT and is fundamental to treatment outcome. There is an established evidence base for the feasibility, acceptability, and effectiveness of mindfulness interventions in autistic individuals, with positive outcomes including decreased rumination (De Bruin et al., 2015), depression, and anxiety (Spek et al., 2013).

There is clinical recommendation that therapeutic input for autistic individuals can be well supported by caregivers and family to maximize generalization to real-life experiences (Kerns et al., 2016; White et al., 2020). In addition to between-session contact and support from a therapist, there is scope and recommendation for involvement of those close to the client to consider their response and management of maladaptive communication, behavior, or risk. This may serve an additional purpose for autistic individuals and allow others to assist with generalization, which is known to be problematic due to the executive functioning (EF) difficulties associated with autism.

DBT is a highly structured and predictable therapy. It involves very clear rules, expectations, and structures both within sessions and across the course of therapy that may be beneficial for autistic individuals due to the preference for predictability and certainty. One of the key aspects of therapeutic contracting in DBT relates to motivation and engagement. It is notable that many autistic individuals may have experienced previous difficulties in therapy and may present as hopeless or frustrated about psychological intervention. DBT allows a focus on contracting expectations for therapy that can address this potential hopelessness.

White and colleagues (2020) outline the importance of self-monitoring, highlighting this as an area that may require specific consideration when working with autistic individuals. They emphasize that increasing self-awareness is a foundational goal and suggest the need for visual tools and support in their utilization. The DBT diary card provides a structured way of increasing self-monitoring between therapy sessions and can be supported by visual aids and therapist contact.

CASE STUDY

Rebecca was a white British 20-year-old female referred to mental health services following a brief psychiatric inpatient admission. Admission followed escalation of self-harming behavior and suicidal ideation. She engaged in comprehensive assessment while she remained an inpatient and then intervention continued after discharge to the community.

Presenting Difficulties

Rebecca presented with a long history of anxiety and aggressive behavior. At the point of referral, there were concerns regarding an escalation of suicidal ideation and self-harm. She was engaging in self-harm via cutting several times per week and frequently expressing suicidal intent. There was a noted escalation in conflict in the home with frequent incidents of aggression from Rebecca toward her mother. This was placing a strain on the family and it was unclear if it was sustainable for Rebecca to remain in the family home.

Rebecca had received a diagnosis of autism when she was 13 years old. Cognitive assessment at this time had highlighted IQ within the average range but identified relative impairments in processing speed and EF.

Assessment and Formulation

Assessment involved clinical interview with Rebecca and her mother and completion of psychometric measures. Her description of her difficulties indicated that she met clinical criteria for depression and anxiety.

While Rebecca was reported to have always had "mood swings" and difficulties with anger, emotional difficulties had become increasingly apparent following Rebecca's transition from education. It was evident that the increasing social and educational demands and a reduction in structure associated with adolescence presented a significant challenge for Rebecca. She found it difficult to maintain employment and had become socially isolated. She had a number of social contacts while in education but these had ceased following her leaving school. Her parents had noticed self-harm since the age of 13 but reported that this had become increasingly concerning over the 12 months prior to referral. She was experiencing difficulties with sleep and parents had also noticed a decline in her personal care.

With regards to biological vulnerability, while Rebecca wasn't able to accurately report on her emotional experiences in detail, she reported that she had a low threshold to becoming angry and felt overwhelmed quickly (high sensitivity), she would often feel out of control and behave aggressively when overwhelmed (high reactivity), and she found it difficult to reduce her levels of arousal. She reported that she found it difficult to manage noisy environments and that she needed time to "take things in." She reported self-harming approximately four times per week on average. With regards to friendships, Rebecca reported that other people had told her she was "intense" and that her mood swings placed strain on relationships. She also found it difficult to understand the intentions of others in relationships and described finding it difficult to assert herself. Her descriptions of relationships indicated that she may have been taken advantage of in relationships, such as lending friends large sums of money that were never repaid.

Her mother reported that she was increasingly frustrated with Rebecca's apparent unwillingness to attend work and felt that her difficulties were largely because of her low motivation and a reliance on her parents to "support her forever." She described how she would try to support Rebecca but felt that any attempt to help was met with frustration and aggression.

Rebecca was very creative and skilled artistically. She was also motivated to travel. Her family was very protective and motivated to support her in therapy.

Table 12-1 BIOPSYCHOSOCIAL FORMULATION OF REBECCA'S DIFFICULTIES

	Biological	**Psychological**	**Social**
Predisposing	Genetic vulnerability to autism Sensory sensitivity	Problems in processing nonsocial information: - Cognitive rigidity - Difficulties in planning and goal setting - Difficulties organizing self - Difficulties shifting attention - Poor time management - Slow processing	Difficulties understanding emotions and intentions of others Difficulties attending to and using social clues (facial expressions, gestures, nonverbal information)
Precipitating	Substance use	Low mood and anxiety	Employment stressors Loss of key peer contact via education
Perpetuating	Poor sleep Substance use	Poor emotion regulation abilities Self-harm as coping mechanism Poor planning and organization abilities	Limited social understanding and skills Financial pressure and lack of independence due to difficulties maintaining employment
Protective		Broadly average IQ	Some previous positive friendships Protective family

Rebecca had had peers when attending college and had been able to maintain the relationships for two years.

The interaction between Rebecca's emotional profile, wider neurodevelopmental needs, and her family environment was fitting with a biosocial model of DBT. A formulation, exploring vulnerabilities, triggers, maintaining factors, and protective aspects, was used to understand her presentation and needs with consideration of biological, psychological, and social factors (see Table 12-1).

DBT Goals

Rebecca's goals for therapy were outlined and discussed within a DBT hierarchy (see Figure 12-1). Simplified and accessible language was used at her request. In discussing her goals, Rebecca found it difficult to think about her future and larger goals. Over the course of engagement, she worked collaboratively with her therapist to make a "future life" visual board that included things she wanted in her

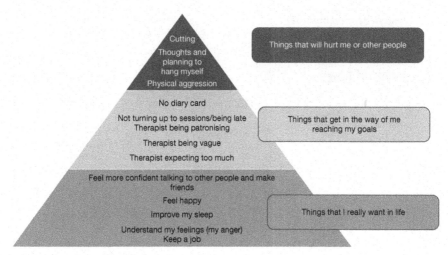

Figure 12-1 Hierarchy of Therapy Goals

future, including social activities and hobbies, close friends, travel, happy family relationships, and a consistent job that utilized her creativity.

Addressing Life-Threatening Behavior

DIARY CARDS
The ability to address risk behavior in therapy relies on the successful reporting of incidents on a diary card. An individualized, simplified diary card was established with Rebecca. However, Rebecca did not complete it and often reported "it was all fine." On discussion, Rebecca reported that she found the task overwhelming and required support. Diary cards were then completed with her therapist during brief, scheduled telephone calls. A visual rating scale was developed and used as a reference during the calls. Rebecca became increasingly able and motivated to complete the diary card independently during the course of therapy with increased emotional understanding and reporting.

CHAIN AND SOLUTION ANALYSIS
Rebecca required individual skill coaching in sessions to support the emotional understanding required to complete a chain analysis. Initial attempts to explore incidents of aggression and self-harm via chain analysis led to several missing links in chains and "don't know" responding.

Sessions were spent exploring her understanding of different emotions, combining coaching and psychoeducation. Rebecca frequently identified her emotional state as "stressed" and responded well to emotional literacy work focusing on her awareness of physiological experience and cognitions. It was helpful to focus on changes in emotional state initially without too much focus on application of verbal labels; this allowed her to more readily apply a regulation strategy

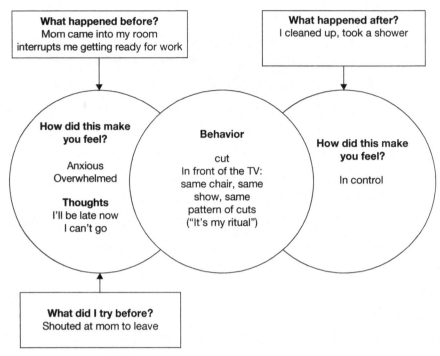

Figure 12-2 Example Chain Analysis

to address physiological arousal in the moment. Through individual sessions and telephone support she was able to broaden her noticing and understanding of basic emotional states that allowed the completion of simplified chain analysis and application of more specific skills and solutions.

Rebecca became increasingly skilled at understanding the relationship between her autistic traits (difficulties understanding emotions of others, sensory sensitivities, poor organizational skills, low processing speed), anger, and self-harm, exploring complex emotions such as guilt and shame following incidents of aggression and self-harm. An example simplified chain analysis is shown in Figure 12-2.

Exploration of potential solutions to chain analysis led to skills from all skills domains with additional consideration of Rebecca's autistic traits. For example, it was possible to address vulnerability factors by addressing sleep hygiene and introducing mindfulness tasks to interrupt her anxious rumination in the evening. Establishing a good sleep routine required additional environmental supports, including alarms to prompt her to initiate a bed routine and ensure she woke up on time. Over the course of therapy, it became evident that her organizational and planning difficulties were often prompting her mother to intervene to provide support when Rebecca was in a heightened emotional state. The problematic interactions were addressed jointly with Rebecca and her mother (see the following section on family work), and DBT and additional skills were suggested

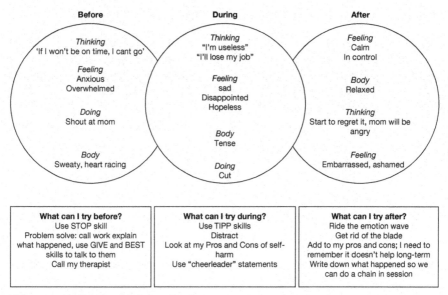

Before	**During**	**After**

Thinking
'If I won't be on time, I cant go'

Feeling
Anxious
Overwhelmed

Doing
Shout at mom

Body
Sweaty, heart racing

Thinking
"I'm useless"
"I'll lose my job"

Feeling
sad
Disappointed
Hopeless

Body
Tense

Doing
Cut

Feeling
Calm
In control

Body
Relaxed

Thinking
Start to regret it, mom will be angry

Feeling
Embarrassed, ashamed

What can I try before?	**What can I try during?**	**What can I try after?**
Use STOP skill	Use TIPP skills	Ride the emotion wave
Problem solve: call work explain	Distract	Get rid of the blade
what happened, use GIVE and BEST	Look at my Pros and Cons of self-	Add to my pros and cons; I need to
skills to talk to them	harm	remember it doesn't help long-term
Call my therapist	Use "cheerleader" statements	Write down what happened so we
		can do a chain in session

Figure 12-3 Chain and Solution Analysis

in relation to her difficulties recognizing and understanding emotions in others, noticing emotions, managing distress, problem solving, and effective communication. A chain and solution analysis is shown in Figure 12-3. While many skills may be suggested to individuals in exploring solutions to crises within typical DBT therapy, care was taken not to overwhelm Rebecca with strategies. Repetition and practice were important in her effective acquisition of skills, and her repertoire of strategies was increased gradually over the course of therapy. Each individual session was recorded and shared with Rebecca and learning summaries were provided visually to enable her to revisit session material easily.

Skills Group

Rebecca attended a DBT skills group to support her individualized learning and skill development. The group did not include others with autism and materials in the group were not adapted in any way. While providing an opportunity to increase social contact, the skills group also provided a platform for her to challenge anxieties regarding social acceptability. Anxiety and relationships were identified as behaviors interfering with quality of life, and, in the absence of risk behaviors, individual therapy provided an opportunity to explore social difficulties and role play effective social skills which could then be practiced in group. In addition, skills group made explicit use of role play and provided a safe environment to practice skills. Rebecca was offered a number of additional individual skills sessions to support her learning and acquisition of skills. Skills group content and adapted skills support are outlined in Table 12-2.

Table 12-2 SUMMARY OF SKILLS GROUP AND REQUIRED ADDITIONAL SKILLS

Skill Module	Group Content	Autism Adaptations Delivered in Individual Sessions
Mindfulness	Wise mind "How" skills "What" skills	Brief mindfulness tasks focused on external experiences Meditation on soles of the feet practice in session
Emotion regulation	Understanding and naming emotions What makes it hard to regulate emotions Emotion myths Model for describing emotions Ways to describe emotions Check the facts Opposite action Problem solving Building positive emotions Cope ahead Taking care of your body Tackling sleep	Increased focus on emotional literacy and understanding and naming emotions in self and others Emotion recognition visual aid Feelings thermometer Understanding the triggers to emotions Recognizing emotions in others, learning about facial expressions, posture, and gesture Accumulating positive emotions—increased support and planning Sleep hygiene
Distress tolerance	STOP skills Pros and cons of managing distress Change your body chemistry Distract Self soothe Body scan IMPROVE the moment	Recognizing physiological sensations using in-session tasks
Interpersonal effectiveness	Obtaining objectives: DEAR MAN Keeping a relationship: GIVE Keeping self-respect: FAST Saying no Building relationships Mindfulness of others Walking the middle path	Noticing rigidity/inflexibility of thought Teaching communication styles: "The assertiveness continuum" Exploring empathy and theory of mind and psychoeducation on cognitive and emotional empathy Explicit role plays and social tasks set in individual sessions for practicing in skills groups In-vivo feedback on social skills

Generalizing Skills

TELEPHONE COACHING

Following a period of time engaging in scheduled therapist-initiated telephone support, telephone coaching became increasingly helpful as Rebecca became able to call her therapist when "stressed out" and to provide information regarding the antecedents to distress, working with the therapist to identify her emotional state and relating this back to situation triggers and thoughts. This expanded further over the course of therapy to focus on appropriate action and management of the emotion with implementation of skills. Rebecca also benefitted from telephone support to check in on her self-care skills and behavioral activation to increase positive emotional experiences.

FAMILY INVOLVEMENT

Given the prioritization of aggression on her hierarchy and the role of interactions with her mother in her self-harm, Rebecca decided to share session materials with her mother and worked toward a number of joint sessions. Role plays and assertiveness scripts were developed in individual sessions to prepare for joint sessions and enabled Rebecca to practice effective communication and prepare ahead for potentially difficult conversations. Rebecca's effective communication of her insights into her risk behavior allowed them to explore alternative ways of managing trigger situations in the home, and these were negotiated using skills from the interpersonal effectiveness module.

It was evident that Rebecca had difficulties in her interactions with her mother and it was noted that she often misinterpreted her mother's communication as hostile. It was notable that Rebecca's distress often occurred within the context of her general social cognition impairment, such as difficulty recognizing, and often misinterpreting, others' emotions and frequently misidentifying anxiety in others as anger; this would lead her to respond with aggression. Explicit conversations with her mother were beneficial and she was able to work on identifying "clues" to different emotions and using her "checking the facts" skill when reacting to the emotional expressions of others. There was also consideration of the impact on her processing speed and organizational difficulties and how these were often misinterpreted by the family.

Therapy-Interfering Behaviors

The transparency around therapy-interfering behaviors within DBT was beneficial for Rebecca. She was able to consider and raise issues around communication and understanding within an open dialogue. It was agreed that the therapist would use concise and concrete language and provide discrete choices where open-ended questions might be too difficult. This was planned in order to avoid "don't know" responding and frustration for Rebecca in sessions.

The therapeutic relationship provided a unique opportunity for exploration of social skills and acceptability for Rebecca. Once rapport was established, the therapist was able to provide feedback on her interactions and explore this in therapy. For example, initially in therapy Rebecca 'would text the therapist several times a day without clear purpose. She would then become frustrated if the therapist didn't respond promptly and would become distressed. She would then shut down communication and not answer the telephone. After a number of weeks, this was highlighted as a therapy-interfering behavior that elicited anxiety in the therapist. Rebecca was able to identify that she also did this to her mother and a friend who had commented on her "being needy." She was able to work in therapy to improve her communication skills using aspects of the interpersonal effectiveness skills module.

Quality of Life Goals

A number of Rebecca's "quality of life" goals were addressed within the broader context of therapy via her acquisition of DBT skills and specific psychoeducation. An overview of adaptations employed during therapy are outlined in Table 12-3.

Table 12-3 SUMMARY OF ADAPTATIONS

Mode	Adaptation
Individual therapy	Shorter, more frequent sessions
	Reduced session content/slower pace; focusing on a reduced number of key learning points and skills and repetition of these Use of visual/written information
	Offering choices/scaffolding responses, for example when completing chain analyses and limiting reliance on individual to "generate" responses
	Telephone contact to support diary card completion
	Use of rapport and feedback in relationship
	Use of special interests to increase engagement
	Inclusion of psychoeducation around autism
Telephone coaching	Graded progression from scheduled, therapist-initiated contact to client-initiated contact during crises in consideration of problems with self-management seen in autistic individuals
	Coaching on emotional understanding and increasing awareness
DBT consult	Psychoeducation for clinicians on autism
	Inclusion of autism experts within teams or access to consultation from autism experts

CLINICAL REFLECTIONS

A key consideration, that cannot be overlooked, is the impact of neuropsychological differences in autism and the contribution of these to difficulties in ER. For example, there may be less scope for increasing flexibility of thought and managing "all or nothing" thinking, but therapy can focus on increasing awareness of inflexibility through mindfulness of thought. The biosocial model provides a helpful framework through which to explore, understand, and accept these differences.

The importance of the therapeutic relationship in teaching social skills is well established. Research has repeatedly attested to the importance of the therapeutic relationship through which the subtle (and invisible) nuances of social situations are made visible (e.g., Ramsay et al., 2005). The relationship also provides space for modeling ER and provides opportunities for individuals to experience emotional attunement and validation from others. This may have been limited in previous interpersonal experiences due to impairments in communicating affect and the lack of nonverbal communication of emotions (through gesture, posturing, and facial expression), making it difficult for others to notice, acknowledge, or respond appropriately to distress. The concept of "radical genuineness" (the highest level of validation) is helpful when thinking about the importance of the relationship when working with autistic individuals. When the therapist is radically genuine, they respond and interact with the individual as a human and equal; responding to and naming the "obvious" while not taking themselves too seriously.

Parent/carer involvement is central to supporting the generalization and sustainability of interventions for autistic individuals. This is in consideration of the lifelong nature of autism and need for support and/or "coaching" beyond 12 months of therapy. Parent/carer involvement in skills groups is routine in child and adolescent DBT programs (Rathus & Miller, 2002), and in our experience this can be a helpful adjunct when working with autistic adults, given continued support offered by parents/carers through adulthood.

Distress is not always visible, and autistic clients may discuss risk behaviors in a very "matter of a fact" way, which can lead to them being disbelieved or to their distress being minimized. There can also be a perceived lack of empathic responding to others, leading clients to be viewed as "callous" or "unemotional" and then responded to in this way, which further adds to their existing experiences of emotional invalidation. This highlights the importance of the DBT consult to support therapists to explore communications of distress and to reflect on their own biases and expectations to ensure that they respond effectively.

In conclusion, DBT provides an excellent opportunity to work with autistic individuals experiencing risk in way that addresses underlying needs while providing structure, containment, and endless potential for adaptation and creativity.

REFERENCES

Beck, K. B., & Conner, C. M., Breitenfeldt, K., Northrup, J., White, S. W., Mazefsky, C. A. (2020). Assessment and treatment of emotion regulation impairment in autism spectrum disorder across the life span. *Child and Adolescent Psychiatric Clinics of North America, 29*(3), 527–542.

Cai, R. Y., Richdale, A., Uljarevic, M., Dissanayake, C., & Samson, A. C. (2018). Emotion regulation in autism spectrum disorder: Where we are and where we need to go. *Autism Research, 11*, 962–978.

Charlton, A. S., Smith, I. C., Mazefsky, C. A., & White, S. W. (2020). The role of emotion regulation on co-occurring psychopathology in emerging adults with ASD. *Journal of Autism and Developmental Disorders, 50*(7), 2585–2592.

Conner, C. M., White, S., Beck, K., Golt, J., Smith, I., & Mazefsky, C. (2019). Improving emotion regulation ability in autism: The emotional awareness and skills enhancement (EASE) program. *Autism, 23*(5) 1273–1287.

Cooper, K., Loades, M. E., & Russell, A. (2018). Adapting psychological therapies for autism. *Research in Autism Spectrum Disorders, 45*, 43–50.

De Bruin, E. I., Blom, R., Smit, F. M., van Steensel, F. J., & Bogels, S. M. (2015). MYmind: Mindfulness training for youngsters with autism spectrum disorders and their parents. *Autism, 19*(8), 906–914.

England-Mason, G. (2020). Emotion regulation as a transdiagnostic feature in children with neurodevelopmental disorders. *Current Developmental Disorders Reports, 7*, 1–9.

Hartmann, K., Urbano, M. Manser, K., & Okwara, L. (2012). Modified dialectical behavior therapy to improve emotion regulation in autism spectrum disorders. *Autism Spectrum Disorders: New Research* (pp. 41–72).

Hartmann, K., Urbano, M. R., Raffaele, C. T., Kreiser, N. L., Williams, T. V., Qualls, L. R., & Elkins, D. E. (2019). Outcomes of an emotion regulation intervention group in young adults with autism spectrum disorder. *Bulletin of the Menninger Clinic, 83*(3), 259–277.

Hedley, D., & Uljarevic, M. (2018). Systematic review of suicide in autism spectrum disorder: Current trends and implications. *Current Developmental Disorders Reports, 5*(1), 65–76.

Ingamells, B., & Morrissey, C. (2014). *I can feel good: Skills training for people with intellectual disabilities and problems managing emotions.* Pavilion Publishing and Media.

Kerns, C., Roux, A., Connell, J., & Shattuck, P. (2016). Adapting cognitive behavioral techniques to address anxiety and depression in cognitively able emerging adults on the autism spectrum. *Cognitive and Behavioral Practice, 23*(3), 329–340.

Kliem, S., Kroger, C., & Kosfelder, J. (2010). Dialectical behavior therapy for borderline personality disorder: A meta-analysis using mixed-effects modelling. *Journal of Consulting and Clinical Psychology, 78*(6), 936–951.

Lecavalier, L., Leone, S., & Wiltz, J. (2006). The impact of behaviour problems on caregiver stress in young people with autism spectrum disorders. *Journal of Intellectual Disabilities Research, 50*(3), 172–183.

Linehan, M. M. (1993). *Cognitive-behavioral treatment of borderline personality disorder.* Guilford Press.

Linehan, M., Schmidt, H., Dimeff, L. A., Craft, J. C., Kanter, J., & Comtois, K. A. (1999). Dialectical behavior therapy for patients with borderline personality disorder and drug-dependence. *The American Journal on Addictions, 8*(4), 279–292.

Lynch, T. R., Morse, J. Q., Mendelson, T & Robins, C. J. (2003). Dialectical behaviour therapy for depressed older adults: A randomized pilot study. *American Journal of Geriatric Psychiatry, 11*(1), 33–45.

Mazefsky, C. A., Herrington, J., Siegel, M., Scarpa, A., Maddox, B. B., Scahill, L., & White, S. W. (2013). The role of emotion regulation in autism spectrum disorder. *Journal of the American Academy of Child and Adolescent Psychiatry, 52*(7), 679–688.

Mazefsky, C. A., & White, S., W. (2014). Emotion regulation: Concepts and practice in autism spectrum disorder. *Child and Adolescent Psychiatric Clinics of North America, 23*(1), 15–24.

McNair, L., Woodrow, C., & Hare, D. (2017). Dialectical behaviour therapy (DBT) with people with intellectual disabilities: A systematic review and narrative analysis. *Journal of Applied Research in Intellectual Disabilities, 30*(5), 787–804.

Nasri, B., Castenfors, M., Fredlund, P., Ginsberg, Y., Lindefors, N., & Kaldo, V. (2020). Group treatment for adults with ADHD based on a novel combination of cognitive and dialectical behaviour interventions: A feasibility study. *Journal of Attention Disorders, 24*(6), 904–917.

Postorino, V., Fatta, L. M., Sanges, V., Giovagnoli, G., De Peppo, L., Vicari, S., & Mazzone, L. (2016). Intellectual disability in autism spectrum disorder: Investigation of prevalence in an Italian sample of children and adolescents. *Research in Developmental Disabilities, 48*, 193–201.

Ramsay, J. R., Brodkin, E. S., Cohen, M. R., Listerud, J., Rostain, A. L., & Ekman, E. (2005). "Better strangers": Using the relationship in psychotherapy for adult patients with Asperger syndrome. *Psychotherapy: Theory, Research, Practice, Training, 42*(4), 483.

Rathus, J. H., & Miller, A. L. (2002). Dialectical behavior therapy adapted for suicidal adolescents. *Suicide and Life-Threatening Behaviour, 32*(2), 146–157.

Rathus, J., & Miller, A. (2014). *DBT° skills manual for adolescents*. Guildford Press.

Reyes, N., Pickard, K., & Reaven, J. (2019). Emotion regulation: A treatment target for autism spectrum disorder. *Bulletin of the Menninger Clinic, 83*, 205–234.

Rosenfeld, B., Galietta, M., Ivanoff, A., Garcia-Mansilla, A., Martinez, R., Fava, J., Fineran, V., & Green, D. (2007). Dialectical behavior therapy for the treatment of stalking offenders. *International Journal of Forensic Mental Health, 6*(2), 95–103.

Sakdalan, J. A., Shaw, J., & Collier, V. (2010). Staying in the here and now: A pilot study on the use of dialectical behaviour therapy group skills training for forensic clients with intellectual disability. *Journal of Intellectual Disability Research, 54*, 568–572.

Sampl, S., Wakai, S., & Trestman, R. L. (2010). Translating evidence-based practices from community to corrections: An example of implementing DBT-CM. *Journal of Behavior Analysis of Offender & Victim: Treatment & Prevention, 2*(2), 114–123.

Segers, M., & Rawana, J. (2014). What do we know about suicidality in autism spectrum disorders? A systematic review. *Autism Research, 7*(4), 507–521.

Stevens. T, Peng, L., & Barnard- Brak, L. (2016). The comorbidity of ADHD in children diagnosed with autism spectrum disorder. *Research in Autism Spectrum Disorders, 31*, 11–18.

Spek, A. A., van Ham, N. C., & Nyklíček, I. (2013). Mindfulness-based therapy in adults with an autism spectrum disorder: A randomized controlled trial. *Research in Developmental Disabilities, 34*(1), 246–253.

Thompson, R. (2011). Emotion and emotion regulation: Two sides of the developing coin. *Emotion Review, 3*, 53–61.

Walters, S., Loades, M., & Russell, A. (2016). A systematic review of effective modifications to cognitive behavioural therapy for young people with autism spectrum disorders. *Review Journal of Autism and Developmental Disorders, 3*, 137–153.

White, S. W., Conner, C., Beck, K & Mazefsky, C. (2020). Clinical update: The implementation of evidence-based emotion regulation treatment for clients with autism. *Evidence-Based Practice in Child and Adolescent Mental Health*, 6(1), 1–10.

White, S. W., Mazefsky, C. A., Dichter, G. S., Chiu, P. H., Richey, J. A., & Ollendick, T. H. (2014). Social-cognitive, physiological, and neural mechanisms underlying emotion regulation impairments: Understanding anxiety in autism spectrum disorder. *International Journal of Developmental Neuroscience, 39*, 22–36.

13

Schema Therapy

RICHARD VUIJK, HANNIE VAN GENDEREN, HILDE M. GEURTS,
AND ARNOUD ARNTZ ■

KEY CONSIDERATIONS

- There is a strong association between autism spectrum disorder (ASD) and dysfunctional personality traits (rigidity, low self-directedness), as well as between ASD and personality disorder (PD), specifically cluster-A (paranoid, schizoid, schizotypal) and cluster-C (avoidant, dependent, obsessive-compulsive) PDs.
- Both ASD and PD are associated with a long-term pattern of difficulties in interpersonal functioning. ASD is characterized by a persistent social disability. PD is characterized by interpersonal difficulties based on a combination of temperament difficulties and early problematic relationships with others, attachment pathology, and/or stressful situations or events.
- ASD is also associated with positive personality attributes.
- Schema therapy is a well-suited and effective treatment for people with chronic mental disorders, including PD, eating disorders, and chronic depression.
- Schema therapy does not differ markedly for people with ASD, compared to people without ASD. Taking into account the "dos and don'ts" and the autism-specific needs and challenges, as well as factoring in personality strengths, we believe schema therapy can be a potential effective treatment for PD in people with ASD.

INTRODUCTION TO SCHEMA THERAPY

Schema therapy (ST) is an innovative, integrative therapeutic approach originally developed by Jeffrey Young as an extension of traditional cognitive behavioral treatments (Young et al., 2003). The schema approach draws from cognitive behavioral therapy (CBT), attachment theory, psychodynamic concepts, and emotion-focused therapies. ST is particularly well-suited and effective for people with chronic mental disorders, including personality disorders (PDs), eating disorders, and chronic depression (Bamelis et al., 2014; Renner et al., 2013; Sempérteguia et al., 2013; Simpson et al., 2010).

A central tenet of ST, drawn from CBT, is that everyone develops schemas during childhood. A schema is an organized knowledge structure that develops in early life and manifests in certain behaviors, feelings, and thoughts. Dysfunctional schemas (such as social alienation, social undesirability, failure, hypercriticalness, subjugation) develop when some core emotional needs (safety, acceptance, nurturance, autonomy, self-appreciation, self-expression, and realistic limits) are not met during formative years. This may be due to shortcomings in the child's environment, or in combination with traumatic events (such as emotional, physical, or sexual abuse, or being bullied) in interaction with the child's temperament. A coping response in combination with a schema results in a so-called schema mode, which describes the momentary emotional-cognitive-behavioral state of the person. A schema mode (such as vulnerable child, happy child, compliant surrender, detached self-soother, demanding parent) is a set of schemas and processes, that, in certain situations, determine the thoughts, feelings, and actions of the person.

ST focuses on changing dysfunctional schemas and maladaptive modes into more flexible and less extreme schemas/modes, and developing adequate coping strategies so that clients develop a more positive image of themselves and others, as well as a more nuanced view of the world around them. First, the therapist and client create a case conceptualization based upon the schemas and modes. Next, in the treatment phase, therapists make use of experiential, cognitive, and behavioral techniques, influencing the client through three channels: feeling (experiential), thinking (cognitive), and doing (behavioral). The experiential techniques (including imagery rescripting, chairwork dialogue, historical role play) seem to be the most crucial mechanisms of change, as they appear to change the schemas and modes on an emotional, as well as cognitive, level. The application of ST techniques can only be successful once a certain level of trust and attachment to the therapist is formed. The therapeutic relationship can be described as limited reparenting, whereby the therapist goes into this relationship as if they are a parent figure for the client.

AUTISM SPECTRUM DISORDER: PERSONALITY ATTRIBUTES

An increasing number of studies have examined autism spectrum disorder (ASD) and comorbid personality pathology. A literature review by Vuijk, Deen, Sizoo, and Arntz (2018) showed strong indications for personality pathology in adults with ASD, such that ASD appeared to be significantly associated with several temperament and character dimensions, and with major PDs. Some adults with ASD, for example, were found to have an introverted, rigid, and passive-dependent temperament and a risk for deficits in character development with low self-directedness and cooperativeness. The majority of adults with ASD do not have a co-occurring PD, but prevalence of PD appears to be higher than in neurotypical adults. The prevalence of meeting criteria for a PD ranges from 48% to 62% among adults with ASD drawn from clinical samples (Hofvander et al., 2009; Lugnegård et al., 2012). Results of a meta-analysis (Vuijk et al., 2018) indicated that the most common PDs were paranoid (24%), schizoid (24%), schizotypal (14%), avoidant (23%), and obsessive-compulsive (32%). To summarize, there is a strong association between ASD and dysfunctional personality traits, as well as between ASD and PD, specifically cluster-A (paranoid, schizoid, schizotypal) and cluster-C (avoidant, dependent, obsessive-compulsive) PDs.

Both ASD and PD are associated with a long-term pattern of difficulties in interpersonal functioning. ASD is characterized by persistent impairments in social communication and social interaction; in other words, a persistent social disability or a neurodevelopmental condition with a focus on problems in the social domain. PD is not characterized by a persistent social disability, but by interpersonal difficulties, based on a combination of temperament difficulties and early problematic relationships with others, attachment pathology, and/or stressful situations or events. Each of the DSM-5 personality disorders describe particular types of interpersonal difficulties. For example, when having an avoidant PD, contact is disturbed by feelings of inadequacy and hypersensitivity to being negatively evaluated. In our case study we will meet Christian, diagnosed with ASD (during childhood) and in adult life, with comorbid avoidant PD features: for him, ASD means a challenge and difficulty in interpreting verbal and nonverbal communication, reading other people's emotions, and expressing his own emotions. In his childhood his parents and peers did not always know how to deal with his ASD. In childhood, negative reactions of others were a real burden and a serious cause of stress for him: he developed low self-esteem and a pattern of fear of being negatively evaluated. The combination of the negative reactions and his thoughts and feelings shaped his personality in an avoidant way.

Importantly, research shows that ASD is also associated with positive personality attributes. In a study examining character strengths in adults with ASD, intellectual open-mindedness (i.e., thinking things through, examining aspects from all sides), authenticity, love of learning, creativity, and fairness were found to be the most frequent signature strengths (Kirchner et al., 2016).

ASD AND SCHEMA THERAPY

People with ASD may have a vulnerability to maladaptive schema development, partly because of their different ways of processing information about others, the self, and nonsocial information, often resulting in social difficulties as well as difficulties with self-management (Gaus, 2019). For example, children with ASD might be at risk of being misunderstood, excluded, and maltreated because of their ASD and/or the impact of symptoms. Such early experiences are well-known risk factors for deficits in character development and the development of PDs. Adults with ASD have scored significantly higher on all the early dysfunctional schemas, apart from self-sacrifice and approval/recognition seeking, compared to typically developing adults (Oshima et al., 2015). Early dysfunctional schemas have also appeared to account for poorer general mental health in nonclinical adults with autism spectrum traits (Oshima et al., 2014).

The increased recognition of personality pathology in adults with ASD implies the need for interventions for personality pathology in this population. To date, very few studies have examined the acceptability and effectiveness of psychosocial interventions for PD in adults with ASD. A naturalistic multiple case study (N = 8, aged 20 to 35, four males, four females) indicated that individual ST is applicable as a treatment for adults with ASD and comorbid psychiatric conditions narratively showing positive changes in quality of life, symptoms of ASD, cognitive schemas, and schema modes (Oshima et al., 2018). However, a lack of specific details and limited documentation of methodology and statistical analysis renders difficult to interpret the positive changes in this study. A specific ST program for adults with ASD and comorbid PDs has been developed and investigated by Vuijk and Arntz (2017). As far as we know, this is the first study investigating ST in adults with ASD and comorbid PD(s). Results of this study are promising, showing a significant decrease of dysfunctional core beliefs, PD traits, psychopathological symptoms, an increase of the functional schema mode of happy child and an improvement in social responsiveness. These results are expected to be published in 2021.

For several reasons, ST might be a useful therapy for adults with ASD and comorbid PD. First, there is increasing empirical support for this therapy as a valuable treatment for PDs, as described in the beginning of this chapter. Second, the therapeutic relationship is active, consistent, supportive, and directive with regard to both content and process, which we consider helpful for people with ASD who are more often characterized by low self-directedness as compared to the general population. Third, ST is a structured and focused psychotherapy, suitable for people with ASD, who often seem to benefit from this way of working. Thus, the approach common in ST (i.e., step by step, focused on a theme, structured by explanation and psychoeducation, and goal-directed) is likely to be of use for people with ASD. An ST modified for autism spectrum conditions (ST-MASC) was developed by Bulluss (2019). This model provides a framework and an extension of the regular ST elements in which autism-driven coping responses and autism-specific needs are incorporated and conceptualized. The model provides illustrative examples of how some people with ASD cope with their core autistic features living in a neurotypical world, using ST terms originally developed to describe how people can dysfunctionally cope with maladaptive schema activation: by surrendering, overcompensating, or avoiding. This can be understood in terms of eye contact, for example: (a) the coping response of surrendering for the tendency of limited eye contact is, for instance, staring at the floor or past people;

(b) the coping response of overcompensating is focusing too much on making eye contact or staring at times; and (c) an avoidant coping response is avoiding situations involving face to face interaction, resulting in isolation. Autism-specific needs are, for instance, the freedom to focus on interests and a stable and reliable base for routine, predictability, and sameness.

SCHEMA THERAPY FOR PEOPLE WITH ASD: CLINICAL CONSIDERATIONS

When starting ST, there are some "dos and don'ts" for a therapist treating PD in people with ASD:

- As a therapist, first take care to set clear expectations about the role of the therapist and the client, setting a realistic pace, using language effectively, validating the client's experience and providing constructive feedback (Gaus, 2019).
- At the beginning of every ST session review psychoeducation of the ST concepts and the specific interventions in order to set clear expectations for clients with ASD. After an intervention, it is helpful to explain or discuss in detail what has been done and what it means for the client's here-and-now situation.
- When cognitive restructuring dysfunctional core beliefs or schema modes, post-its (on the wall or on the chair when doing chair dialogues) can make beliefs or modes more visible and concrete in the here-and-now for clients with ASD.
- People with ASD often say they have never had the opportunity to explore difficult and challenging personal situations and getting constructive feedback on their thoughts and feelings. A man with ASD, avoidant PD, and traumatic memories caused by being bullied for 10 years in his childhood by other children was treated with ST: his reaction after imagery rescripting sessions was that the trauma had been solved because he had verbalized the trauma in therapy. For him, the trauma was easier to deal with in his daily life.
- For people with ASD, experiential interventions can be a challenge. For example, a woman with ASD and obsessive-compulsive PD could not imagine herself as a child. The therapist solved this as follows: he let her imagine a general family situation at a dinner table with a father, a mother, and a little child. After the intervention she discovered that in the imagery rescripting she had brought up her own family situation and she was the little child. Explaining, translating, and discussing afterwards can lead to expression of new functional beliefs about one's self.

Another example is a man with ASD and schizoid PD who said when starting imagery rescripting, "I do not feel, but I think. I have a clear and detailed picture how it used to be when I was a child: I do have no feelings, but only thoughts about it." The therapist can validate the client's attempt to imagine: he did it in a cognitive way. He finally expressed new functional core beliefs (of the past) and could change his actual situation by improved cognitive mentalizing. ST does not differ substantially for people with ASD compared to people with other mental disorders.

> The psychotherapist needs to be fluent in "Aspergerese"; in other words, to recognize that autism is a different way of thinking—almost a different culture—and be able to translate the concepts and components of the therapy to someone with this different way of thinking. (Gaus, 2019, p. ix)

Taking into account the "dos and don'ts," the autism-specific needs and challenges, as well factoring in personality strengths, we believe ST can be a potential effective treatment for PD in people with ASD.

CASE STUDY: CHRISTIAN

Demographic Information

LIVING SITUATION
Christian is a 52-year-old Dutch man. He lives alone, has no partner and no children. He worked for 23 years as a high school teacher in mathematics. Last year, he was dismissed: he was unable to deal with the major changes in the Dutch system for high school education. Currently, he works as a volunteer in a group home for elderly people one day a week, serving coffee and tea.

Christian is a member of a Dutch network for, and led by, adults with ASD, visiting its activities once a month. Further, he spends a lot of time home alone.

HISTORY
Christian is an only child. His father worked as a teacher in Latin language at high school. His mother was a nurse in a children's hospital. After high school Christian obtained his master's degree in mathematics at university.

During childhood, there was a lot of order and discipline at home. He experienced challenges in understanding others and playing with other children. His parents did not encourage him to join other children, so he seldom dared to participate: as a child, he felt afraid of his peers' negative reactions toward him, which he considered were due to him not knowing how to interact with them. He had a strong desire for interaction, but did not feel that he possessed the knowledge or skills to do this adeptly. In his childhood, he was a member of the scout movement. When he participated in scouting activities, he was often a loner in the group and rarely involved in activities or plays. These experiences contributed to him feeling unlikable and unwanted, and he developed core beliefs relating to being different, not good enough, and bound to be alone. He developed a pattern of low self-esteem and avoidance of interpersonal contact, due to fear of disapproval and rejection.

Presenting Problems

After being dismissed from his teaching post, Christian visited his general practitioner (family doctor), reporting depressed feelings and social anxiety. He was referred to a center specializing in providing diagnostic assessments and interventions for adults with ASD.

His key presenting difficulties were low self-esteem, a substantial need for order and interpersonal control, fear of negative evaluation, and a depressed mood. In addition, his ASD-specific challenges related to trying to understand what others mean: he often needed extra time to process what he hears, sees and feels when having contact with others.

In his manner, Christian presented as very kind. He regularly sought clarification regarding the actual meaning of remarks made by the therapist. He also asked for a clear and structured way of communicating and required time to provide what he felt was the right answer.

Assessment and Diagnosis

Mental disorders were assessed at intake in a structured, organized, ASD-friendly way. After the assessment, his ASD was confirmed and Christian was additionally diagnosed with depressive disorder, social anxiety disorder, and avoidant PD features. Pharmacological treatment, CBT, and ST were indicated.

Individualized Treatment Plan

GOALS

First, depressive disorder and social anxiety disorder were treated with antidepressants and CBT focusing on scheduling enjoyable activities, physical exercise, relaxation skills, in-vivo exposure, and cognitive interventions. After a period of 4 months of treatment, ST was introduced to enhance Christian's ability to challenge dysfunctional core beliefs (schemas), coping styles, and schema modes; to increase functional coping styles and schema modes; and to help meet basic emotional needs.

Christian hoped to increase his competence and confidence in social situations, thereby feeling less anxiety and stress in these situations. He wanted to express new beliefs about himself, such as "I am capable and competent" and "I am good enough to be loved by others." He also wanted emotional memories to feel less intense.

ST for Christian consisted of four phases: (a) five sessions exploring current and past functioning, psychological symptoms, dysfunctional core beliefs, and schema modes; (b) 15 weekly sessions of cognitive-behavioral interventions; (c) 15 weekly sessions of experiential interventions; and (d) 10 monthly follow-up booster sessions.

Experiential Interventions

Imagery rescripting and chairwork dialogues are powerful experiential techniques. Imagery rescripting uses the power of imagination and visualization to identify and change meaningful and traumatic orders in the past, resulting in transformation in the present. Chairwork dialogues give a chair to the schema modes in the individual so that they can enact or re-enact scenes from the past, the present, or the future. To make these interventions more accessible for people with ASD, like Christian, the therapist takes into account the "dos and don'ts" and the autism-specific needs and challenges mentioned earlier in this chapter. Here, we exemplify two experiential interventions by outlining one of Christian's imagery rescripting sessions and chairwork dialogue sessions, helping him to bring about actual behavioral change and less intense emotions and memories. Christian described a recent situation in which he felt completely ignored by his colleague volunteers at the elderly home. At team meetings, he never felt able to say what he wanted to say, at the right time, as conversations moved on too quickly for him.

IMAGERY RESCRIPTING

THERAPIST (T): Christian, can you close your eyes and imagine the meeting from last week?

PATIENT (P): Yes, I am sitting in the meeting room, we are having a meeting with all 10 of the volunteers. Everyone is talking and mentioning things they want to say. Everyone except me.

T: And what do you feel?

P: I feel frustrated.

T: Stay with that frustration for a moment. Can you feel it right now?

P: Yes, I feel it in my shoulders.

T: I want you to concentrate on that feeling. The situation with your colleagues. Let it go. Go back to your childhood and see if a situation comes in mind in which you are also frustrated as a little child.

[Christian is thinking.]

T: And do you have an image?

P: I am at scouting, and again, I am standing on the sidelines, I am not participating in building a tent and nobody asks me to join in. Even the leaders do not pay attention to me. I want to join, but I do not know how.

T: Is it okay, if I enter the image and talk to the leaders to support you?

P: Yes, that's okay.

T: [To the leaders] I would like you to know that little Christian is standing all alone and he wants to join. Can you please involve him in building the tent?

[To Christian] Is this okay for you, Christian?

P: Well, I am not convinced the leaders will listen to you.

T: Then, I will repeat it again and in a louder voice. [Therapist repeats the message to the leaders with a louder voice.]

P: Ah, that feels better. I can see that one of the leaders is coming up to me and asks me to join building the tent.

T: Okay, Christian, take a minute to enjoy the event. When you are okay with it, you may open your eyes and return to the therapy room. How do you feel?

P: This was for me the first time that someone [the therapist who came in the imagery exercise] was giving me support. It feels very good.

T: How can this exercise help you when being together with your colleagues?

P: [Christian is thinking.]
Well I think, I have to speak the manager before the meeting and ask her to give me some time to say something during the meeting.

T: That sounds good.

P: Yes, but I am not sure how I can ask her, how I have to do this.

T: Let us give it a try: we can practice this in a role play.

Chairwork Dialogue

Christian was now confronted with two scenarios: "Do I still say nothing at team meetings or do I say what I want to say?" He felt very nervous thinking about this dilemma, having a voice in his mind telling him he would not succeed. The therapist invited him to a three-chair dialogue to give voice to what he was currently feeling and experiencing. In one chair he gave voice to his vulnerable child mode ("I feel ashamed of myself when starting conversation in a group"), in the second chair he gave voice to his demanding parent mode ("You will not succeed"), and in the third chair he gave voice to his healthy adult mode ("I know you find this scary, because you are not used to saying what you want to say at team meetings, but I know you will succeed. It is ok if you don't speak in perfect sentences. It is much more important that you speak up than that you strive for perfection, because then you are much more likely to say nothing").

The therapist guided him through the dialogue by asking him to take place vice-versa in the chairs, especially repeating and strengthening the functional words and thoughts that came up in Christian's mind. Christian switched several times from chairs, having a dialogue between his shame and social anxiety (vulnerable child mode), his highest standards and self-criticism (demanding parent mode), and his growing assertiveness and self-confidence (healthy adult mode), in the end resulting in less tense feelings and more realistic and confident thoughts about himself regarding the team meetings.

Evaluation of Treatment

At follow-up Christian reported that he found ST a long and intensive treatment. During the therapy, he often wondered if all the interventions and the talking could glean a positive outcome. ST was confronting, yet in the end, he realized that it facilitated new functional core beliefs about himself (such as "I am different, but I am good enough the way I am"; "I am confident enough in saying what I want to say"), better self-esteem, less anxious feelings and thoughts, and more skills to manage social interaction.

CONCLUSION

We believe ST might be a potential treatment for PD in people with ASD, when also taking into account the autism-specific needs and challenges and making use of the personality strengths. Randomized effectiveness studies are needed. Promising results of a first study examining ST in people with ASD and comorbid PD (Vuijk & Arntz, 2017) are expected in the near future.

REFERENCES

American Psychiatric Association (APA) (2013). *Diagnostic and statistical manual of mental disorders (5th ed.)*. Arlington, VA: American Psychiatric Association.

Bamelis, L. L. M., Evers, M. A. A., Spinhoven, P., & Arntz, A. (2014). Results of a multicentered randomized controlled trial on the clinical effectiveness of schema therapy for personality disorders. *American Journal of Psychiatry, 171*(3), 305–322.

Bulluss, E. K. (2019). Modified schema therapy as a needs based treatment for complex comorbidities in adults with autism spectrum conditions. *Australian Clinical Psychologist, 1*, 1–7.

Gaus, V. L. (2019). *Cognitive-behavioral therapy for adults with autism spectrum disorder* (2nd ed.). Guilford Press.

Hofvander, B., Delorme, R., Chaste, P., Nydén, A., Wentz, E., Ståhlberg, O., Herbrecht, E., Stopin, A., Anckarsäter, H., Gillberg, C., Råstam, M., & Leboyer, M. (2009). Psychiatric and psychosocial problems in adults with normal-intelligence autism spectrum disorders. *BMC Psychiatry, 9*, 35.

Kirchner, J., Ruch, W., & Dziobek, I. (2016). Brief report: Character strengths in adults with autism spectrum disorder without intellectual impairment. *Journal of Autism and Developmental Disorders, 46*(10), 3330–3337.

Lugnegård, T., Hallerbäck, M. U., & Gillberg, C. (2012). Personality disorders and autism spectrum disorders: What are the connections? *Comprehensive Psychiatry, 53*(4), 333–340.

Oshima, F., Iwasa, K., Nishinaka, H., & Shimizu, E. (2015). Early maladaptive schemas and autism spectrum disorder in adults. *Journal of Evidence-Based Psychotherapies, 15*(2), 191–205.

Oshima., F., Nishinaka, H., Iwasa, K., Ito, E., & Shimizu, E. (2014). Autism spectrum traits in adults affect mental health status via early maladaptive schemas. *Psychology Research, 4*(5), 336–344.

Oshima, F., Shaw, I., Ohtani, T., Iwasa, K., Nishinaka, H., Nakagawa, A., & Shimizu, E. (2018). Individual schema therapy for high-functioning autism spectrum disorder with comorbid psychiatric conditions in young adults: Results of a naturalistic multiple case study. *Journal of Brain Science, 48*, 43–69.

Renner, F., Arntz, A., Leeuw, I., & Huibers, M. (2013). Treatment for chronic depression using schema therapy. *Clinical Psychology Science and Practice, 20*(2), 166–180.

Sempertegui, G. A., Karreman, A., Arntz, A., & Bekker, M. H. (2013). Schema therapy for borderline personality disorder: A comprehensive review of its empirical foundations, effectiveness and implementation possibilities. *Clinical Psychology Review, 33*(3), 426–447.

Simpson, S. G., Morrow, E., van Vreeswijk, M., & Reid, C. (2010). Group schema therapy for eating disorders: A pilot study. *Frontiers in Psychology, 1*, 182.

Vuijk, R., & Arntz, A. (2017). Schema therapy as treatment for adults with autism spectrum disorder and comorbid personality disorder: Protocol of a multiple-baseline case series study testing cognitive-behavioral and experiential interventions. *Contemporary Clinical Trials Communications, 5*(2), 80–85.

Vuijk, R., Deen, M., Sizoo, B., & Arntz, A. (2018). Temperament, character and personality disorders in adults with autism spectrum disorder: A systematic literature review and meta-analysis. *Review Journal of Autism and Developmental Disorders, 5*, 176–197.

Young, J. E., Klosko, J. S., & Weishaar, M. E. (2003). *Schema therapy: A practitioner's guide.* Guilford Press.

14

Compassion-Focused Therapy

JAMES ACLAND AND DEBBIE SPAIN ■

KEY CONSIDERATIONS

- Psychosocial and systemic risk factors increase vulnerability for high levels of self-criticism and shame.
- Shame, self-criticism, and impaired capacity to self-soothe and regulate emotions can mediate the effectiveness of traditional talking therapies.
- Compassion-focused therapy (CFT) encourages people to move from a position of inward criticism and judgment toward a stance of self-kindness, compassion, warmth, empathy, and care.
- CFT interventions include psychoeducation; formulation; development of self-soothing strategies and emotion recognition and regulation skills; imagery and belief work; deliberate compassionate exercises; and mindfulness practice.

OVERVIEW

Compassion-focused therapy (CFT) is a third-wave psychological therapy, informed by evolutionary and social psychology, neuropsychology and attachment theories, cognitive behavior therapy (CBT), and Buddhist and mindfulness principles. CFT developed as an approach for people struggling to form secure attachments with others and presenting with shame-based difficulties and high levels of self-criticism, who did not respond favorably to more traditional talking therapies (Gilbert, 2009a). CFT principally aims to (a) support people to develop the capacity to self-soothe more effectively, and have empathy and acceptance for their "suffering"; (b) help people to move from a position of self-criticism, self-condemnation, and blame toward a stance of kindness, compassion, warmth, and care toward themselves; and (c) be more compassionate toward others and feel able to accept others' compassion toward them (Gilbert, 2009a, 2009b). People are encouraged to develop the strength to move toward suffering and the wisdom to alleviate this by learning what might help, in the moment and longer-term. CFT also involves acquiring mindfulness skills to jump out of any loops that can maintain suffering, and to build up compassionate qualities.

There are three main elements to self-compassion: (a) self-kindness versus self-judgment (adopting a curious approach to oneself, rather than self-judgment and criticism); (b) common humanity versus isolation (the view that we share common experiences and are *all* part of humanity, rather than being alone); and (c) mindfulness versus overidentification (the idea that balanced thoughts are better than overidentifying with specific thoughts).

CFT seeks to "depersonalise and de-shame by helping the client to understand how their brain regulates emotion" (Beaumont & Hollins-Martin, 2015, p. 22). This is informed by a theoretical evolutionary model categorizing emotions into threat, drive, and soothing systems (see Figure 14-1). The threat system is designed to react quickly to internal and external triggers and gives rise to negative emotions (e.g., anger, anxiety, disgust). The drive system encourages a search for "important rewards and resources" (e.g., food, alliances); when activated, people experience excitement and pleasure. The soothing system kicks in at times of safety and rest, evident through contentment and peacefulness, and it facilitates affiliative relationships (Gilbert & Choden, 2014). The three systems are deemed both necessary and important for helping humans thrive; that is, we need to be primed to respond rapidly to danger, to feel perpetually motivated toward meeting our basic needs, and to have downtime when we can rest, recuperate and develop relationships with others who might help us mitigate threat and discover opportunities. Yet for some people, these systems are unbalanced: specifically, the threat system is overactive and the soothing system is underactive (e.g., due to

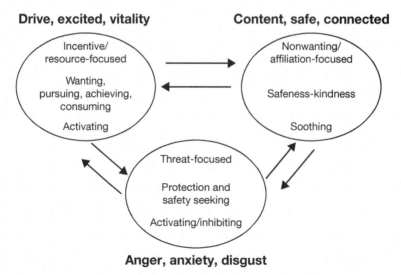

Figure 14-1 Gilbert, The Compassionate Mind (2009), reprinted with permission from Little Brown Book Group

adversity or trauma; Gilbert, 2009b). CFT helps people to understand how and why this might be and to redress this imbalance. Partly, this is informed by the notion of having a "tricky brain," with "old" and "new" components: the old brain is responsible for basic drives and the new brain processes more complex information (Gilbert, 2014).

SELF-COMPASSION OF PEOPLE WITH AUTISM

Scant research has examined compassion in people with autism. One study by Howes and colleagues (2020) investigated self-compassion and autistic traits in 176 neurotypical university students (60% male, mean age 24.5 years, range 18–71 years old). Participants completed demographic questions (e.g., about sex, age); the autism quotient (AQ; Baron-Cohen et al., 2001), which is a 50-item self-report measure of autism traits; and the self-compassion scale (SCS; Neff 2003), which is a 26-item self-report questionnaire of positive and negative facets of compassion. Positive facets of compassion were significantly negatively correlated with the AQ, and negative aspects of compassion were significantly positively correlated with the AQ. In a related study, Galvin and colleagues (2020) asked 164 students (42% male, mean age 24.2 years, range 18–51 years old) to complete the AQ, SCS, and hospital anxiety and depression scale (Zigmond & Snaith, 1983). Self-compassion was found to mediate relationships between autism, anxiety, and depression, providing support for the hypothesis that self-compassion may be associated with, or predict, mental health symptoms (MacBeth & Gumley, 2012).

RISK FACTORS FOR SELF-CRITICISM AND SHAME-BASED DIFFICULTIES IN PEOPLE WITH AUTISM

Several factors might increase the susceptibility of people with autism to developing self-criticism and shame. First, many people with autism experience peer victimization, rejection, and ostracism (Maiano et al., 2016; Weiss & Fardella, 2018). Victimization negatively affects people's sense of safety and security, socially and relationally. Additionally, people with autism may have few positive relationships (Petrina et al., 2014), thereby impacting their capacity to develop social confidence. Second, people with autism tend to do less well educationally and occupationally, relative to their abilities (Kirby et al., 2016). Over time, this may reinforce negative self-beliefs (e.g., about performance). Third, people with autism experience disproportionately high rates of internalizing disorders, including anxiety disorders and depression (Lai et al., 2019), and these are commonly associated with poorer self-esteem in neurotypical samples (Sowislo & Orth, 2013). Prevalence rates of posttraumatic stress disorder (PTSD) are also high (Rumball, 2019). Shame—including perceptions that others view a person as inferior, faulty, or inadequate, and comparable self-beliefs—are common experiences for people with PTSD (Lee et al., 2001). Fourth, failure to attain an autism diagnosis until later life can contribute to a sense of "not knowing" (e.g., why some situations/interactions are difficult), giving rise to core beliefs about being different or inferior (Spain et al., 2020), and increasing vulnerability to shame-based difficulties. Fifth, evidence suggests that some people with autism deliberately mask autistic traits (Hull et al. 2017). Indirectly, this may increase concerns about being different and not fitting in, exacerbating self-focused attention and self-condemnation. Lastly, people with autism commonly fall between gaps in health services (Murphy et al., 2018) and frequently report being told they are "too complex" for generic health services. This plausibly incurs feelings of rejection, further augmenting concerns about being different or defective. Taken together, psychosocial and systemic factors affecting people with autism across the lifespan potentially precipitate and perpetuate negative core beliefs and high levels of self-criticism and shame.

CFT IN PRACTICE

CFT typically includes formulation, functional analysis, exploring the narrative of past experiences to deepen a sense of compassion (and its flow from ourselves to and from others, and to ourselves), imagery exercises, acting approaches, and belief work. Some techniques are shared with CBT, schema therapy and mindfulness-based approaches. As CFT is not protocol-driven, this allows for an individualized approach, transdiagnostically. See Table 14-1 for common CFT strategies.

OUTCOME MEASURES

Compassion-focused outcomes can be measured via self-report questionnaires, such as the fear of compassion scale (FOCS; Gilbert et al., 2011), which has three subscales assessing fears of compassion for self, from others, and for others. If someone experiences difficulty answering questions about others' thoughts (as can be the case for people with autism), the social comparison scale (SCS; Allan & Gilbert, 1995) has been a useful guide to assessing perceived social standing without having to infer too much from others. Clinically, this has often indicated improvement in feeling equal and included with others, while allowing a person to be different.

THE EVIDENCE BASE FOR COMPASSION-FOCUSED INTERVENTIONS

CFT and other compassion-focused approaches are empirically supported in neurotypical samples. For instance, data summarized in a recent systematic review of 14 studies (Leaviss & Uttley, 2015) and recent meta-analysis of 21 studies

Table 14-1 Compassion Focused Therapy: An Overview of Therapy Phases, Interventions, and Techniques

Phases of CFT	Purpose of Intervention and Examples of Techniques	Autism-Relevant Adaptations
Psychoeducation: the flow of life	**Why:** introduce CFT model; outline evolutionary explanation for, and de-shaming of, present difficulties (e.g., "not your fault," "we did not choose to be born here, now, in this context")	• clarify whether shame is associated with thoughts about social interaction • identify strengths • note that people with autism may have been the driving force in Stone Age cave paintings and helped to build pyramids
Psychoeducation: three-systems model	**Why:** introduce CFT model, explore the three-affect systems and notion that we have "tricky brains"; this can enhance flow of compassion to others as it raises the possibility that we all have different models of ourselves	• reduce complexity of language • use different colors or circle sizes to represent three systems
Developing self-soothing strategies	**Why:** learn how to activate and regulate the soothing system **How:** practice deep-rhythm breathing; relaxation strategies; imagery exercises (e.g., safe/calm place, compassionate coloring; listen to relaxing music; participate in calming activities	• embed reasonable adjustments in self-soothing activities (e.g., to the temperature, sound, light) • list enjoyable activities people can do alone or with others
Enhancing emotion recognition skills	**Why:** enhance recognition; highlight bidirectional relationships between emotions, behaviors, and responses, in the self and others **How:** psychoeducation; behavioral experiments or tasks testing out experiences of, and reactions to, positive emotions; explore evolutionary explanations for each emotion and alternative behaviors	• enhance emotional literacy • use mindfulness to notice urges of different emotions • develop idiosyncratic scales to depict gradations of emotions (and associated physiological arousal) • draw pictures of different emotions to help externalize these

Addressing fear of compassion	**Why:** address compassion-interfering thoughts/beliefs (e.g., being compassionate is a sign of weakness), and primary emotions activated by compassion responses (e.g., worry/ fear activated by kindness) **How:** Socratic conversations about past experiences and the meaning of these; cognitive interventions to target less helpful assumptions and beliefs	• provide psychoeducation about primary and secondary emotions • inquire about thoughts of meeting others; explore self-criticism as a potential attempt to change themselves or others; validate the emotions that arise from experiencing this • allow more time for behavioral experimentation • use visual/written summaries
Compassionate functional analysis	**Why:** identify links between: (a) influential experiences and events predisposing to shame-based difficulties, (b) key fears, (c) safety behaviors, and (d) intended and unintended consequences **How:** functional analysis	• provide examples if people struggle to identify consequences • repeat for different situations
Learning and practicing: caring commitment	**Why:** to experience compassion in three behavioral attributes; to begin noticing suffering in oneself and others **How:** compassionate memory techniques; develop a "care box," comprising objects that evoke calm or calm/relaxed memories	• use sensorily adapted mindfulness to notice and slow down responses of getting stuck in, or avoiding, distress • Socratic exploration of how others know we are suffering • use time-limited special interests to feel safe • include sensorily pleasurable objects in a "care box"
Learning and practicing: strength	**Why:** to turn toward suffering and understand unintended consequences of turning away from suffering **How:** soothing-rhythm breathing and safe-place imagery to increase tolerance of powerful emotions; mountain meditation exercise	• incorporate new, helpful reflections into imagery or role play to show strength • compare different postures in detail, using the mountain meditation exercise • with consent, ask family to note changes in posture between sessions
Learning and practicing: wisdom	**Why:** to have choice over how to live, approach suffering and alleviate this **How:** inner best friend exercise (treating/talking to yourself as you would a best friend); generate positive self-statements	• summaries positive statements on cue cards • use Socratic dialogue about how to connect to others via less expressed emotions (i.e., when suffering)

(continued)

Table 14-1 CONTINUED

Phases of CFT	Purpose of Intervention and Examples of Techniques	Autism-Relevant Adaptations
Putting it all together	**Why**: develop an image of the self that is "equal, included and different" **How**: consolidation of previously mentioned interventions	• explore each of the three qualities described, from the perspectives of (i) receiving these, (ii) giving these to others, and (iii) observing these between others • compile a flashcard of warning signs of becoming socially exhausted, and ways of getting adjustments
Developing social skills	**Why**: enhance knowledge, skills and confidence in developing adaptive, secure affiliative relationships; consider whether self-criticism or shame impact upon interactions/relationships **How**: psychoeducation; chairwork to explore different roles within different relationships; systemically informed conversations about important past and current relationships	• clarify understanding of social relationships • consider drawing social circles with the person in the middle, family in a circle around them, and moving in circles further out, to identify friends, colleagues, acquaintances and strangers; make this visual—different colored circles representing different types of relationship and responses to them • use systemic techniques to explore personal narratives and meaning making about autism
Enhancing assertiveness	**Why**: to manage the wider context of adjustments needed for people to live well in work, relationships, health appointments, and other situations **How**: chairwork; role play; imagery exercises	• identify scenarios involving disclosing the autism diagnosis, to whom, and what this felt like • discuss thoughts/beliefs and emotions about masking—and the degree to which this may link to the formulation
Managing therapy endings	**Why**: for people to be empowered to make choices over how they live **How**: make a therapy blueprint; problem solve potential setbacks; compassionate letter writing	• plan for gradual tapering of sessions • compile diagrammatic therapy blueprint or video/audio recordings of key points (use the therapist's voice if this helps)

Adapted from Cowles et al., 2020; Gilbert 2009a, 2009b.

(Kirby et al., 2017) have indicated that CFT is associated with improved self-compassion, mood, anxiety, stress, and self-esteem, as well as reduced self-criticism.

No studies, to our knowledge, have described CFT for people with autism. A few studies have examined effectiveness and/or acceptability of CFT for adults with intellectual disabilities a proportion of whom also had autism), individually (Cooper & Frearson, 2017; Cowles et al., 2020) and in six session groups (Clapton et al., 2018; Goad & Parker, 2020; Hardiman et al., 2018). Given the co-occurrence of intellectual disabilities and autism (Emerson & Baines, 2010) and potential commonalities in some risk factors for mental health symptoms, brief review of these studies here seems appropriate. Interventions have principally sought to enhance self-compassion, general mental health, trauma-related symptoms, and low mood. Standard CFT interventions were offered, with some adaptations, notably: (a) reducing complexity of psychoeducation; (b) more simplistic formulation; (c) slower session pacing; (d) less abstract information; (e) use of visual aids (e.g., diagrams, workbooks); (f) frequent repetition and practice; (g) involving family/caregivers to prompt homework completion and reinforce ideas; and (h) embedding compassion-focused principles at home. Results indicated subjective and/or objective improvements in mood, anxiety, self-criticism, and general functioning. Qualitative feedback indicated some participants found therapy to be de-shaming and normalizing: they realized they had shared experiences and difficulties and felt together with, rather than separate to, others.

CASE STUDY

Background

Clara was in her thirties when she was referred to the service. She had previously been diagnosed with depression, obsessive compulsive disorder (OCD), and borderline personality disorder, prior to receiving an autism diagnosis, in her late twenties.

She grew up with her mother, described as quiet, and her father, described as inexpressive and uncompromising. He often insulted Clara, especially when she was seeking help (e.g., with homework), and "walked out" of the family home during her teens. She recalled enjoying school formalities (e.g., studying, completing coursework about circumscribed interests), yet she found transitions between classrooms and subjects, and unstructured interactions, difficult. Break times were unpredictable and overwhelming, so she often hid in the bathrooms. She was physically, verbally, and financially harassed. She perceived her peers "got on" well, whereas she felt at a loss, not knowing what to say or how to join in, and on the periphery of groups.

As an adult, Clara lived with her mother and was relatively independent. She maintained a restricted diet, primarily due to sensory aversions. Her sleep/wake cycle was slightly reversed and she typically felt fatigued. She often felt distressed, managing this by hair pulling and making impulsive online purchases. Her social network was limited. She was closest to her mother, mainly communicating with others via email and internet forums. In-person interactions were strained due to difficulties with understanding social rules and cues and problems engaging reciprocally. Conversations could be short and stilted, or could result in monologuing about topics of interest to her. Clara coped with social interactions by learning to emulate others and mentally scripting conversations, which is conceptualized by some as camouflaging. While this partially helped to reduce uncertainty in social situations, it also required substantial mental energy and incurred fatigue. Consequently, Clara rested most evenings, thereby missing out on potential opportunities for social contact. She worked as an administrator, reliably and consistently. As at school, unstructured times and social activities (e.g., lunch breaks, work socials) were problematic. She experienced some interpersonal difficulties at work, resulting in her feeling bullied, stressed and low. She subsequently presented to mental health services and was diagnosed with autism.

Assessment

Given the history of difficult interpersonal experiences, sense of isolation, and tendency for camouflaging, assessment took five sessions. Overall, this was to (a) enhance Clara's capacity to feel more at ease with expressing more authentic thoughts, feelings, and behaviors; (b) encourage development of engagement and trust, which is requisite for subsequent shame-based discussions; and (c) allow for habituation to the location, context, and therapist.

The assessment focused on standard therapy domains and CFT-specific themes, including:

- Autism diagnosis: how she referred to, and made sense of (a) traits before diagnosis, (b) at the time of diagnosis, (c) during life transitions, and (d) presently;
- Family support: if and how family members were supportive during childhood and now;
- Relationships: her interest in other people, and having friendships or relationships;
- Alexithymia: if and how she described emotions;
- Relating to self and others: if, when, and how she noticed she was different from others, and how this influenced her behavior;
- Other-to-self relating: what she thought others thought of her, across contexts;
- Self-to-other relating: what she thought about others when socializing; and
- Self-to-self relating: what she thought about herself.

Within initial sessions, the therapist aimed to convey and model a sense of understanding and compassion toward Clara. This involved clarifying how best to engage; for example, confirming environmental/sensory considerations, ascertaining her preferences for sustaining eye contact (or not), building time into sessions for Clara to acclimatize to the context and as discussion topics changed, and asking her to say if she needed more time to process information or if question/remarks lacked clarity. Focusing on these steps was also intended to encourage a shift from the threat system to the soothing system, in order for Clara to have a different experience to the many other social situations in which she felt the need to deliberately try to "fit in." Overall, talking with openness and curiosity about someone's preferences and capacity to influence their context helps to normalize the process of acquiring reasonable adjustments is a key aspect of CFT for people with autism.

Formulation

Formulation aimed to better understand Clara's intentions in social situations; for example, did she try to fit in so as to feel connected to others? Did she try to manage these situations to increase a sense of certainty over everyday life? Did she enjoy time away from others? Latterly, the formulation focused on establishing unintended internal and external consequences of actions (e.g., internal, how she viewed anxiety, sadness, memories, or herself as a person; and external, such as rejection, criticism, and losses).

Functional analysis helped Clara identify earlier experiences of trying to feel connected with others that had been marred by negative core beliefs about herself and others (e.g., that they were punitive, dismissive, more able; see Figure 14-2, adapted from Gilbert & Irons, 2015). Moreover, the effort of trying to fit in and self-monitor during interactions exacerbated fatigue and perpetuated worry. A tendency for black-and-white thinking helped her to accomplish work adeptly, yet it affected social interactions. Difficulties with mentalizing others' speech and actions also "hijacked" her strength in details; she often noticed inconsistencies in her interactions, resulting in self-criticism (e.g., for not being perfect). Importantly, part of the formulation also involved noting strengths: Clara showed dedication, loyalty, a detailed and focused style that helped her understand complex processes and see the beauty in objects others overlooked. She also had a profound empathy for people she related to.

Goals

Historically, Clara's goals largely focused on trying to "fit in" and be "the same" as others (e.g., learning to maintain eye contact and to make socially desirable comments). Yet, working toward these exacerbated a sense of difference and shame, indirectly giving more credence to negative beliefs.

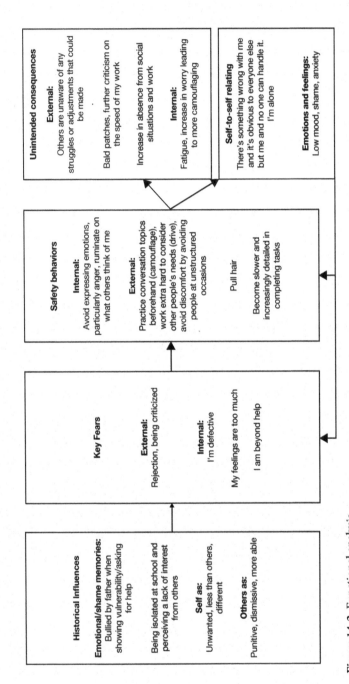

Historical Influences

Emotional/shame memories: Bullied by father when showing vulnerability/asking for help

Being isolated at school and perceiving a lack of interest from others

Self as: Unwanted, less than others, different

Others as: Punitive, dismissive, more able

Key Fears

External: Rejection, being criticized

Internal: I'm defective

My feelings are too much

I am beyond help

Safety behaviors

Internal: Avoid expressing emotions, particularly anger, ruminate on what others think of me

External: Practice conversation topics beforehand (camouflage), work extra hard to consider other people's needs (drive), avoid discomfort by avoiding people at unstructured occasions

Pull hair

Become slower and increasingly detailed in completing tasks

Unintended consequences

External: Others are unaware of any struggles or adjustments that could be made

Bald patches, further criticism on the speed of my work

Increase in absence from social situations and work

Internal: Fatigue, increase in worry leading to more camouflaging

Self-to-self relating There's something wrong with me and it's obvious to everyone else but me and no one can handle it. I'm alone

Emotions and feelings: Low mood, shame, anxiety

Figure 14-2 Functional analysis

Clara's therapy goals were to:

- Improve her mood and anxiety
- Request reasonable adjustments at work and in public
- Increase social confidence and develop relationships
- Feel more able to enjoy engaging in highly detailed, nonsocial interests, with and without others

At times, goal setting in CFT can be complicated. Therapists may have to weigh the advantages and constraints of working on specific goals and building engagement through collaborating in the present moment, while finding out more about a person's difficulties and values in the process. Many adults with autism have internalized perceived failures educationally, socially, and occupationally, giving rise to worries about, memories of, and a lack of confidence in, striving toward outcomes they would ideally like to pursue.

Therapy

Overall, CFT for people with autism is intended to create a space for "live" practice for each of the features of compassion—strength, caring commitment, and wisdom—whereby they feel able to ask for autism-relevant reasonable adjustments. This is the most important foundation to build a life equal to others, be included with others, dare to be different from others, and allow for (and appreciate) each other's neurodiversity.

Clara attended 20 CFT sessions, the standard number of sessions offered at the service, focusing on:

- Psychoeducation: the shaping of our experiences—the flow of life; three-systems model of emotion
- Development of soothing strategies
- Labelling of emotions in the body
- Compassionate functional analysis
- Learning and practicing: (a) caring commitment, (b) strength, and (c) wisdom
- Social and assertiveness skills development

Several adaptations were incorporated to make CFT more accessible (see Table 14-1 for autism-relevant adaptations). These also involved: (a) fewer imagery exercises focused on the compassionate other and compassionate self; and (b) combining the three qualities of compassion with questions from different perspectives, to practice experiencing compassion (i.e., caring commitment, strength, and wisdom, all from receiving, giving, and observing perspectives).

Outcomes

Overall, Clara felt more confident in "being myself" after 20 sessions. She reported far less drive to "fit in," and felt more able and "safe" to do more tasks she enjoyed, resulting in her starting new hobbies that involved group classes. This increased her social network. She began telling others when she felt overwhelmed socially, and why. She disclosed her autism diagnosis at work, enabling her to access reasonable adjustments.

Clara's scores on the FOCS changed from 25 to seven points in fears of compassion for others, 38 to 17 for fears of compassion from others, and 33 to six points in compassion from herself to herself. This supported her view that she was managing her threat more helpfully across the domains and that her highest fear was fear of compassion from others. While scores reduced reliably in a clinical sense, fear of compassion remained higher than the other domains, supporting the need for reasonable adjustments and skillful pacing in her social interactions.

THERAPIST CONSIDERATIONS

As with all therapeutic approaches, there are some considerations for therapists using CFT with clients who have autism.

- Many people with autism work extremely hard, using their drive system to manage threats in everyday life. Understandably, when they trust therapists sufficiently to work on these areas, therapists can feel a pull to work extremely hard too. This can be to avoid the sadness that often occurs when receiving and adjusting to a diagnosis of autism.
- Slowly explore interventions. Be curious about clients' emotions and any avoidance or subtle expressions of shame. This helps people apply the techniques "live" and feel able to take a positive risk to make a change, despite the much higher short-term discomfort this brings.
- Changing topic is difficult for some people, and results in reliance on saying "I don't know." Labelling this can provide an early example into the importance of using the quality of strength to gain reasonable adjustments.
- Be mindful of individuals attending sessions but not doing homework. Clarify if there is any pressure from family members, partners, or employers for the person to change. The person may feel shame from not knowing how to do a task or have a prediction they will "fail." This is an opportunity to use functional analysis and build the relevant skills for CFT. It is also possible to delve into the experiences that shaped this prediction. Be mindful of responding to these fears and resultant avoidance or defensiveness, in an open, fallible way, to

help both therapist and individual experience safety to learn through mistakes.

- Model the flow of compassion: it is vitally important to help people engage with different ways of responding to their emotions. This can be done by modeling the variety of techniques listed.

CONCLUSIONS

People with autism commonly experience transdiagnostic symptoms, including self-criticism and shame-based difficulties, rendering engagement in more traditional talking therapies, and with therapists, problematic. Empirical support for CFT in neurotypical adults and adults with an intellectual disability is growing. Clinically, we have found that many adults with autism find that CFT interventions and techniques resonate with them, subject to incorporating adaptations and encouraging requests for (reasonable) adjustments. We suggest that further sustained research is required to understand links between compassion and mental health in people with autism and the effectiveness of CFT for this clinical population.

REFERENCES

Allan, S., & Gilbert, P. (1995). A social comparison scale: Psychometric properties and relationship to psychopathology. *Personality and Individual Differences, 19*(3), 293–299.

Baron-Cohen, S., Wheelwright, S., Skinner, R., Martin, J., & Clubley, E. (2001). The autism-spectrum quotient (AQ). Evidence from Asperger syndrome/high-functioning autism, males and females, scientists and mathematicians. *Journal of Autism & Developmental Disorders, 31*(1), 5–17.

Beaumont, E., & Hollins Martin, C. (2015). A narrative review exploring the effectiveness of compassion-focused therapy. *Counselling Psychology Review, 30*(1), 21–32.

Clapton, N., Williams, J., Griffith, G., & Jones, R. (2018). "Finding the person you really are . . . on the inside": compassion focused therapy for adults with intellectual disabilities. *Journal of Intellectual Disabilities, 22*(2), 135–153.

Cooper, R., & Frearson, J. (2017). Adapting compassion focused therapy for an adult with a learning disability: A case study. *British Journal of Learning Disabilities, 45*(2), 142–150.

Cowles, M., Randle-Phillips, C., & Medley, A. (2020). Compassion-focused therapy for trauma in people with intellectual disabilities: A conceptual review. *Journal of Intellectual Disabilities, 24*(2), 212–232.

Emerson, E., & Baines, S. (2010). *The estimated prevalence of autism among adults with learning disabilities in England.* Improving Health and Lives: Learning Disabilities Observatory, Durham.

Galvin, J., Howes, A., McCarthy, B., & Richards, G. (2020). Self-compassion as a mediator of the association between autistic traits and depressive/anxious symptomatology. *Autism*, epub. doi.org/10.1177/1362361320966853

Gilbert, P. (2009a). Introducing compassion-focused therapy. *Advances in Psychiatric Treatment*, 15(3), 199–208.

Gilbert, P. (2009b). The nature and basis for compassion focused therapy. *Hellenic Journal of Psychology*, 6(20), 273–291.

Gilbert, P. (2014). The origins and nature of compassion focused therapy. *British Journal of Clinical Psychology*, 53(1), 6–41.

Gilbert, P., & Choden (2014). *Mindful compassion: How the science of compassion can help you understand your emotions, live in the present, and connect deeply with others.* New Harbinger Publications.

Gilbert, P., & Irons, C. (2015). Compassion focused therapy. In S. Palmer (Ed.), *The beginner's guide to counselling & psychotherapy* (pp. 127–139). SAGE Publications Ltd.

Gilbert, P., McEwan, K., Matos, M., & Rivis, A. (2011). Fears of compassion: Development of three self-report measures. *Psychology and Psychotherapy: Theory, Research and Practice*, 84(3), 239–255.

Goad, E. J., & Parker, K. (2020). Compassion-focused therapy groups for people with intellectual disabilities: An extended pilot study. *Journal of Intellectual Disabilities*, epub. doi.org/10.1177/1744629520925953

Hardiman, M., Willmoth, C., & Walsh, J. (2018). CFT & people with intellectual disabilities. *Advances in Mental Health and Intellectual Disabilities*, 12(1), 44–56.

Howes, A., Richards, G, & Galvin, J. (2020). A preliminary investigation into the relationship between autistic traits and self-compassion. *Psychological Reports*, epub. doi.org/10.1177/0033294120957244

Hull, L., Petrides, K., Allison, C., Smith, P., Baron-Cohen, S., Lai, M. C., & Mandy, W. (20176). "Putting on my best normal": Social camouflaging in adults with autism spectrum conditions. *Journal of Autism and Developmental Disorders*, 47(8), 2519–2534.

Kirby, A., Baranek, G., & Fox, L. (2016). Longitudinal predictors of outcomes for adults with autism spectrum disorder: Systematic review. *OTJR: Occupation, Participation and Health*, 36(2), 55–64.

Kirby, J., Tellegen, C., & Steindl, S. (2017). A meta-analysis of compassion-based interventions: Current state of knowledge and future directions. *Behavior Therapy*, 48(6), 778–792.

Lai, M., Kassee, C., Besney, R., Bonato, S., Hull, L., Mandy, W., Szatmari, P., & Ameis, S. (2019). Prevalence of co-occurring mental health diagnoses in the autism population: A systematic review and meta-analysis. *The Lancet Psychiatry*, 6(10), 819–829.

Leaviss, J., & Uttley, L. (2015). Psychotherapeutic benefits of compassion-focused therapy: An early systematic review. *Psychological Medicine*, 45(5), 927–945.

Lee, D., Scragg, P., & Turner, S. (2001). The role of shame and guilt in traumatic events: A clinical model of shame-based and guilt-based PTSD. *British Journal of Medical Psychology*, 74(4), 451–466.

MacBeth, A., & Gumley, A. (2012). Exploring compassion: A meta-analysis of the association between self-compassion and psychopathology. *Clinical Psychology Review*, 32(6), 545–552.

Maiano, C., Normand, C., Salvas, M., Moullec, G., & Aimé, A. (2016). Prevalence of school bullying among youth with autism spectrum disorders: A systematic review and meta-analysis. *Autism Research, 9*(6), 601–615.

Murphy, D., Glaser, K., Hayward, H., Eklund, H., Cadman, T., Findon, J., Woodhouse, E., Ashwood, K., Beecham, J., Bolton, P., McEwen, F., Wilson, E., Ecker, C., Wong, I., Simonoff, E., Russell, A., McCarthy, J., Chaplin, E., Young, S., & Asherson, P. (2018). Crossing the divide: A longitudinal study of effective treatments for people with autism and attention deficit hyperactivity disorder across the lifespan. *Programme Grants for Applied Research, 6*(2), 1–240.

Neff, K. (2003). The development and validation of a scale to measure self-compassion. *Self and Identity, 2*(3), 223–250.

Petrina, N., Carter, M., & Stephenson, J. (2014). The nature of friendship in children with autism spectrum disorders: A systematic review. *Research in Autism Spectrum Disorders, 8*(2), 111–126.

Rumball, F. (2019). A systematic review of the assessment and treatment of posttraumatic stress disorder in individuals with autism spectrum disorders. *Review Journal of Autism and Developmental Disorders, 6*(3), 294–324.

Sowislo, J., & Orth, U. (2013). Does low self-esteem predict depression and anxiety? A meta-analysis of longitudinal studies. *Psychological Bulletin, 139*(1), 213.

Spain, D., Zıvralı Yarar, E., & Happé, F. (2020). Social anxiety in adults with autism: A qualitative study. *International Journal of Qualitative Studies on Health and Well-Being, 15*(1), 1803669.

Weiss, J., & Fardella, M. (2018). Victimization and perpetration experiences of adults with autism. *Frontiers in* Psychiatry, *9*, 203.

Zigmond, A. S., & Snaith, R. P. (1983). The hospital anxiety and depression scale. *Acta Psychiatrica Scandinavica, 67*(6), 361–370.

15

Eye Movement Desensitization and Reprocessing Therapy

NAOMI FISHER AND CAROLINE VAN DIEST ■

KEY CONSIDERATIONS

- EMDR can be an effective therapy for autistic adults.
- Therapists need to be flexible in their approach, responding to the individual in front of them and formulating their experiences.
- Living an autistic life can be highly stressful even without experiencing a major trauma, and EMDR can be used to alleviate this.
- Adaptations to EMDR include simplifying the cognitive demands of the protocol, mapping from emotions and body sensations, working from the here and now, being more directive, and using some of the adaptations developed for use with children.
- EMDR should never be used to make a person's behavior more convenient, and the function of a behavior should always be part of the formulation.

OVERVIEW

Eye movement desensitization and reprocessing (EMDR) therapy is a psychotherapy which is recognized by the National Institute for Health and Clinical Excellence (NICE) and the World Health Organization (WHO) as an effective treatment for posttraumatic stress disorder (PTSD). It was developed by the American clinical psychologist Francine Shapiro in the 1980s (Shapiro, 1989). EMDR therapy is powerful and should only be attempted after having attended an accredited training program and under appropriate supervision.

In this chapter we describe EMDR and the adaptive information processing model, and we briefly summarise the evidence base for EMDR in general and autistic populations. We will use a case example to demonstrate how EMDR can be used with autistic people. This is an illustrative example rather than a specific individual.

WHAT IS EMDR?

EMDR is a structured psychotherapy underpinned by a trauma-informed model. The conceptual framework suggests that psychological problems in the present day can be caused or influenced by distressing (and therefore "unprocessed") memories of the past. The adaptive information processing model (AIP; Shapiro, 2007) suggests that memories for most life events are naturally integrated into an individual's existing memory networks, becoming part of their autobiographical memory store. This is referred to as "adaptive information processing." These "processed" memories are recalled without significant distress in the present day, even if the event remembered was distressing at the time. Many people can remember that they were anxious when taking exams without actually re-experiencing the physical and emotional sensations of anxiety.

When a person is highly physiologically aroused, memories are not integrated in the same way. They can continue to cause distress and to influence behavior. An unprocessed memory could result in a person avoiding driving, because when they get into a car, they re-experience the terror of an earlier road traffic accident.

Recently, there has been an increased awareness of the way in which trauma plays a part in the etiology of a range of experiences and behaviors beyond those typically associated with PTSD. These include psychosis (Varese et al., 2012), eating problems, people diagnosed with personality disorder, substance misuse, depression. and anxiety. In all of these cases, EMDR could potentially be helpful.

EMDR therapy targets unprocessed memories directly. This is done using dual attention. The person connects to their distress while engaging in some form of bilateral stimulation (BLS). This is typically either eye movements, alternate tapping (e.g., on the back of the person's hands or knees), or auditory clicks. EMDR can be used remotely with a therapist, where BLS is delivered through self-tapping or by an app. The use of bilateral stimulation (BLS) to facilitate processing is a unique element of EMDR.

The standard EMDR protocol consists of eight phases. These include assessment and history taking, with trauma processing happening from phase three onwards, and the protocol ends with closure exercises. The protocol is a framework rather than a manual. The therapist uses it to establish a safe and containing structure for the client. During EMDR, clients typically experience a change in their relationship with the memory, with more adaptive material emerging as well as the traumatic memory becoming less distressing.

The strongest evidence for the efficacy of EMDR is with PTSD, but EMDR is increasingly considered a transdiagnostic approach. Given recent concerns about the lack of reliability of diagnostic categories and the findings of shared genetic risk factors between mental health conditions (Caspi et al., 2014; Hengartner & Lehmann, 2017; Insel, 2010), it seems arbitrary to restrict access to a therapy by a diagnosis. From an information-processing perspective, there is no reason why the nature of a life event should dictate treatment. It is the nature of the psychological response to an event that matters.

FORMULATION: TRAUMA AND AUTISM SPECTRUM DISORDER

The distinction between focusing on *what* happened to someone and focusing on *a person's response* to whatever happened may be particularly important for autistic people. The writings of autistic people tell us that, for some, the events of a typical life can be intensely stressful (Poe, 2019; Ratcliffe, 2020; Rowe, 2013; Williams, 1998). "Trauma memories" are created during times of high physiological arousal, something which many writers with autistic describe feeling as they go about their everyday lives. Many autistic people attempt to compensate for their differences, but this comes at a cost. Years of sustained effort can cause burnout or mental fatigue.

Autistic people may also experience frequent adverse events. Vulnerability for unhealthy relationships is increased, as are risk factors for depression, anxiety, and suicidal ideation (Livingston et al., 2019). Autistic people may be more likely to experience bullying, hostility, and social exclusion (Kerns et al., 2015). There is also suggestion in the research (and much anecdotal evidence) that events that are seen to be mildly annoying by many people can be perceived as extremely distressing or traumatic by autistic people (Taylor & Gotham, 2016). This could include nondisabled people parking in a disabled parking space, someone breaking an agreement, or an appointment starting late.

Taken together, these can result in a person feeling and behaving as if they are traumatized, even when they have not experienced an event which would generally be classified as a "trauma." Figure 15-1 summarizes this within an ecological model. In this model, disability and distress are not an inevitable consequence of difference. A person interacts with the world in a bidirectional fashion, meaning that both individual characteristics and the response of society to those characteristics affects outcome.

This means that therapists should look beyond what they consider to be "traumatic events," and instead examine the meaning of a wide range of adverse events or stressors in a person's life. This should inform their formulation, an essential part of EMDR therapy.

EFFECTIVENESS OF EMDR IN THE GENERAL POPULATION

Several meta-analyses have shown that EMDR is an effective treatment for PTSD in adults (Chen et al., 2015; Khan et al., 2018; Novo Navarro et al., 2018) and children (Rodenburg et al., 2009). A systematic review of randomized controlled trials (RCTs) of EMDR found that it is useful for a range of mental health problems including phobias, substance misuse, depression, and panic disorder (Valiente-Gomez et al., 2017).

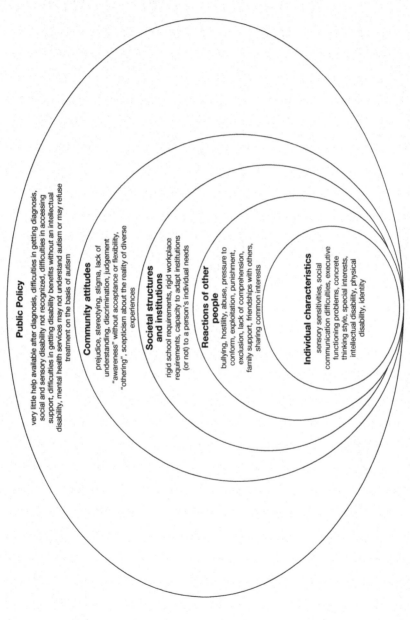

Public Policy
very little help available after diagnosis, difficulties in getting diagnosis, social and sensory disability not recognized, difficulties in accessing support, difficulties in getting disability benefits without an intellectual disability, mental health services may not understand autism or may refuse treatment on the basis of autism

Community attitudes
prejudice, stereotyping, stigma, lack of understanding, discrimination, judgement "awareness" without acceptance or flexibility, "othering", scepticism about the reality of diverse experiences

Societal structures and institutions
rigid school requirements, rigid workplace requirements, capacity to adapt institutions (or not) to a person's individual needs

Reactions of other people
bullying, hostility, abuse, pressure to conform, exploitation, punishment, exclusion, lack of comprehension, family support, friendships with others, sharing common interests

Individual characteristics
sensory sensitivities, social communication difficulties, executive functioning problems, concrete thinking style, special interests, intellectual disability, physical disability, identity

Figure 15-1 An Ecological Model of Autism: Individual Characteristics Are Only One Part of the Experience of Being Autistic

HOW DOES EMDR WORK?

There are several hypotheses as to the mechanism of EMDR. There is good evidence that bilateral stimulation, such as eye movements, taxes the working memory (Van Den Hout & Engelhard, 2012) and that using eye movements while activating an emotionally charged memory results in the memory becoming less emotional and vivid (Van Den Hout et al., 2013). Other hypotheses focus on the alternating nature of the eye movements, with some suggesting that eye movements produce a state similar to REM sleep (Stickgold, 2002), while others propose that it enhances communication between the hemispheres of the brain, which enhances the retrieval of episodic memories (Propper & Christman, 2008).

It is likely that EMDR works via multiple mechanisms. The working-memory hypothesis alone does not account for the "reprocessing" aspect of EMDR, whereby a new, more adaptive (consolidated) way of thinking about the event emerges (Solomon & Shapiro, 2008).

EFFECTIVENESS OF EMDR FOR AUTISTIC PEOPLE

There is limited research on EMDR and autism, although clinically this is a growth area. The earliest work consisted of case studies. These demonstrated that EMDR could be effective with autistic adults who also had intellectual disabilities (Barol & Seubert, 2010). The adaptations made included additional resources, visualization, metaphor, narrative techniques, and directive interventions. Some people required the target to be somatic or emotional experiences rather than a specific memory. Three of the four participants processed current stressors. They reported that each participant managed affect better following EMDR. These examples show how EMDR can be used even when a client does not link their distress to past experiences.

Kosatka and Ona (2014) used intensive EMDR (three times per week over 3 weeks) with a 21-year-old female with a diagnosis of Asperger's syndrome without intellectual disability. After eight sessions of EMDR, her PTSD symptom score was significantly reduced to below clinical levels and maintained at 8-month follow-up. Her functioning significantly improved overall, raising the possibility that some challenges were due to trauma and not Asperger's syndrome.

The first larger scale study of EMDR with autistic people used a within-study case control design, with adult participants acting as their own controls while receiving treatment as usual (Lobregt-van Buuren et al., 2018). Twenty-one participants completed this study with an average of seven sessions of EMDR. The study used the Dutch EMDR protocol for children (which reduces the demands as compared to the standard protocol). They found a significant reduction in PTSD symptoms, psychological distress, and autistic features including social motivation and communication. Participants were less impaired in their daily life after EMDR and results were maintained at 6–8 week follow up.

Morris-Smith and Silvestre describe using EMDR with 10 children on the autistic spectrum, eight of whom showed improvement (Morris-Smith & Silvestre, 2014).

They propose that autistic children can be traumatized by daily living experiences (which could include being bumped into in the playground, or being told off by a teacher) due to their difficulties in making sense of the social world. They emphasized how proactive and flexible therapists need to be in doing this work.

Most recently, Leuning has used EMDR with autistic children in order to target stressful daily life experiences. Her study is unpublished but has been presented at conferences. After 10 weekly sessions of EMDR some participants showed improvements in their social awareness and perceived stress scores. There was some reduction in self-reported autism symptoms (Leuning, 2020).

A reduction in autistic features, including social communication and motivation following EMDR, is found across several studies (Kosatka & Ona, 2014; Leuning, 2020; Lobregt-van Buuren et al., 2018; Morris-Smith & Silvestre, 2014). This is surprising. It is possible that some behaviors which are perceived to be symptoms of autism may be due to unresolved stress responses. These behaviors could include obsessional and repetitive behavior, social anxiety, separation anxiety, demand avoidance, challenging behavior, and sleep problems. Given the difficulties experienced by many autistic people, unresolved stress responses and trauma may be a frequent part of the presentation.

CASE STUDY: "MY FEAR KEEPS ME SAFE"

The last part of this chapter is a case example. Through it, we will highlight how the EMDR protocol can be adapted to make it more accessible.

Background

Donny was a 34-year-old man with a diagnosis of autism and a mild intellectual disability. He lived in a group home while his parents lived nearby.

Donny presented with needle phobia. He had a history of food intolerance from childhood. In order to avoid a reaction, he had severely restricted his diet. His parents felt allergy testing (which involved a needle) might help to expand his diet. Donny could not allow a needle close to him, kicking and fighting anyone who tried to suggest it.

At assessment, Donny found it hard providing details about the past. His mother was invited to attend history-taking sessions. She reported that Donny was bullied at primary school. His food intolerances were not yet diagnosed, and he had often felt sick. Doctors assumed that his stomach aches were due to unwillingness to attend school and encouraged his parents to keep sending him.

Donny had tried to escape from school several times. He remembered finding the school's response to this (isolation in the head teachers' office) terrifying as he had had no idea when he would be allowed to leave. Diagnosed with autism at the age of 10, he moved to a specialist secondary school. Here he felt unsafe due to the disruptive behavior of other students.

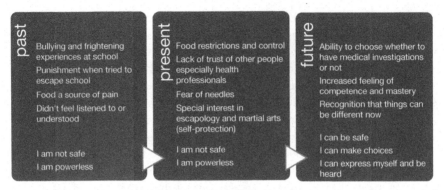

Figure 15-2 The Three-Pronged Approach: Donny's Experiences in the Past, Present, and Hoped-For Future

Donny had a special interest in self-defense and escapology. He was an expert in escape room puzzles and spent his free time devising his own escape games, building working models in a shed at the bottom of his parents' garden. He was a keen member of a local karate club. He worked at a local warehouse and knew all the potential routes out of the building, should a problem ever arise.

During assessment, an EMDR therapist will be looking for areas of strength and resilience which could be used as resources. Special interests can be a rich source of resource imagery as well as a way for a therapist to establish a therapeutic relationship. Part of the assessment should include asking for details of a person's special interests, and what it is specifically that they find engaging. Family members may need to be involved at this stage and systemic issues should be considered.

Case Conceptualization

The therapist's formulation was that Donny's apparent "phobia" was in fact part of a bigger picture where he felt unsafe and powerless. His intense responses to needles was just one part of this.

Figure 15-2 builds on the simple framework to create a more elaborate formulation, identifying targets for EMDR processing. The hypothesis was that Donny had learnt that he was powerless and unsafe during his childhood. These feelings were being triggered by how pressured he felt to have allergy testing and by the way in which health professionals related to him (see Box 15-1).

Intervention

Before EMDR processing starts, the preparation phase establishes the therapeutic relationship and develops self-soothing skills, as well as systemic interventions. The adaptations made are summarized in Box 15-1.

Preparation Phase

The first task was to form a therapeutic alliance and to agree on collaborative goals. The therapist started by finding out what really interested Donny. Donny became enthusiastic as he showed the therapist several prototype escape room games he had created. These, together with videos of himself at karate, were used to create resource imagery. Donny practiced feeling powerful and competent as he solved an escape room puzzle in his head and visualized doing karate.

The therapist realized that Donny's needle phobia was important because he feared that without it he would be pressured into allergy testing. She talked to his parents and they agreed that Donny would retain control over whether he had the tests even if his phobia was resolved. Donny agreed he would be safer if he could make informed choices regarding injections without feeling so fearful.

Donny and the therapist worked on creating a "calm place" which he could imagine to self-soothe. He chose his workshop. For many people, their calm place may be most effective if it is active rather than static. Each session ended with Donny describing an escape room puzzle he was designing in his workshop, something he found calming and positive. If a person has trouble with visualization, a photo or video can be used which they can store on their phone. Others may want to draw, model, or use a soft toy or animal. The purpose of the "calm place" is to access feelings of safety and therapists can be creative in how they achieve this.

EMDR Processing

The therapist started with the standard EMDR protocol which she modified in response to Donny's needs.

Donny initially reported no emotional connection to his memories from childhood and so the decision was taken to start with recent events. A visit to the allergy clinic was chosen. During the visit, Donny had become very distressed and had corralled himself in a corner to protect himself. Emotional activation of a target memory is an essential part of the EMDR protocol. Therapists may need to be adaptable in order to help their client connect with their emotions, including being flexible about what is chosen as a target.

The protocol requires a person to hold in mind a traumatic memory and identify the negative belief they have about themselves which still feels true now. Donny found the challenge of holding the past in mind while identifying present day beliefs extremely difficult. The therapist adapted by asking him about his feelings and sensations. He described terror, and the therapist asked if "I'm not safe" fitted with the memory. Donny confirmed that it did. In the standard protocol, this "negative cognition" usually comes from the client. Suggesting a negative cognition is an adaptation used with those who find it hard to verbalize their thoughts.

Box 15-1

CASE CONCEPTUALIZATION WITH THE AIP MODEL

Past experiences: Donny found school difficult and perceived it as a hostile environment. Social and sensory problems meant he was confused and overwhelmed for much of primary school. He tried to escape but was punished for it, which was traumatic. Diagnosis came at the end of primary school when he transferred to a secondary school for those with mild to moderate intellectual disabilities.

Secondary school was difficult due to the behavior of the other students. He became anxious about what he was eating as he felt unwell for much of the time. Health problems were dismissed by doctors until he was almost adult, when he was diagnosed with intolerances to dairy and legumes. Family attachments were strong and positive.

Unprocessed memories: 1. Punishment by head teacher at age 9 by being isolated in his office. 2. Visiting doctor aged 8 and being diagnosed as malingering. 3. Physical violence by other students at secondary school. 4. Bullying at primary school. 5. More recent memories of visiting allergy clinics.

All these events were linked by the underlying negative belief "*I am not safe.*" Related to this was another belief: "*I am powerless.*"

Present day consequences: Donny lives his life as if he is not safe. He is lacking trust in health professionals. He is restricting food choices with health and social consequences, as he cannot eat away from home and will only eat very few foods. His feelings of powerlessness mean that he does not believe that his voice will be heard and his opinions taken into account. He has an ongoing feeling of lack of safety and the necessity to protect himself. All of this means that he does not have confidence that he will be safe without the intense threat response which has been labelled a "needle phobia."

Strengths and resilience: Donny's special interests are linked to keeping himself safe, escapology, and martial arts. He is extremely talented at devising escape room puzzles. He has positive relationships with family and makes friends through his special interests. His interests provide a feeling of safety, connection to others, and a chance to develop competence and mastery. Donny is in a stable living situation where he is happy and holds down a job.

Goals/future: Donny's family want him to have allergy testing to expand his diet. Donny wants to be able to make his own decisions about allergy testing and other important decisions in his life. The therapist would like to help Donny feel safer and more in control of his life.

Processing began with the allergy clinic memory. Donny rated the distress associated with the memory as a 9/10 using a visual scale, an adaptation often used with children. The therapist used eye movements, which Donny initially found difficult but was able to follow after some practice. When processing became blocked, the therapist asked him to "float back" to an earlier time when he had felt the same. When therapists intervene in the processing, this is called a "cognitive

Box 15-2

Adaptations Made at Each Stage of Donny's EMDR Therapy

Preparation:

Therapeutic relationship established using interests as basis for communication and conversation.

Resource imagery developed from special interests (competency, control and mastery).

Calm place established from interests and explored in the here and now, using videos and pictures as cues.

Psychoeducation regarding being heard, expressing self, and making choices.

Context The importance of the symptoms was explored and discussed with Donny and his family.

Processing:

The standard EMDR protocol was initially used but a recent event was used as the target since Donny connected more easily with this.

Adaptations were made as necessary (e.g. the assessment phase was somewhat simplified in a way which is often used with children). Sessions were sometimes shorter than usual, to avoid overwhelming Donny.

Donny found it hard to identify cognitions and to distinguish between how his thoughts about himself in relation to a past memory, and his thoughts about his life now.

The therapist helped Donny make the connection between how he had felt more recently and how he had felt in the past by explicitly asking about this. She suggested possible thoughts based on how Donny described his emotions.

Cognitive interweaves were used with a special focus on avoiding non-literal use of language.

The therapist used sessions of talking interspersed with the EMDR sessions to talk about what Donny was remembering and to identify new target memories.

Donny required support in verbalising his negative belief in relation to the traumatic event (I am not safe) but was well able to identify his emotions. This enabled the therapist to guess at the negative belief. Other people may be able to identify body sensations or thoughts but not emotions. It is not always necessary to name emotions as long as a body sensation can be identified and emotional activation has occurred.

Eye movements were used as Donny tolerated these well. Distress levels were collected using a visual scale.

Donny's distress reduced but his beliefs related to the memory did not become more adaptive, and so further adaptations were made. These included proactive introduction of imagery into the processing and use of the EMDR Storytelling technique (Logie et al 2020).

Outcome:

Adaptive Beliefs Donny reported adaptive thoughts such as "I can choose what I do now, it was different when I was young" and 'I am safe now, they can't make me do things'.

Systemic change Donny's family committed to fully involving him in decisions about his healthcare and to respect his right to say no. Donny therefore felt safer in his ability to consent and refuse treatment.

Behavioural change Donny was able to have the allergy testing without problems. Goals for therapy had been met and discharge was requested.

---

interweave." These interweaves are usually very brief and can include a question or the introduction of new information. However, with autistic clients interweaves can be a source of confusion if they are not carefully considered. Language may be understood literally, meaning that phrases commonly used in the EMDR process such as "go with that" may not make sense to the client (who might think, "Go where? Why do I need to go anywhere?"). Clearer alternatives can be used.

Donny did not understand what was meant by "float back," (a term he associated with swimming) so the therapist asked "Does the way you feel now remind you of times in the past?" Donny then recalled a memory of being isolated in the head teacher's office. The therapist told him to notice that and continued with the BLS.

Despite what looked like effective processing, Donny's progress was unusual. He rated his distress as low (0.5/10), but continued to say that he did not feel safe when he thought about that memory. When asked why this was, he said that he could not feel safe when he thought about the allergy clinic, since he actually wasn't safe. His reasoning was that when he went outside, people shouted at him in the street (because his appearance and dress was unusual), making him feel unsafe. His thinking style made it hard for him to distinguish between how he felt now, and how he felt in relation to the memory.

The therapist suspected his beliefs about other people were rooted in other early experiences which he was not linking to spontaneously during processing. They spent a session talking about his childhood. The therapist asked specific questions about Donny's feelings as a child based on his history. Donny talked about a bad memory from secondary school. Another boy had become angry and thrown a desk, narrowly missing Donny's head. Donny was expected to continue to sit next to this boy in class even though he was scared. Donny had felt that he didn't matter and that he was powerless. The therapist felt that Donny's feelings of powerlessness could be related to his feeling unsafe in the present day. She suggested to Donny that part of his brain might have "got stuck" on feeling powerless when he was at school, and that the part hadn't updated even though things had changed. She used the metaphor of one person getting stuck on a puzzle in an escape room, and continuing to work on it even though the time was up and the game over.

The therapist took a more proactive role in the processing than would usually be the case. In particular, she provided more scaffolding to help Donny connect with adaptive memory networks. She spent a session talking about the links between present-day beliefs and past experiences. She used interweaves to link to the past and was more directive and less socratic that usual.

Donny's difficulty in shifting to more adaptive cognitions with this memory then led the therapist to try a narrative technique. A short story describing difficult events in his life (using EMDR story-telling techniques; Logie et al., 2020) was written. This story included all elements of the EMDR protocol, including an adaptive ending. Donny listened to the story while tracking eye movements. The story ended with the central character feeling safer in the knowledge that he could make choices and that the people around him would listen.

Donny engaged well with the story. For the first time he spontaneously expressed some adaptive thoughts, such as "I can choose what I do now, it was different when I was young" and "I am safe now, they can't make me do things."

Further sessions were planned after a holiday. However, following the break an email from Donny's mother arrived. Donny had completed the allergy testing, thanked the therapist for her help, and decided that further sessions were not required. A closure session was offered but Donny did not feel it was necessary. An abrupt or unplanned ending can, in our experience, be a feature of working with some autistic people. This is perhaps due to honesty about their preference to stop once their goals have been achieved, when others might feel a social pressure to continue.

CONCLUSION

This case study illustrates how flexible EMDR therapists need to be when working with autistic individuals, and how an apparently simple phobia presentation may be linked with earlier events. For Donny, the experience of growing up autistic and an intellectual disability had shaped the way he felt about the world.

Donny's phobia was important to him because it enabled him to say no, and he had had experiences in the past where his voice was ignored. It was necessary to get agreement from everyone involved in Donny's life that that a resolved phobia would not be used as a reason to pressure him to submit to testing. Donny ended EMDR therapy feeling that he had more power in the present than he had had in the past. He used this power to end the therapy on his terms.

Donny's case illustrates the importance of seeing an individual in context, particularly those who may have limited autonomy. It is important that the therapist does not take on the agenda of the client's family or support team without asking what the client individually wants. EMDR should not be used as a way to make people's behavior more convenient to others when their behavior might have an important function.

SUMMARY

EMDR is a promising therapy for autistic people. Access to EMDR therapy may be an issue due to a tendency by services to see anxiety and challenging behavior as autistic traits, rather than reactions to adverse experiences. To use EMDR effectively, we need to widen our perspective on trauma, focusing on how people experience the events of their lives, and then adapt the protocol as necessary to enable them to process. Formulation is essential, and the therapist will need be ready to adapt to each person's individual needs as they go along.

REFERENCES

Barol, B. I., & Seubert, A. (2010). Stepping stones: EMDR treatment of individuals with intellectual and developmental disabilities and challenging behavior. *Journal of EMDR Practice and Research, 4*(4), 156–169.

Caspi, A., Houts, R. M., Belsky, D. W., Goldman-Mellor, S. J., Harrington, H., Israel, S., Meier, M. H., Ramrakha, S., Shalev, I., Poulton, R., & Moffitt, T. E. (2014). The p factor: One general psychopathology factor in the structure of psychiatric disorders? *Clinical Psychological Science, 2*(2), 119–137.

Chen, L., Zhang, G., Hu, M., & Liang, X. (2015). Eye movement desensitization and reprocessing versus cognitive-behavioral therapy for adult posttraumatic stress disorder: Systematic review and meta-analysis. *Journal of Nervous and Mental Disease, 203*(6), 443–451.

Hengartner, M. P., & Lehmann, S. N. (2017). Why psychiatric research must abandon traditional diagnostic classification and adopt a fully dimensional scope: Two solutions to a persistent problem. *Frontiers in Psychiatry, 8,* 101.

Insel, T., Cuthbert, B., Garvey, M., Heinssen, R., Pine, D. S., Quinn, K., & Wang, P. (2010). Research domain criteria (RDoC): Toward a new classification framework for research on mental disorders. *American Journal of Psychiatry, 167*(7), 748–751.

Kerns, C. M., Newschaffer, C. J., & Berkowitz, S. J. (2015). Traumatic childhood events and autism spectrum disorder. *Journal of Autism and Developmental Disorders, 45,* 3475–3486.

Khan, A. M., Dar, S., Ahmed, R., Bachu, R., Adnan, M., & Kotapati, V. P. (2018). Cognitive behavioral therapy versus eye movement desensitization and reprocessing in patients with post-traumatic stress disorder: Systematic review and meta-analysis of randomized clinical trials. *Cureus, 10*(9), e3250.

Kosatka, D., & Ona, C. (2014). Eye Movement Desensitization and Reprocessing in a Patient with Asperger's Disorder: Case Report. *Journal of EMDR Practice and Research, 8*(1).

Livingston, L., Shah, P., & Happe, F. (2019). Compensatory strategies below the behavioural surface in autism. A qualitative study. *Lancet Psychiatry, 6,* 766–777.

Leuning, E. (2020). *The efficacy of EMDR in youngsters with autism (EYE-catcher)* [Paper presentation]. EMDR Congress, The Netherlands.

Logie, R., Bowers, M., Dent, A., Elliott, J., O'Connor, M & Russell, A. (2020). *A guide to the storytelling (narrative) approach to EMDR therapy.* Trauma Aid UK.

Morris-Smith, J., & Silvestre, M. (2014). Autistic spectrum disorders. In *EMDR for the next generation: Healing children and families.* Academic Publishing International Ltd.

Novo Navarro P., Landin-Romero, R., Guardiola-Wanden-Berghe, R., Moreno-Alcázar, A., Valiente-Gómez, A., Lupo, W., García, F., Fernández, I., Pérez, V., & Amann, B.

L. (2018). 25 years of eye movement desensitization and reprocessing (EMDR): The EMDR therapy protocol, hypotheses of its mechanism of action and a systematic review of its efficacy in the treatment of post-traumatic stress disorder. *Rev Psiquiatr Salud Ment (Engl. Ed.)*, *11*(2), 101–114.

Poe, C. A. (2019). *How to be autistic*. Myriad Editions.

Propper, R., & Christman, S. (2008). Interhemispheric Interaction and Saccadic Horizontal Eye Movements, Implications for Episodic Memory, EMDR, and PTSD. *Journal of EMDR Practice and Research*, *2*(4).

Ratcliffe A. (2020). *Our autistic lives: Personal accounts from autistic adults around the world aged 20–70+*. Jessica Kingsley Publishers

Rowe, A. (2013). *The girl with the curly hair: Asperger's and Me*. Lonely Mind Books.

Rodenburg, R., Benjamin, A., de Roos, C., Meijer, A. M., & Stams, G. J. (2009). Efficacy of EMDR in children: a meta-analysis. *Clinical Psychology Review*, *29*(7), 599–606.

Shapiro, F. (1989). Eye movement desensitization. *Journal of Behavior Therapy and Experimental Psychiatry*, *20*, 211–217.

Shapiro, F. (2007). EMDR, adaptive information processing, and case conceptualization. *Journal of EMDR Practice and Research*, *1*, 68–87.

Stickgold, R. (2002). EMDR: A putative neurobiological mechanism of action. *Journal of Clinical Psychology*, *58*, 61–75.

Solomon, R. M., & Shapiro, F. (2008). EMDR and the adaptive information processing model: Potential mechanisms of change. *Journal of EMDR Practice and Research*, *2*(4), 315–325. https://doi.org/10.1891/1933-3196.2.4.315

Taylor, J. L., & Gotham, K. O. (2016). Cumulative life events, traumatic experiences, and psychiatric symptomatology in transition-aged youth with autism spectrum disorder. *Journal of Developmental Disorders*, *8*, 28.

Valiente-Gomes, A., Moreno-Alcazar, A., Treen, D., Cedron, C., Colom, F, Perez, V., & Amann, B. L. (2017). EMDR beyond PTSD: A systematic literature review. *Frontiers in Psychology*, *8*, 1668.

Van den Berg, D. P., de Bont, P. A., van der Vleugel, B. M., de Roos, C., de Jongh, A., Van Minnen, A., & van der Gaag, M. (2015). Prolonged exposure vs eye movement desensitization and reprocessing vs waiting list for posttraumatic stress disorder in patients with a psychotic disorder a randomized clinical trial. *JAMA Psychiatry*, *2*, 259–267.

Van den Hout, M. A., & Engelhard, I. M. (2012). How does EMDR work? *Journal of Experimental Psychopathology*, 724–738.

Van den Hout, M. A, Bartelski, N., & Engelhard, I. M. (2013). On EMDR: Eye movements during retrieval reduce subjective vividness and objective memory accessibility during future recall, *Cognition and Emotion*, *27*(1), 177–183.

Varese, F., Smeets, F., Drukker, M., Lieverse, R., Lataster, T., Viechtbauer, W., Read, J., van Os, J., & Bentall, R. P. (2012). Childhood adversities increase the risk of psychosis: A meta-analysis of patient-control, prospective-and cross-sectional cohort studies. *Schizophrenia Bulletin*, *38*(4), 661–671.

Williams, D. (1998). *Nobody nowhere: The remarkable autobiography of an autistic girl*. Jessica Kingsley Publishers Ltd.

16

Group-Based Interventions

PETER E. LANGDON, ADAM ROBERTSON, AND
THECLA FELLAS ■

KEY CONSIDERATIONS

- Fear of stigma and discrimination may lead some individuals to avoid taking part in groups.
- Strategies to promote group cohesion are likely to lead to better outcomes from group work.
- Specific adaptations are required for autistic adults when taking part in group work. This can include adaptations to the physical environment, the structure and routine of groups, and the pace and style of communication. Further adaptations are needed to the content of the group, depending upon its purpose. For example, if you are running an anxiety-management group, you may need to provide further teaching about emotions, autism, and mental health.
- Collaboratively running groups with autistic adults may help overcome some of the barriers faced when accessing groups by increasing a sense of belonging and improving group cohesion.

GROUP-BASED INTERVENTIONS FOR AUTISTIC ADULTS

Group-based psychological therapies and interventions have been shown to be effective for a range of mental health problems such as depression (Huntley et al., 2012; McDermut et al., 2001), symptoms of psychosis (Burlingame et al., 2020), insomnia (Koffel et al., 2015), anxiety (Barkowski et al., 2020), including social anxiety (Barkowski et al., 2016), and skills teaching, such as social skills teaching with those who have psychosis (Pfammatter et al., 2006). While this evidence is positive, there is also some evidence that individually delivered psychological therapy, relative to group-based approaches, may be associated with more positive outcomes immediately after treatment, and while the dropout rate tends to be lower within individual treatment relative to group-based treatment (Cuijpers et al., 2008), some of the treatment benefits associated with individual therapy may lessen over time relative to group-based therapy (Cuijpers et al., 2008; Huntley et al., 2012). Others have suggested that individually delivered psychological therapies may be associated with larger effect sizes for some with developmental disabilities, and specifically adults with intellectual disabilities (Vereenooghe & Langdon, 2013). There are several challenges associated with offering group-based psychological therapies, especially considering tentative evidence to suggest that in some circumstances individual therapy may be preferential, and many of these challenges are markedly relevant to autistic people.

THE CHALLENGES ASSOCIATED WITH GROUP-BASED PSYCHOLOGICAL THERAPY

Strauss, Spangenberg, Brähler, and Bormann (2015), drawing upon ideas that group-based interventions may be unpopular and avoided by those seeking help for mental health problems because of issues associated with disclosure, uneasiness, and anxiety (Hahn, 2009), surveyed a large sample of adults in an attempt to understand factors that impact upon willingness to engage in group psychotherapy. They reported that women had more positive attitudes and greater knowledge toward group psychotherapy relative to men. Further, while there were some positive attitudes toward group psychotherapy, some reported anxiety, and concerns about rejection within groups, with it being noted that those reporting positive experiences were those who had more experience of group psychotherapy. They noted that those who preferred groups tended to have fewer difficulties with anxiety, depression, and emotional burnout, which may lead to an assumption that groups may not be the most preferential method for those with more severe mental health difficulties.

Related to this, an important construct that is relevant to our understanding of the utilization of group psychotherapy is stigma. This can act as a substantial barrier to seeking help for mental health problems, as individuals avoid seeking help due to fear of being labelled in a pejorative manner. Autistic people experience stigma, and although there is some evidence to suggest that self-stigma rates may be lower for those with autism, stigmatizing societal conceptualizations of autism continue and may affect mental health, including the mental health of families and caregivers (Bachmann et al., 2019; Botha et al., 2020; Dubreucq et al., 2020; Papadopoulos et al., 2019). Corrigan (2004) argued that one of the reasons that people do not seek help for their mental health problems is an attempt to hide their problems from others because of stigma and discrimination, as behavior seen as unusual is judged negatively. Individuals seek to avoid being portrayed as part of a group that is stereotyped to avoid negative emotional reactions and judgments from others, and consequently they avoid seeking help that may assist them in recovery. Such attitudes, stigma, and discrimination can be internalized and have a negative impact upon an individual's view of themselves, exacerbating their distress, increasing their avoidance of help, and increasing their belief that they are low-value individuals, often provoking shame. Corrigan (2004) conceptualized stigma as a substantial public health concern.

Within group-based psychotherapy, individuals may avoid taking part because of stigma and associated fears that they may be judged negatively by other participants or their communities. Individuals may avoid disclosure, experience anxiety, fear rejection, and express concerns that other group members may disclose their personal information outside of the group. Vogel, Wade, and Hackler (2007) demonstrated that public stigma about mental health predicted self-stigma, which had a negative impact upon attitudes toward counseling. Both self-stigma and attitudes about counseling mediated the relationship between wider stigma and help seeking.

Nevertheless, group-based psychotherapies are often construed as more cost-effective due to a reduction in therapist costs, but the evidence for this is mixed (Tucker & Oei, 2007). There is evidence that internet-delivered therapy is more cost-effective than group-based approaches for social anxiety disorder (Hedman et al., 2011), which has been demonstrated in a further study where a range of individually delivered cognitive behavior therapies (CBT) was shown to be the most cost effective (Mavranezouli et al., 2015). Group-based psychotherapies are often seen as offering an opportunity for participants to develop a sense of belonging and relating to a group of others with shared experiences, allowing for additional opportunities to learn and feel connected.

Burlingame, McClendon, and Yang (2018) demonstrated that group cohesion within group psychotherapy accounts for positive treatment outcome across a range of studies. They discussed some of the challenges associated with defining group cohesion, which often includes reference to acceptance, interpersonal factors, well-being, attendance, attrition, the use of nonverbal communication, and engagement. More broadly, it refers to the quality of the relationships between therapists and group members and the relationships between group members with reference to concepts such as warmth, genuineness, and emotional bond. Burlingame et al. (2018) reported that participant sex, age, or diagnosis did not explain the relationship between cohesion and treatment outcome within groups, while an interpersonal orientation among therapists did, and to a lesser degree this was the case for therapists who adopted another orientation such as psychodynamic or cognitive-behavioral. A positive relationship between cohesion and treatment outcome was also seen within studies where increased focus was given to enhancing cohesion within sessions. Further, they also demonstrated that groups made up of volunteers or those that were task-focused (i.e., problem solving, goal focused, and not psychological therapy) tended to have a stronger positive relationship between cohesion and outcome relative to psychotherapy and support groups. The relationship was also stronger for groups where there was a focus upon interaction within the group and the group comprised those with similar diagnoses, while an increasing number of sessions was also associated with a stronger relationship. Specifically, those groups with 20 or more sessions fared better; the relationship decreased as the number of sessions decreased. Finally, they found that group size moderated the relationship between cohesion and positive outcomes; specifically, groups comprising five to nine participants had the largest positive relationship between cohesion and treatment outcome, while smaller and larger groups did not.

GROUP-BASED PSYCHOLOGICAL THERAPY
FOR ADULTS WITH AUTISM SPECTRUM DISORDER

Group-based interventions for autistic adults have been commonplace within many countries as clinicians, educators, and others attempt to help autistic people who have mental health problems and associated challenges related to autism. Autism is associated with difficulties with social communication and interaction, as well as restricted and repetitive behaviors, and many have attempted to help autistic people with social interaction through the provision of group-based interventions. Often, the premise, considering the intervention is delivered within a group, is that it provides an opportunity for individuals to meet others, form relationships, and practice social skills. There are other group-based interventions which focus more upon mental health, with anxiety being of particular interest, as difficulties with anxiety are frequently experienced by autistic people (Lai et al., 2019). Again, groups themselves have been conceptualized as a way of exposing individuals to feared social situations, allowing for anxiety to be induced while encouraging the development of skills through teaching and vicarious and direct learning.

Many factors such as social functioning, skills, and motivation (Bellini, 2004, 2006; Factor et al., 2016; Kamp-Becker et al., 2009); a lack of flexibility and an insistence upon sameness (Black et al., 2017; Hollocks et al., 2014; Wallace et al., 2016); sensory issues (Black et al., 2017; Uljarevic et al., 2016); and intolerance of uncertainty (Vasa et al., 2018; Wigham et al., 2015) have direct implications for the therapeutic process. Often, specific adaptations are needed for therapy or group-based interventions to promote inclusion considering the difficulties that are faced by autistic people. This can include: (a) adapting the physical environment to minimize the impact of sensory issues, such as problems with lights, temperature, and sound, and working with group members to help develop an understanding of the role that sensory issues have in their experience of anxiety and avoidance; (b) adapting the structure and routine of the group to meet the needs of autistic people by making sure it is clear and focused and sharing agendas with group members in advance so that they know the topics that are to be discussed and how the sessions will be run; and (c) adapting the pace and communication used during the sessions to meet the needs of autistic people (e.g., avoiding the use of complex verbal and abstract information). This would also include making sure that therapists, session leaders, and group members are well versed in the idiosyncratic nature of speech that is used by some autistic people. The inclusion of visual aids, role play, and technology can be helpful to encourage engagement and skill acquisition. Therapist or group leaders may need to be more direct in their communication with autistic people within group sessions to avoid misunderstandings. Further, some focus will be needed, considering the nature of the group intervention, upon teaching about emotions, autism, and mental health. Group members may wish to share information about their interests with others. There may be some group members who will readily wish to hear about the interests of others, while other group members may find this challenging and difficult. Scheduling time within groups to talk about interests can be helpful. Depending upon the nature of the group and participants, it may be helpful to include parents or carers who may be able to support individuals further outside of sessions. If there are tasks to be completed outside of sessions, it is important to be flexible and considerate about the nature of this work and the medium used to help participants to understand and complete tasks. This could be providing information in audio or visual form, or where possible making use of technology such as mobile telephones and computers, as well as carers or supporters. Computer-based cognitive remediation therapy, which includes taking part in both a social-cognitive group and computer-based training, has been shown to be more effective than supportive therapy in improving attention, processing speed, affective management, social cognition, and subsequent employment (Eack et al., 2018). Further, therapists and group facilitators will need to consider the marked heterogeneity among group members, which can impact upon the therapeutic process and the group. For example, some individuals may prefer the room to be warm, while others prefer a cool room, and this may lead to conflict. Some participants may wish to talk only about circumscribed interests, while others may need time to engage in sensory stimulation, or others may experience strong emotional reactions and need time to process what is happening and manage their emotion. There may be miscommunication within sessions, which may lead to conflict. This can be related to language problems and difficulties with understanding social communication, while for others, when using a manualized intervention, they may feel that their individual needs are not being addressed effectively and increased flexibility may be required at times. Many of the changes that have been made to CBT when used with autistic people have been described (Walters et al., 2016).

Recently, Adams and Young (2020) undertook a systematic review of studies that described factors that promote or interfere with psychological treatment for autistic people, synthesizing a helpful list of factors that have implications for the provision of group-based interventions for autistic people. Their findings indicated that therapists or professionals who lack knowledge about autism, interventions that are not tailored to meet the needs of autistic people, increasing waiting lists, not understanding how to access interventions within the care system, not meeting service criteria or being referred between services, difficulties with communication that are likely related to autism, difficulties with scheduling and finding time to take part, and finding it difficult to trust professionals, among other reasons, were all likely barriers faced by autistic people when trying to access psychological therapies. At the same time, they identified that consistency of service provision, including having the same therapist and regular sessions, were helpful, as was the willingness of services to make adaptations to meet the needs of autistic people. Together, these findings strongly support the argument that services need to adapt their provision to meet the needs of autistic people, which would include autistic-tailored or specific mental health interventions.

There is evidence that group-delivered social skill teaching for autistic youth is helpful and effect sizes have been reported to be large based on self-report measures, but small for parent- or observer-based ratings of outcome (Gates et al., 2017). This is the reverse to what has been reported for CBT with autistic youth and adults, where effect sizes based upon self-report measures were small and informant- and therapist-rated outcomes were associated with medium effect sizes (Weston et al., 2016). There are similarities and differences between group-based interventions that aim to improve social skills and interaction and group-based CBT for autistic people. For example, many social skills programs involve psychoeducation about social skills, emotions, nonverbal and verbal communication, and relationships, along with the inclusion of role play and specific tasks in and outside of group sessions (Ashman et al., 2017), where there is a focus upon tasks and teaching, with some programs also making use of video modeling. Other groups focused upon social skills may also incorporate aspects of CBT, for example teaching about cognitive mediation, how to challenge unhelpful ways of thinking, and the inclusion of some behavioral interventions (Spain et al., 2017). Social skills programs that do and do not explicitly include components of CBT have been described elsewhere, including programs where parents are included (Cappadocia & Weiss, 2011), and these interventions, associated outcome measures, and characteristics have been summarized (McMahon et al., 2013; Miller et al., 2014). There have been some trials comparing group CBT and group recreational activity where there was no difference in outcome, but attrition was reported to be lower within group CBT, with autistic people who received CBT rating well-being as more increased (Hesselmark et al., 2014).

SOCIAL GROUPS

There has been an increase in self-help groups or groups that have been developed, led, and run by autistic people for autistic people, sometimes with additional support from health and social care professionals. Many of these groups are run within the charitable sector, and an example of such a group is one run by Asperger East Anglia, a charity in the east of England. For many who make use of the services offered by the charity, the only opportunity to meet others socially is within these social groups. These flagship groups tend to be popular and attendance is frequently high. At the moment, there are over 50 members registered to take part. The charity has also experienced an increase in the number of autistic adults seeking social support due to increased feelings of loneliness and isolation, which is thought to be related to the COVID-19 pandemic.

Prior to the COVID-19 pandemic and the associated restrictions, the social groups met in person every 2 weeks for 2 hours on the same day and at the same time. Each group was specifically organized around a planned activity, and decisions about the activities were made by the people attending the group. Many of the planned activities had a fun and light-hearted theme that aimed to encourage and promote the sharing of experiences, increase social communication, and allow members to practice and develop their social skills. Charity-employed staff helped to organize and assist group members to deliver the chosen activities, which included quiz and bingo nights, talent contests, board games, and evenings where they talked about and shared special interests. A strong focus within the groups was the development of a culture that is both supportive and nonjudgmental, promoting inclusion, reducing stigma, and providing an opportunity for what is hoped to be a positive experience for members.

The most popular organized activities included those that focused heavily upon promoting community inclusion. These included going to the pub, bowling, trampolining, having a meal in a restaurant, attending the theatre, going on bus trip outings, and boat trips on the picturesque and rather pleasant Norfolk broads. The Norfolk broads, also known as the The Broads National Park in England, contains interconnected rivers and lakes that are used for boating. For many, engagement in these activities would not have been possible outside of the social groups. The inclusion that develops within both groups and the community through group participation is of marked value to members. They form and develop relationships with likeminded people who share similar interests and have encountered similar problems. Through the groups, many find acceptance and peer support, which can lead to a reduction in anxiety, and an increase in engagement within local communities through the participation of activities that are rewarding. It is important to mention that the global pandemic has led to these groups being delivered online using videoconferencing software. Staff have noted that this change has not led to a reduction in attendance and the groups have continued to provide a way for many autistic people to connect and share their experiences, increasing opportunities to feel valued and to experience social inclusion.

Autistic adults have said that these groups bring individuals together to share experiences and provide support to one another. The groups are ability focused, taking in the needs of everyone into account, rather than focusing upon disability. Group members have said that the groups allow people to socialize, and this is important for people who find socializing difficult. At the same time, some have said that being part of a group made up of autistic people has meant that many do not worry about having to change their behavior by attempting to make use of eye contact or appropriate body language, as they are surrounded by neurodiverse people. Together, within the group, there is a sense of equality and disability solidarity; individuals come together to lament that they are perceived as inferior to others by some neurotypical individuals. Some have commented that they have a variety of skills to offer an employer and wish to have paid employment, and the group has helped them to realize this and increase their confidence. One individual has said that being part of the group has helped them to escape the "rat race" of the employment market and to appreciate their employment and focus less on materialism. They commented that they have come to learn that real friends judge you on your character. On the negative side, some have commented that the social groups lack diversity, there are fewer women, and not many people from Black, Asian, and minority ethnic communities attend. Sometimes members have made comments that have offended others, which have had to be managed.

Overall, these groups provide an excellent opportunity for autistic adults to learn new skills while promoting social inclusion. The theory underpinning these groups, with a focus upon engagement in activities that are rewarding while also providing an opportunity to practice and develop social skills, is similar to that underpinning behavioral activation, a well-established psychological therapy for depression (Kanter et al., 2010; Veale, 2018). For many autistic people, various aspects of daily living may become associated with negative emotions, leading to avoidance and the development of aversive control. Avoidance of activities may be more likely to lead to a cessation of aversive feelings associated with these activities, otherwise known as negative reinforcement, and a reduced probability that an individual will encounter positive reinforcers. At the same time, and important for autistic people, they may have a restricted or narrowed range of activities that tend to be associated with positive reinforcement, and they may have some difficulties with eliciting positive reinforcement. For example, they may experience less enjoyment from some types of social interaction. However, engagement in activities may restrict further, as avoidance increases, which increases the risk of developing mental health problems, including depression. This can become a vicious cycle of avoidance and increasing restriction of activities, and in turn this avoidance maintains and increases their experiences of low mood and/or anxiety. The positive reinforcement strength and quality previously associated with activities may be reduced. Aversive control can develop where activities that were associated with positive reinforcement are avoided as they are perceived to be aversive (Kaiser et al., 2016). There is some promising evidence that guided self-help, adapted for use with autistic adults and based upon behavioral activation, is a useful treatment for low mood and depression among autistic adults (Russell et al., 2019).

The social groups that are run by Asperger East Anglia encourage adults to work together and collaboratively choose which activities they which to engage in, and together they work effectively to take part in these activities; this engagement and the completion of the activities are likely associated with positive reinforcement, and the peer-related support that is integral to these groups is likely to help encourage participation. As the activities allow for the development of an increasing behavioral repertoire, a previously established cycle of avoidance because of aversive feelings is disrupted, allowing individuals to experience positive reinforcement, which will have positive effects upon their mental health. At the same time, as these groups are run collaboratively with autistic people, some of the barriers to taking part in group-based interventions may be reduced. The groups are made up of volunteers, and the development of a sense of feeling part of community, the development of friendships and bonds, a reduction in hiding problems from others because of stigma and discrimination or concerns that your behavior may be judged negatively, the inclusion of individuals with the same diagnosis, a focus upon interaction, and the scheduling of task-focused sessions are likely to promote positive outcomes though the development of stronger group cohesion (Burlingame et al., 2020). However, the outcomes from these groups have not been formally examined, and while there is evidence to suggest that mutual-help groups are helpful for mental health problems, this literature has not focused upon autistic adults (Pistrang et al., 2008). Investigation is needed into the potential beneficial impact of self-help social groups for autistic people.

GROUP-BASED PSYCHOLOGICAL THERAPIES

On the other hand, there are group-based psychological therapies for autistic adults where the focus is upon attempting to treat mental illness. This includes groups developed and designed for the treatment of anxiety disorders, including obsessive compulsive disorder. An example of such a group was developed for use with autistic adults who have anxiety disorder and used during the PAsSA trial (Doble et al., 2017; Langdon et al., 2013, 2016). The intervention is manualized and is available from the authors.

The intervention involved 24 sessions, and the first three were individual sessions designed to orient an individual to the group sessions, address any concerns, share the timetable and agendas, begin socializing the individual into homework tasks, and work toward building some initial rapport. The 21 group-based sessions and their aims are found in Table 16-1.

Within a single-blind randomized pilot trial of this intervention, the authors demonstrated that the conversion rate was high and the attrition rate was low for participants in the trial. Bearing in mind that this was a pilot trial that was not powered to test the clinical efficacy of the intervention, both those who received the intervention and those within the waiting list improved over time and there was no difference between the two arms in the trial at endpoint. A supplementary analysis using data of only those who attended at least 50% of the treatment sessions was suggestive of an improved treatment response (Langdon et al., 2016).

Notably, participants were interviewed about their experiences taking part in group-based psychological therapy for anxiety. Nearly 60% of participants said that they now knew how to manage anxiety following treatment, and just over half agreed that their anxiety had decreased. Almost 40% agreed that the session time was too short, and they wanted longer and more sessions. Nearly 80% reported that hearing other participants talk about their experiences was helpful, and nearly 80% felt supported by other group members. Seventy-three percent of participants said that they would recommend this therapy to others and agreed that therapy had been helpful. Further interviews with participants

Table 16-1 A DESCRIPTION OF THE GROUP-BASED SESSIONS USED TO TREAT ANXIETY AMONG AUTISTIC ADULTS

Session Number	Aims
1	• Introductions—getting to know one another • Discuss the group rationale and format • Devise the group rules • Assign homework—rating subjective units of distress
2	• Review of the previous session and homework • Psychoeducation about autism and anxiety • Assign homework—rating subjective units of distress
3	• Review of the previous session and homework • More psychoeducation about anxiety • Assign homework—rating subjective units of distress
4	• Review of the previous session and homework • Psychoeducation about cognitive-behavioral therapy and the cognitive model—learning to identify thoughts, feelings, and behaviors • Assign homework—rating subjective units of distress and identifying thoughts, feelings, and behaviors
5	• Review of the previous session and homework • Cognitive mediation training • Cognitive metallization training • Assign homework—rating subjective units of distress and identifying thoughts, feelings, and behaviors
6	• Review of the previous session and homework • Psychoeducation about obsessions, compulsions, and obsessive-compulsive disorder • Assign homework—rating subjective units of distress and identifying thoughts, feelings, and behaviors
7	• Review of the previous session and homework • Introduction to social skills training • Social skills role play • Assign homework—rating subjective units of distress and identifying thoughts, feelings, and behaviors
8	• Review of the previous session and homework • Social skills role play • Assign homework—completion of social situations recording sheets
9	• Review of the previous session and homework • Social skills role play • Program recap • Assign homework—completion of social situations recording sheets
10	• Review of the previous session and homework • Introduction to relaxation • Practicing relaxation • Assign homework—to practice the relaxation techniques over and record

(*continued*)

Table 16-1 CONTINUED

Session Number	Aims
11	• Review of the previous session and homework • Negative automatic thoughts, assumptions, and beliefs • Anxiety and vicious cycles • Assign homework—to practice the relaxation techniques over and record thoughts, assumptions, and beliefs
12	• Review of the previous session and homework • Negative automatic thoughts and thinking errors • Hypervigilance and selective attention • Assign homework—to practice the relaxation techniques over and record thoughts, assumptions, and beliefs
13	• Review of the previous session and homework • Cognitive restructuring • Assign homework—recording thoughts and considering possible, alternative explanations
14	• Review of the previous session and homework • More cognitive restructuring and positive beliefs • Assign homework—recording thoughts and considering possible, alternative explanations
15	• Review of the previous session and homework • Developing hierarchies of fears • Assign homework—recording thoughts and considering possible, alternative explanations
16	• Review of the previous session and homework • Systematic desensitization • Assign homework—practicing and recording systematic desensitization
17	• Review of the previous session and homework • Introducing behavioral experiments • Planning behavioral experiments • Assign homework—practicing and recording systematic desensitization
18	• Review of the previous session and homework • Doing behavioral experiments as a group • Assign homework—practicing and recording systematic desensitization
19	• Review of the previous session and homework • Doing behavioral experiments as a group • Assign homework—practicing and recording systematic desensitization
20	• Review of the previous session and homework • Discussing and reviewing behavioral experiments • Assign homework—practicing and recording systematic desensitization
21	• Review of the previous session and homework • Bringing it all together and becoming your own therapist

and the subsequent analysis indicated that participants who volunteered to take part in the trial did so because they wanted help for their mental health problems and recognized that anxiety was causing them problems. They described a series of positive experiences about taking part in therapy which included interacting with others with shared or similar experiences and learning that others have had similar problems. Some talked about how being in a group helped them to "open up" and share, while others commented about the value of learning new skills and the positive impacts the group had upon their lives. There were some important negative experiences shared with the research team, which included the sessions being too short because they needed longer to "warm up." Others talked about how some participants would talk too much about irrelevant issues, and this tended to be discussions about circumscribed interests, meaning that the therapists needed to sometimes work harder to refocus the group. Some individuals did find the experience of taking part in group therapy challenging and reflected that it was a negative experience for them (Langdon et al., 2016).

Finally, the participants made a series of suggestions for how group-based therapy for autistic adults could be improved. These suggestions included an increased focus upon preparatory work for some, especially those who found group work difficult. There was also a suggestion that a combination of individual and group-based interventions would be helpful as this would allow for individuals to focus more upon their problems with a therapist while working to help support others within the group-based sessions. Most notably, participants communicated that they wanted longer sessions to allow more in-depth work, and the inclusion of technology to help promote learning and the completion of homework tasks was thought likely valuable. Finally, they reported that challenges associated with using public transport, parking, the timings of some groups, and things like poor heating was an issue for them and required careful future planning.

CONCLUSIONS

Group-based interventions for autistic people have tended to focus upon the delivery of interventions for mental illness, social skills teaching, or a combination of the two. Autistic adults present with a variety of needs and groups need to be adapted to promote inclusion and skill acquisition. These adaptations should include a focus upon factors that promote group cohesion and involvement while also ensuring the needs of autistic adults are effectively addressed. There is evidence that social skills groups and interventions based upon CBT are effective, but there has been little exploration of the value and effectiveness of social groups run by autistic people for autistic people. Self-help groups have the potential to smash through barriers faced by autistic people when attempting to access interventions and thus to promote effective community inclusion.

REFERENCES

Adams, D., & Young, K. (2020). A systematic review of the perceived barriers and facilitators to accessing psychological treatment for mental health problems in individuals on the autism spectrum. *Review Journal of Autism and Developmental Disorders*, 1–18.

Ashman, R., Banks, K., Philip, R. C. M., Walley, R., & Stanfield, A. C. (2017). A pilot randomised controlled trial of a group based social skills intervention for adults with autism spectrum disorder. *Research in Autism Spectrum Disorders*, *43–44*, 67–75.

Bachmann, C. J., Hofer, J., Kamp-Becker, I., Kupper, C., Poustka, L., Roepke, S., Roessner, V., Stroth, S., Wolff, N., & Hoffmann, F. (2019). Internalised stigma in adults with autism: A German multi-center survey. *Psychiatry Research, 276*, 94–99.

Barkowski, S., Schwartze, D., Strauss, B., Burlingame, G. M., Barth, J., & Rosendahl, J. (2016). Efficacy of group psychotherapy for social anxiety disorder: A meta-analysis of randomized-controlled trials. *Journal of Anxiety Disorders, 39*, 44–64.

Barkowski, S., Schwartze, D., Strauss, B., Burlingame, G. M., & Rosendahl, J. (2020). Efficacy of group psychotherapy for anxiety disorders: A systematic review and meta-analysis. *Psychotherapy Research, 30*(8), 965–982.

Bellini, S. (2004). Social skill deficits and anxiety in high-functioning adolescents with autism spectrum disorders. *Focus on Autism and Other Developmental Disabilities, 19*(2), 78–86.

Bellini, S. (2006). The development of social anxiety in adolescents with autism spectrum disorders. *Focus on Autism and Other Developmental Disabilities, 21*(3), 138–145.

Black, K. R., Stevenson, R. A., Segers, M., Ncube, B. L., Sun, S. Z., Philipp-Muller, A., Bebko, J. M., Barense, M. D., & Ferber, S. (2017). Linking anxiety and insistence on sameness in autistic children: The role of sensory hypersensitivity. *Journal of Autism and Developmental Disorders, 47*(8), 2459–2470.

Botha, M., Dibb, B., & Frost, D. M. (2020). "Autism is me": An investigation of how autistic individuals make sense of autism and stigma. *Disability & Society*, 1–27.

Burlingame, G. M., McClendon, D. T., & Yang, C. (2018). Cohesion in group therapy: A meta-analysis. *Psychotherapy (Chicago, Ill.), 55*(4), 384–398. doi:10.1037/pst0000173

Burlingame, G. M., Svien, H., Hoppe, L., Hunt, I., & Rosendahl, J. (2020). Group therapy for schizophrenia: A meta-analysis. *Psychotherapy (Chicago, Ill.), 57*(2), 219–236.

Cappadocia, M. C., & Weiss, J. A. (2011). Review of social skills training groups for youth with Asperger syndrome and high functioning autism. *Research in Autism Spectrum Disorders, 5*(1), 70–78.

Corrigan, P. (2004). How stigma interferes with mental health care. *American Psychologist, 59*(7), 614–625.

Cuijpers, P., van Straten, A., & Warmerdam, L. (2008). Are individual and group treatments equally effective in the treatment of depression in adults? A meta-analysis. *The European Journal of Psychiatry, 22*(1), 38–51.

Doble, B., Langdon, P. E., Shepstone, L., Murphy, G. H., Fowler, D., Heavens, D., Malovic, A., Russell, A., Rose, A., Mullineaux, L., & Wilson, E. C. F. (2017). Economic evaluation alongside a randomized controlled crossover trial of modified group cognitive–behavioral therapy for anxiety compared to treatment-as-usual in adults with Asperger syndrome. *MDM Policy & Practice, 2*(2).

Dubreucq, J., Plasse, J., Gabayet, F., Faraldo, M., Blanc, O., Chereau, I., Cervello, S., Couhet, G., Demily, C., Guillard-Bouhet, N., Gouache, B., Jaafari, N., Legrand, G., Legros-Lafarge, E., Pommier, R., Quilès, C., Straub, D., Verdoux, H., Vignaga, F., Massoubre, C., . . . Franck, N. (2020). Self-stigma in serious mental illness and autism spectrum disorder: Results from the REHABase national psychiatric rehabilitation cohort. *European Psychiatry, 63*(1), e13.

Eack, S. M., Hogarty, S. S., Greenwald, D. P., Litschge, M. Y., Porton, S. A., Mazefsky, C. A., & Minshew, N. J. (2018). Cognitive enhancement therapy for adult autism spectrum disorder: Results of an 18-month randomized clinical trial. *Autism Research, 11*(3), 519–530.

Factor, R. S., Condy, E. E., Farley, J. P., & Scarpa, A. (2016). Brief report: Insistence on sameness, anxiety, and social motivation in children with autism spectrum disorder. *Journal of Autism and Developmental Disorders, 46*(7), 2548–2554.

Gates, J. A., Kang, E., & Lerner, M. D. (2017). Efficacy of group social skills interventions for youth with autism spectrum disorder: A systematic review and meta-analysis. *Clinical Psychology Review, 52*, 164–181.

Hahn, W. K. (2009). Ingenuity and uneasiness about group psychotherapy in university counseling centers. *International Journal of Group Psychotherapy, 59*(4), 543–552.

Hedman, E., Andersson, E., Ljotsson, B., Andersson, G., Ruck, C., & Lindefors, N. (2011). Cost-effectiveness of Internet-based cognitive behavior therapy vs. cognitive behavioral group therapy for social anxiety disorder: Results from a randomized controlled trial. *Behaviour Research and Therapy, 49*(11), 729–736.

Hesselmark, E., Plenty, S., & Bejerot, S. (2014). Group cognitive behavioural therapy and group recreational activity for adults with autism spectrum disorders: A preliminary randomized controlled trial. *Autism, 18*(6), 672–683.

Hollocks, M. J., Jones, C. R., Pickles, A., Baird, G., Happe, F., Charman, T., & Simonoff, E. (2014). The association between social cognition and executive functioning and symptoms of anxiety and depression in adolescents with autism spectrum disorders. *Autism Research, 7*(2), 216–228.

Huntley, A. L., Araya, R., & Salisbury, C. (2012). Group psychological therapies for depression in the community: Systematic review and meta-analysis. *British Journal of Psychiatry, 200*(3), 184–190.

Kaiser, R. H., Hubley, S., & Dimidjian, S. (2016). Behavioural activation theory. In Adrian Wells & Peter Fisher (Eds.), *Treating depression: MCT, CBT and third wave therapies* (pp. 221–241). Wiley Blackwell.

Kamp-Becker, I., Ghahreman, M., Smidt, J., & Remschmidt, H. (2009). Dimensional structure of the autism phenotype: Relations between early development and current presentation. *Journal of Autism and Developmental Disorders, 39*(4), 557–571.

Kanter, J. W., Manos, R. C., Bowe, W. M., Baruch, D. E., Busch, A. M., & Rusch, L. C. (2010). What is behavioral activation? A review of the empirical literature. *Clinical Psychology Review, 30*(6), 608–620.

Koffel, E. A., Koffel, J. B., & Gehrman, P. R. (2015). A meta-analysis of group cognitive behavioral therapy for insomnia. *Sleep Medicine Reviews, 19*, 6–16.

Lai, M.-C., Kassee, C., Besney, R., Bonato, S., Hull, L., Mandy, W., Szatmari, P., & Ameis, S. H. (2019). Prevalence of co-occurring mental health diagnoses in the autism population: a systematic review and meta-analysis. *The Lancet Psychiatry, 6*(10), 819–829.

Langdon, P. E., Murphy, G. H., Shepstone, L., Wilson, E. C. F., Fowler, D., Heavens, D., Russell, A., Rose, A., Malovic, A., & Mullineaux, L. (2016). The people with Asperger syndrome and anxiety disorders (PAsSA) trial: A pilot multi-centre single blind randomised trial of group cognitive behavioural therapy. *British Journal of Psychiatry Open, 2*, 179–186.

Langdon, P. E., Murphy, G. H., Wilson, E., Shepstone, L., Fowler, D., Heavens, D., Malovic, A., & Russell, A. (2013). Asperger syndrome and anxiety disorders (PAsSA) treatment trial: A study protocol of a pilot, multicentre, single-blind, randomised crossover trial of group cognitive behavioural therapy. *BMJ open, 3*(7), e003449.

Mavranezouli, I., Mayo-Wilson, E., Dias, S., Kew, K., Clark, D. M., Ades, A. E., & Pilling, S. (2015). The cost effectiveness of psychological and pharmacological interventions for social anxiety disorder: A model-based economic analysis. *PLOS ONE, 10*(10), Article e0140704.

McDermut, W., Miller, I. W., & Brown, R. A. (2001). The efficacy of group psychotherapy for depression: A meta-analysis and review of the empirical research. *Clinical Psychology: Science and Practice, 8*(1), 98–116.

McMahon, C. M., Lerner, M. D., & Britton, N. (2013). Group-based social skills interventions for adolescents with higher-functioning autism spectrum disorder: A review and looking to the future. *Adolescent Health, Medicine, and Therapeutics, 4*, 23–28.

Miller, A., Vernon, T., Wu, V., & Russo, K. (2014). Social skill group interventions for adolescents with autism spectrum disorders: A systematic review. *Review Journal of Autism and Developmental Disorders, 1*(4), 254–265.

Papadopoulos, C., Lodder, A., Constantinou, G., & Randhawa, G. (2019). Systematic review of the relationship between autism stigma and informal caregiver mental health. *Journal of Autism and Developmental Disorders, 49*(4), 1665–1685.

Pfammatter, M., Junghan, U. M., & Brenner, H. D. (2006). Efficacy of psychological therapy in schizophrenia: Conclusions from meta-analyses. *Schizophrenia Bulletin, 32 Suppl 1*, S64–80.

Pistrang, N., Barker, C., & Humphreys, K. (2008). Mutual help groups for mental health problems: A review of effectiveness studies. *American Journal of Community Psychology, 42*(1–2), 110–121.

Russell, A., Gaunt, D., Cooper, K., Horwood, J., Barton, S., Ensum, I., Ingham, B., Parr, J., Metcalfe, C., Rai, D., Kessler, D., & Wiles, N. (2019). Guided self-help for depression in autistic adults: The ADEPT feasibility RCT. *Health Technology Assessment (Winchester, England), 23*(68), 1–94.

Spain, D., Blainey, S. H., & Vaillancourt, K. (2017). Group cognitive behaviour therapy (CBT) for social interaction anxiety in adults with autism spectrum disorders (ASD). *Research in Autism Spectrum Disorders, 41–42,* 20–30.

Strauss, B., Spangenberg, L., Brahler, E., & Bormann, B. (2015). Attitudes towards (psychotherapy) groups: Results of a survey in a representative sample. *International Journal of Group Psychotherapy, 65*(3), 410–430.

Tucker, M., & Oei, T. P. S. (2007). Is group more cost effective than individual cognitive behaviour therapy? The evidence is not solid yet. *Behavioural and Cognitive Psychotherapy, 35,* 77–92.

Uljarevic, M., Lane, A., Kelly, A., & Leekam, S. (2016). Sensory subtypes and anxiety in older children and adolescents with autism spectrum disorder. *Autism Research, 9*(10), 1073–1078.

Vasa, R. A., Kreiser, N. L., Keefer, A., Singh, V., & Mostofsky, S. H. (2018). Relationships between autism spectrum disorder and intolerance of uncertainty. *Autism Research, 11*(4), 636–644.

Veale, D. (2018). Behavioural activation for depression. *Advances in Psychiatric Treatment, 14*(1), 29–36.

Vereenooghe, L., & Langdon, P. E. (2013). Psychological therapies for people with intellectual disabilities: A systematic review and meta-analysis. *Research in Developmental Disabilities, 34,* 4085–4102.

Vogel, D. L., Shechtman, Z., & Wade, N. G. (2010). The role of public and self-stigma in predicting attitudes toward group counseling. *The Counseling Psychologist, 38*(7), 904–922.

Vogel, D. L., Wade, N. G., & Hackler, A. H. (2007). Perceived public stigma and the willingness to seek counseling: The mediating roles of self-stigma and attitudes toward counseling. *Journal of Counseling Psychology, 54*(1), 40–50.

Wallace, G. L., Kenworthy, L., Pugliese, C. E., Popal, H. S., White, E. I., Brodsky, E., & Martin, A. (2016). Real-world executive functions in adults with autism spectrum disorder: Profiles of impairment and associations with adaptive functioning and co-morbid anxiety and depression. *Journal of Autism and Developmental Disorders, 46*(3), 1071–1083.

Walters, S., Loades, M., & Russell, A. (2016). A systematic review of effective modifications to cognitive behavioural therapy for young people with autism spectrum disorders. *Review Journal of Autism and Developmental Disorders, 3*(2), 137–153.

Weston, L., Hodgekins, J., & Langdon, P. E. (2016). Effectiveness of cognitive behavioural therapy with people who have autistic spectrum disorders: A systematic review and meta-analysis. *Clinical Psychology Review, 49,* 41–54.

Wigham, S., Rodgers, J., South, M., McConachie, H., & Freeston, M. (2015). The interplay between sensory processing abnormalities, intolerance of uncertainty, anxiety and restricted and repetitive behaviours in autism spectrum disorder. *Journal of Autism and Developmental Disorders, 45*(4), 943–952.

17

Offender-Focused Interventions

DAVID MURPHY ■

KEY CONSIDERATIONS

- Regardless of whether features of autism are directly linked to their offending, offenders with autism present with difficulties and needs that can pose a challenge for mainstream forensic services.
- Offenders with autism can benefit from offence-focused interventions, yet the factors influencing engagement and outcome remain poorly understood.
- Without appropriate adaptation and consideration of autism, any offence-focused intervention will likely be unsuccessful in terms of engagement and outcomes.
- Offence-focused interventions rarely operate in isolation and can be influenced by all those who work with individuals, necessitating organizational awareness of autism.

OVERVIEW

While individuals with autism are no more likely to engage in law-breaking behaviors than those without autism (and may actually more likely be victims of crime; (King & Murphy, 2014), it is generally accepted that the combination of an individual's specific difficulties (often directly related to their autism, such as a tendency toward literal thinking, focusing on specific details at the expense of appreciating the wider context, perspective-taking difficulties, preoccupations, sensory sensitivities, and emotional regulation [ER] difficulties) in particular environmental circumstances may increase their vulnerability toward engaging in some form of law-breaking behavior and subsequent involvement with the criminal justice system (CJS). Such circumstances typically involve high-stress situations involving a lack of structure to life, social isolation and alienation, transition periods, and being used by other more able peers. Law-breaking behavior may also take many forms such as interpersonal violence, pursuing deviant preoccupations, arson, inappropriate sexual conduct and behavior, harassment and stalking, or involvement with extremism ideology.

In terms of prevalence within the CJS, methodological differences between studies (with many restricted to single settings and differences in how autism has been screened or diagnosed) make it is difficult to ascertain an exact number of individuals with autism within specific forensic services. However, the consensus view is that individuals with autism are likely to be overrepresented in many secure settings, including UK high-secure psychiatric care, the most secure level of psychiatric care where admission is determined by whether individuals represent an immediate and grave risk to others (Murphy et al., 2017), and UK prisons (Underwood et al., 2016); as well as prisons in the US (Fazio et al., 2012) and Sweden (Billstedt et al., 2017). It is also suspected that such estimates are likely to be an underestimate of the actual figure, especially considering atypical cases (i.e., individuals who display some features of autism but who may not necessarily fulfil all of the diagnostic criteria), as well as those who are likely to have autism but who refuse to engage with diagnostic assessments.

Once within the CJS, individuals with autism also present with difficulties and needs that pose a challenge to conventional services (Allely, 2015; Higgs & Carter, 2015; Murphy, 2010b). Such challenges can be present at all stages of CJS (Browning & Caulfield, 2011), including initial interviews with the police, attending court and subsequent management in custodial settings, secure psychiatric environments, or in community services. Regardless of the relevance of an individual's autism to their offending, engaging offenders who have autism with interventions that aim to reduce risks for future offending also present specific challenges. There is also the high prevalence of co-occurring conditions in this population, such as other neurodevelopmental disorders (notably attention deficit/hyperactivity disorder [ADHD], intellectual disabilities), psychiatric disorders such as psychosis, personality disorders, and, for some, psychopathy. An initial step in guiding an appropriate offence-focused intervention is completing a risk assessment with an individual (Murphy, 2019; Shine & Cooper, 2016). Indeed, a good risk assessment should include a formulation of an individual's autism, its relevance to offending, and potential targets for intervention or management.

INDIVIDUAL, GROUP, AND ORGANIZATIONAL OFFENCE-FOCUSED INTERVENTIONS

Within the UK, regardless of whether the forensic setting is a prison, specialist autism unit, or generic forensic psychiatric setting, the management of individuals with autism has been significantly influenced by growing professional awareness and governmental legislation. For example, the Autism Act (2009), followed by other pieces of legislation, including the Think Autism Strategy (Department of Health, 2014), the Adult Autism Strategy: Statutory Guidance

(2015), and Transforming Care (2017) have placed autism on the agenda of most institutions and established a duty to provide appropriate diagnostic assessments and staff training. A review of neurodiversity in UK prisons (Criminal Justice Joint Inspection, 2021) and the policy paper outlining a national strategy for autistic children, young people and adults (Department of Health and Social Care, 2021) have also both highlighted the need to develop a 'neurodiverse' informed model of care and to have made demonstrable progress in the assessment and management of individuals with autism in UK prisons and the criminal justice system. Although not specifically targeted just at the needs of individuals with autism, the Equalities Act (2010) within the UK has also had some impact in ensuring "reasonable adjustments" are made to make environments, procedures, and opportunities more "autism friendly." Internationally, similar legislation has also had a significant influence on how individuals with autism are assessed and managed, such as the Combating Autism Act (2006) in the US. The United Nations Convention on the Rights of Persons with Disabilities (U.N. General Assembly, 2007) also serves a function in protecting the rights of offenders with autism.

In terms of promoting organization awareness of autism and complying with these pieces of legislation, within high secure psychiatric care the author provides general autism awareness training to all staff who have direct patient contact. In addition to providing information on the current understanding of what autism is, including the characteristic difficulties and features, the training introduces the so-called SPELL guidelines, which place emphasis on a Structured approach, a Positive approach, Empathy, Low arousal, and Links with other professionals (National Autistic Society, 2013). The aim of the SPELL approach is to encourage staff to work with an individual's strengths and reduce the likelihood of problem behaviors by making the immediate environment and any interactions more autism friendly. Although the impact of such training on the management of patients with autism remains to be evaluated, there is the general view that training is valued and that it should be mandatory, as assessed via a staff survey (Murphy & Broyd, 2019; Murphy & McMorrow, 2015). These findings are particularly relevant in the context of the proposal by the UK government that all National Health Service clinical staff should receive some form of compulsory autism awareness training (Department of Health, 2019). This recommendation is also interesting within forensic settings where the importance of having an awareness of autism among staff is not a new idea. Over 20 years ago, Wing (1997) highlighted that the crucial elements for appropriate care of individuals with Asperger's syndrome in forensic settings lie in carefully structuring the environment and daily program and in training staff in the psychological strategies to be used. Wing also noted that some, perhaps most, of those who commit violent or other serious offences may require long-term care and supervision in a secure environment, with the emphasis "that in the right kind of environment, the individual may behave in an exemplary way, but if he or she is moved to a setting that does not provide the right type of program, the criminal behavior may very well reoccur" (p. 256). In terms of a wider awareness of autism across the CJS, it is also noteworthy that autism awareness training is now common among many police forces both in the UK and internationally.

In terms of prison settings, experience assessing individuals with autism suggests that while there has been an increased awareness of autism among many staff, and several prisons have been accredited by the UK National Autistic Society (e.g., Lewis et al., 2013), there remains considerable uncertainty with regard to how best to therapeutically address an individual's needs, with individuals themselves reporting limited opportunities to engage with rehabilitation programs (Robertson & McGillivray, 2015). At the time of writing there are no accredited group programs for any offending behavior available specifically for individuals with autism detained in forensic settings. While some adapted versions of the sex offender treatment programs designed for individuals with intellectual difficulties (SOTSEC-ID, 2010) have been developed, outcomes for individuals with autism in these groups do not appear promising because they often function at a much higher level compared to others and present with different needs (Haaven, 2006). Indeed, some research also suggests that men with autism who have noncontact sexual offending histories and have completed such groups may actually have higher recidivism rates (Heaton & Murphy, 2013). Possible explanations for this higher recidivism rate may be due to such offences having a higher rate regardless of the presence of autism, but also perhaps because of a failure to address deviant preoccupations and the social difficulties present in some individuals with autism. Participation in mainstream offender groups within prison settings may also be problematic, where individuals with autism may experience sensory overload and exclusion (Higgs & Carter, 2015). However, while within forensic psychiatric settings it remains debatable as to whether it is harmful to include individuals with autism in mainstream groups, there is an argument that some individuals with autism benefit from participating in mixed groups by hearing different points of view and listening to other individuals' experiences. The qualitative reports by some individuals with autism seen by the author in a HSPC setting suggest that mixed-membership groups are useful. For example, dialectical behavior therapy (DBT) devised by Linehan (1993) and applied to forensic psychiatric care (Moulden et al., 2020) shows promise in that it aims to promote positive coping and change unhelpful behaviors through recognizing the cognitive and emotional triggers that increase stress. Although empirical research is lacking, key factors that influence outcomes with such groups appear to include facilitator awareness of the difficulties associated with having autism and facilitator sensitivity to making appropriate adjustments, as well as the sensitivity of other group members to such difficulties.

Evidence for the effectiveness of individual psychological work addressing the offending behaviors of individuals who have autism also remains to be explored in any depth. Cognitive behavior therapy (CBT) and other psychological approaches (such as mindfulness-based approaches) that are adapted for any cognitive and communication difficulties have been found to be useful interventions for adults who have autism in nonforensic contexts (Spain et al., 2016), but there has been limited exploration of how psychological therapies can address offence-specific behaviors in autism. In a systematic review, Melvin, Langdon, and Murphy (2017) identified four quantitative studies and nine case studies describing interventions and outcomes for offenders with autism. Among the studies identified, sexual offending was the most common offence (58%), followed by interpersonal violence (19%), arson (15%), manslaughter (11%), theft (8%), and firearms and a bomb hoax (4% each). No single therapeutic approach was followed between studies and there were differences in how outcome was assessed. Some studies also included individuals with co-occurring intellectual difficulties and psychiatric disorders. Unsurprisingly, it was concluded from this review that there were too many significant differences between studies in terms of an individual's presenting difficulties, offending behaviors, and specific interventions used, to prevent any generalization of findings.

Clinical experience with several individuals has found that if a CBT approach is used to address risk or criminological issues among offenders with autism (such as improving victim empathy and an appreciation of consequences), clear realistic goals need to be identified and specific further adaptations need to be made allowing for the presence of any cognitive, communication, sensory, and ER difficulties, as well as for any comorbid psychiatric disorder (Murphy, 2010a). For many individuals a "personalized" education plan about their autism can also be helpful as a way of improving their understanding of past and current difficulties. For example, one individual described being able to "outthink" his autism as a result of being aware of what his difficulties had been in the past. However, while many individuals with autism do respond to individual psychological interventions (such as developing general problem-solving skills; working on basic social inference skills; encouraging appropriate assertiveness; reducing individual social anxieties; shifting preoccupations, obsessive thoughts, and negative ruminations; and developing perspective-taking skills), it may be unrealistic to expect significant changes in cognitive style compared to other offenders who do not have autism. Engagement with those individuals who present with significant egocentricity, who take limited personal responsibility, and who reject their diagnosis can be particularly problematic. For example, Hare (2013) has suggested that a primary goal in CBT with autism should be not to focus on cognitive changes, but more to concentrate on behavioral changes that increase an individual's ability to function in everyday life, while being aware of difficulties in challenging dysfunctional cognitions and beliefs that may be present. As with many individuals with autism, some specific therapeutic adaptations may also be required with the pace of therapy, providing individuals with sufficient time to process information and to work on "Asperger's time" (Gaus, 2007, p. 73). Such adaptations to processing information may be particularly prominent in forensic settings where comorbid psychosis can be an issue. For many offenders with autism there is also a role for pharmacological interventions that can assist with anxiety and comorbid neurodevelopmental (such as ADHD) or psychiatric disorders, as well as with the experience of any auditory hallucinations or delusional ideas linked to offending that may be present (Kelbrick & Radley 2013).

Other interventions within secure settings can include occupational therapy and further education, which can have a positive impact on increasing social inclusion and self-esteem, as well as opportunities to learn new skills. The application of a restorative justice approach with offenders who have autism in HSPC is also beginning to be explored (Tapp et al., 2020).

Beyond detention, there remains a lack of research examining what difficulties individuals with autism experience during the transition back to the community from custodial settings. Leaving prison and returning back to the community can be difficult for many individuals, but it may be particularly difficult for individuals with autism who might experience particular issues dealing with change in routine and the reduced structure (Royal College of Psychiatry, 2006). Within the UK, where prison to community services are available, it has been found that accessing these for many individuals with autism is confusing and that success depends on a coordinated multi-agency approach including health, social care and justice (Prison Reform Trust, 2018).

CASE STUDY

Robert, aged 30 years with a history of early neglect and physical abuse, was admitted to HSPC due to concerns within medium-secure care that he was at risk of attempting to abscond and immediate threats of violence to nursing staff, whom he perceived as abusing his rights. Robert's original index offence (the offence leading to his conviction and detainment in forensic services) was for sending explosive devices to a probation officer whom he believed had wrongly portrayed him as a pedophile (where the reality was that there was no evidence to support the probation officer's this view). Prior to his admission, Robert had never been assessed for autism and had received a diagnosis of an antisocial personality disorder and possible psychosis (based on assumed paranoid ideas about probation services). A formulation of difficulties and multidisciplinary "treatment" plan was devised following a detailed and extended assessment of Robert's presenting difficulties and history, including a comprehensive neuropsychological assessment (focusing on identifying thinking style), an autism diagnostic assessment (following the observation of intolerance to noise and a need for routines, predictability, and preoccupations), and a detailed risk assessment. The formulation was based on the findings that Robert's early experience of neglect and physical abuse, in combination with his thinking style, associated with having autism. Notably, his literal thinking, perspective-taking difficulties, focus on details, as well as his social isolation and low self-esteem, led to his mistrust of authority and his vulnerability toward making negative interpretations of others, grudge bearing, and defensive/aggressive reaction. Robert's management plan included individual psychoeducation exploring his experience and acceptance of the autism diagnosis, as well as individual autism-adapted CBT to address his tendency to form negative interpretations of others' actions and comments and to react in a defensive way. A collaborative risk management plan was also devised, including encouraging prosocial interests and opportunities to promote self-esteem through further education and work activities. A psychiatric assessment and management plan also led to the exclusion of a psychosis and the introduction of a short-term low-dose mood stabilizer medication. The SPELL guidelines were also encouraged to be followed by all staff involved in Robert's management.

In terms of outcome, Robert was initially reluctant to accept the diagnosis of autism and externalized responsibility for all perceived wrongdoings onto others. However, with some initial motivational work, over several sessions it was possible to encourage Robert to acknowledge the diagnosis, to challenge his negative bias in thinking and consider alternative perspectives, and to view his thinking style (literal with a tendency to focus on details) as an advantage in many situations. More adaptive ways of challenging the perceived negative comments of others were also developed, including a shared collaborative formulation of understanding the risks for interpreting and acting on perceived wrongdoing (linked with his early experiences of neglect and abuse), along with the development of protective factors (such as improved self-esteem through education, positive relationships, social inclusion, and valued work activities).Working in combination to address dysfunctional thinking patterns, to reframe negative early experiences and grudge bearing, and to work toward positive goals, these interventions led Robert to move back to medium-secure care and eventually to transfer back into community care. Of particular significance was the shift in the formulation of Robert's difficulties by those involved in his management, viewing him in terms of autism and trauma informed rather than a personality disorder.

CONCLUSIONS AND FUTURE RESEARCH

The development and evaluation of offence-focused interventions for individuals with autism will continue to evolve. Although there are no "validated" treatment programs for addressing the offending behavior of individuals with autism, clinical experience suggests many offenders with autism can benefit from a range of interventions. Indirect interventions in the form of staff and organization awareness of autism—how staff interact with and make reasonable adjustments for someone with autism—can also have a significant influence in addressing offence behaviors and reducing future risk for re-offending. The variation in therapeutic engagement and outcomes following offence-focused interventions should not be surprising; while offenders with autism share the same diagnosis, every individual presents with different life circumstances; profiles of functioning; age-related factors (where CBT with a 18-year-old offender can be quite different from a 48-year-old offender), including perhaps delayed or different patterns of brain maturation (Ecker et al., 2015); and possible gender identity issues (George & Stokes, 2018). Our understanding of how all these factors might influence individual engagement and outcome following interventions remains poor. A similar degree of uncertainty of influence is also present regarding therapist characteristics and any "autism-specific adaptions" to interventions.

A key target for future research on offender-focused interventions for au-tism should focus on attempting to understand the factors that influence an individual's capacity to engage with interventions, including matching specific interventions to individual presentations and how best to define outcomes. For example, individuals with good verbal abilities and capacity to considerer al-ternative perspectives may engage well with CBT as well as mindfulness. Other individuals with high levels of motivation and personal curiosity might also benefit from psychoeducational approaches. While typologies of offenders with autism have been suggested based on the presence or absence of psychosis and psychopathy (e.g., Alexander et al., 2016) and which have been proposed would guide interventions, these alone can potentially oversimplify presentations and fail to appreciate the diversity within autism (notably within different aspects of social and nonsocial cognition, social naivete, need for routine and predictability, emotional regulation, and sensory sensitivities). The potential role of "severity" of autism in determining capacity to benefit from interventions has also been suggested (Melvin et al., 2017). However, this raises questions around what aspect of autism is used to define severity (such as the specific features associated with autism, or the overall general level of functioning or support required, however this is defined), where any cut-off of ability or dysfunction might be, and the influ-ence of any co-occurring neurodevelopmental and psychiatric difficulties. As with many offenders, the role of past traumas in understanding presenting difficulties may be particularly significant in autism, where some have suggested an associa-tion between past traumas and an increased risk of violence (Im, 2016). Running alongside an autism-sensitive approach to offender management, a trauma-in-formed approach to care may also be required (Fuld, 2018).

Of particular importance with regard to determining an individual's capacity to engage and benefit from any intervention appears to be their cognitive style. Clinical experience suggests that many individuals with autism who present with more flexible thinking and relatively less egocentricity engage very well with therapeutic interventions addressing a range of issues that are sensitive to their autism. In contrast, individuals who present with significant social cognition difficulties and extreme literal thinking, as well as perhaps a greater degree of co-occurring intellectual difficulties, struggle to benefit from "insight orientated" psychological or occupational interventions (Murphy, 2010a) and require a more environmental and behavioral approach directed by staff. Individuals with autism and co-occurring psychopathy can also be particularly difficult to engage with any direct offence-focused intervention. Regardless of what specific offence-focused interventions are followed, these do not operate in isolation and typically form part of a coordinated multi-agency and multiprofessional approach to individual management. Indeed, the most economically and clinically effective method of addressing the needs of offenders with autism remains the promotion of awareness of autism among all those involved with their management. Although there is no specific research evidence devoted to examining how organizational awareness of autism specifically improves the outcomes of offenders with autism or the impact on reducing recidivism, staff surveys of probation, prison, and secure psychiatric care facilities consistently find most staff feel underskilled with regard to how they work with individuals who have autism and that training is valued. Clearly any service or intervention that is sensitive to, and makes reasonable adjustments for, an individual's autism is more likely to result in positive outcomes than those that do not. It is also possible that having staff with autism-sensitive qualities (including autism knowledge and "empathy" toward an individual's difficulties) is particularly beneficial in encouraging positive outcomes (Worthington, 2016). In terms of promoting positive outcomes for offenders with autism detained within forensic psychiatric settings, it also remains to be established whether secure specialist autism services result in better "outcomes" for individuals than more generic secure units that aim to be autism sensitive. As has been suggested by one study examining patient experiences in HSPC, some individuals with autism report a preference to be around mixed patient groups rather than just those with autism (Murphy & Mullens, 2017).

Of significance is the observation that most research exploring interventions addressing the offending behavior of individuals with autism has been with men. While this no doubt reflects the prevalence of offenders with autism, there is a need to explore whether women with autism who enter the CJS have additional vulnerabilities and needs that require different interventions (Ashworth et al., 2020; Markham, 2019). Other offender subgroups including ethnic minorities may also have specific needs that need to be considered during assessment and subsequent interventions. In terms of potential future offender-focused interventions, especially so in a post-COVID-19 world, the use of new technologies in therapies and risk assessments such as computer simulation and virtual reality are likely to play an increasingly important role (Benbouriche et al., 2014). This may be especially so with the relatively easy accessibility and low cost now associated with such technologies, as well as the potential to manipulate and replicate a wide range of variables.

REFERENCES

Alexander, R., Langdon, P., Chester, V., Barnoux, M., Gunaratna, I., & Hoare, S. (2016). Heterogeneity within autism spectrum disorder in forensic mental health: the introduction of typologies. *Advances in Autism, 2*(4), 201–209.

Allely, C. (2015). Autism spectrum disorders in the criminal justice system: Police interviewing, the courtroom, and the prison environment. In *Recent Advances in Autism* (pp. 1 – 13). SM Group.

Ashworth, S., Bamford, J., & Tully, R. (2020). The effectiveness of a CBT based intervention for depression symptoms with a female forensic inpatient with cognitive disability and autism. *Journal of Forensic Psychiatry and Psychology*, 31,(3), 432–454.

Autism Act. (2009). Accessed at www.legislation.gov.uk/ukpga/2009/15/contents

Benbouriche, M., Nolet, K., Trottier, D., & Renaud, P. (2014, April 9–11). Virtual reality applications in forensic psychiatry. *Proceedings of the Virtual Reality International Conference*. Laval Virtual (VRIC 14), Laval, France.

Billstedt, E., Anckarsater, H., Wallinius, M., & Hofvander, B. (2017). Neurodevelopmental disorders in young violent offenders: Overlap and background characteristics. *Psychiatry Research*, *252*, 234–241.

Browning, A., & Caulfield, L. (2011). The prevalence and treatment of people with Asperger's syndrome in the criminal justice system. *Criminology and Criminal Justice*, *11*, 165.

Combating Autism Act of 2006, Pub. Law No 109-416 (2006). http://www.amchp.org/Policy-Advocacy/Documents/Combating%20Autism%20Act%20Summary%204-08.pdf

Criminal Justice Joint Inspections (2021). Neurodiversity in the criminal justice system: a review of evidence. https://www.justiceinspectorates.gov.uk/cjji/wp-content/uploads/sites/2/2021/07/Neurodiversity-evidence-review-web-2021.pdf

Department of Health. (2014). *Think autism: Fulfilling and rewarding lives. The strategy for adults with autism in England: An update.* https://assets.publishing.service.gov.uk/government/uploads/system/uploads/attachment_data/file/299866/Autism_Strategy.pdf

Department of Health. (2019). "Right to be heard": The Government's response to the consultation on learning disability and autism training for health and care staff. Published the 5th November: https://assets.publishing.service.gov.uk/government/uploads/system/uploads/attachment_data/file/844356/autism-and-learning-disability-training-for-staff-consultation-response.pdf

Department of Health and Social Care (2021). The national strategy for autistic children, young people and adults: 2021 to 2026. https://www.gov.uk/government/publications/national-strategy-for-autistic-children-young-people-and-adults-2021-to-2026/the-national-strategy-for-autistic-children-young-people-and-adults-2021-to-2026

Ecker, C., Bookheimer, S., & Murphy, D. (2015). Neuroimaging in autism spectrum disorder: Brain structure and function across the lifespan. *Neurology*, *14*(11), 1121–1134.

Equality Act. (2010). Equality Act 2010. www.gov.uk/guidance/equality-act-2010-guidance

Fazio, R. L., Pietz, C. A., & Denney, R. L. (2012). An estimate of the prevalence of autism spectrum disorders in an incarcerated population. *Open Access Journal of Forensic Psychology*, *4*, 69–80.

Fuld, S. (2018). Autism spectrum disorder: The impact of stressful and traumatic life events and implications for clinical practice. *Clinical Social Work Journal*, *46*, 210–219.

Gaus, V. (2007). *Cognitive behavioural therapy for adult Asperger syndrome.* Guildford Press.

George, R., & Stokes, M. (2018). Gender identity and sexual orientation in autism spectrum disorder. *Autism*, *22*(8), 970–982.

Hare, D. J. (2013). Developing psychotherapeutic interventions with people with autism spectrum disorders. In J. L. Taylor, W. R. Lindsay, & R. Hastings (Eds.), *Psychological therapies for adults with intellectual* disabilities (pp. 193–206). John Wiley & Sons.

Haaven, J. (2006). Suggested treatment outline using the old me/new me model. In G. Blasingame (Ed.), Practical treatment strategies for forensic clients with severe and sexual behaviour problems among persons with developmental disabilities. Wood N. Barnes/Safer Society Press.

Heaton, K., & Murphy, G. (2013). Men with intellectual disabilities who have attended sex offender treatment groups: A follow up. *Journal of Applied Research in Intellectual Disabilities, 26*(5), 489–500.

Higgs, T., & Carter, A. (2015). Autism spectrum disorder and sexual offending: Responsivity in forensic interventions. *Aggression and Violent Behaviour, 22*, 112–119.

Im, D. (2016). Trauma as a contributor to violence in autism spectrum disorder. *Journal of the American Academy of Psychiatry, 44*(2), 184–192.

Kelbrick, M., & Radley, J. (2013). Forensic rehabilitation in Asperger syndrome: A case report. *Journal of Intellectual Disabilities and Offending Behaviour, 4, 1–2,* 60–64(5).

King, C., & Murphy, G. (2014). A systematic review of people with autism spectrum disorder and the criminal justice system. *Journal of Autism and Developmental Disorders, 44,* 2717–2733.

Lewis, A., Pritchet, R., Hughes, C., & Turner, K. (2013). Development and implementation of autism standards for prisons. *Journal of Intellectual Disabilities and Offending Behaviour, 6*(2), 68–80.

Linehan, M. (1993). *Cognitive behavioural treatment of borderline personality disorder: Diagnosis and treatment of mental disorders.* Guildford Press.

Markham, S. (2019). Diagnosis and treatment of ASD in women in secure and forensic hospitals. *Advances in Autism, 5*(1), 64–76.

Melvin, C., Langdon, P., & Murphy, G. (2017). Treatment effectiveness for offenders with autism spectrum conditions: A systematic review. *Psychology, Crime & Law, 23*(8), 748–776.

Moulden, H., Mamak, M., & Chaimowitz, G. (2020). A preliminary evaluation of the effectiveness of dialectical behaviour therapy in a forensic psychiatric setting. *Criminal Behaviour and Mental Health, 30,* 141–150.

Murphy, D. (2010a). Extreme violence in a young man with an autistic spectrum disorder: Assessment and intervention within high security psychiatric care. *Journal of Forensic Psychiatry and Psychology, 21*(3), 462–477.

Murphy, D. (2010b). Invited commentary. Understanding offenders with autism spectrum disorders: What can forensic services do? Commentary on Asperger syndrome and criminal behaviour. *Advances in Psychiatric Treatment, 16*(1), 44–46.

Murphy, D. (2019). Risk assessment and management. In E. Chaplin, D. Spain, & J. McCarthy (Eds.), *Clinicians' guide to mental health conditions in adults with autism spectrum disorders.* Jessica Kingsley Publishers.

Murphy, D., & Broyd, J. (2019). Evaluation of autism awareness training for staff in high secure psychiatric care hospital. *Advances in Autism, 6(1),* 35–47.

Murphy, D., Bush, E. L., & Puzzo, I. (2017). Incompatibilities and seclusions among individuals with an autism spectrum disorder detained in high secure psychiatric care. *Journal of Intellectual Disabilities and Offending Behaviour, 8*(4), 188–200.

Murphy, D., & McMorrow, K. (2015). View of autism spectrum conditions held by staff working in a high secure psychiatric hospital. *Journal of Forensic Practice, 17*(3), 231–240.

Murphy, D., & Mullens, H. (2017). Examining the experiences and quality of life of patients with an autism spectrum disorder detained in high secure psychiatric care. *Advances in Autism, 3*(1), 3–14.

Prison Reform Trust. (2018). Behaviour that challenges: Planning services for people with learning disabilities and or autism who sexually offend. http://www.

prisonreformtrust.org.uk/Portals/0/Documents/Behaviour%20that%20challenges.
pdf

Robertson, C., & McGillivray, J. (2015). Autism behind bars: a review of the research literature and discussion of key issues. *The Journal of Forensic Psychiatry and Psychology, 26*(6), 719–736.

Royal College of Psychiatrists. (2006). *Psychiatric services for adolescents and adults with Asperger syndrome and other autistic spectrum disorder.*

Sex Offender Treatment Services Collaborative–Intellectual Disabilities (SOTSEC-ID). (2010). Effectiveness of group cognitive behavioural treatment for men with intellectual disabilities at risk of sexual offending. *Journal of Applied Research in Intellectual Disabilities, 23,* 537–551.

Shine, J., & Cooper-Evans, S. (2016). Developing an autism specific framework for forensic case formulation. *Journal of Intellectual Disabilities and Offending Behaviour, 7*(3), 127–139.

Spain, D., O'Neil, L., Harwood, L., & Chaplin, E. (2016). Psychological interventions for adults with ASD: Clinical approaches. *Advances in Autism, 2*(1), 24–30.

Tapp, J., Moore, E., Stephenson, M., & Cull, D. (2020). The image has been changed in my mind: A case of restorative justice in a forensic mental health setting. *Journal of Forensic Practice, 22*(4), 213–222.

Underwood, L., McCarthy, J., Chaplin, E., Forrester, A., Mills, R., & Murphy, D. (2016). Autism spectrum disorder traits among prisoners. *Advances in Autism, 2*(3), 106–117.

U.N. General Assembly. (2007, 24 January). Convention on the Rights of Persons with Disabilities: resolution/adopted by the general assembly. A/RES/61/106. www.reworld.org/docid/45f973632.html.

Wing, L. (1997). Asperger's syndrome: Management requires diagnosis. *Journal of Forensic Psychiatry, 2*(8), 253–257.

Worthington, R. (2016). What are the key skills that staff require to support adults on the autism spectrum effectively? *Forensic Update Compendium 2016,* 61–69.

18

Pharmacological Interventions

TOMOYA HIROTA AND BRYAN H. KING ■

KEY CONSIDERATIONS

- Psychiatric conditions occur among autistic adults more frequently in comparison to the non-autistic population.
- Similar to autistic children and adolescents, psychotropic medication treatment in autistic adults is indicated for psychiatric conditions, but not for core autistic symptoms.
- Psychotropic medication can be an important adjunct treatment to therapy when autistic adults suffer from moderate to severe psychiatric conditions and have functional impairments.
- Medication needs to be used judiciously by balancing benefits and risks/ side effects.
- The level of evidence supporting each psychotropic medication for autistic adults is weaker than that for autistic youth due to the paucity of controlled studies.
- Polypharmacy is common in this population in clinical practice and deserves careful scrutiny; reduction of medication requires systematic approaches by experienced clinicians.

OVERVIEW

This chapter highlights themes related to psychiatric medication treatment (psychopharmacotherapy) in autistic adults. Compared to scientific data and resources about psychopharmacotherapy in autistic children and adolescents (AACAP Autism Parents' Medication Guide Work Group, 2016; Mohiuddin & Ghaziuddin, 2013), those for adult populations are scarce. Autism persists into adulthood, and autistic-related difficulties are lifelong. Typically, autistic individuals require ongoing support and treatment, which can include medication.

Indeed, studies have reported that psychotropic medication use in autistic adults is higher than in the non-autistic population (Cvejic et al., 2018). Nearly 60% are found to be on at least one psychotropic medication (Alfageh et al., 2020; Buck et al., 2014; Cvejic et al., 2018). These psychotropic medications span a broad range of categories, as described in detail later in this chapter. Among all of these, the antidepressant class is the most commonly prescribed across studies. These findings underscore that psychopharmacotherapy can be an important treatment option for autistic adults.

In this chapter, we will cover the following topics: the role of pharmacotherapy in autistic adults; psychiatric problems that co-occur in autistic adults; a brief overview of the medication classes commonly used in autistic adults and available evidence; challenges in pharmacotherapy in this population; and future implications.

THE ROLE OF PSYCHOPHARMACOTHERAPY IN AUTISTIC ADULTS

Indications for Pharmacotherapy

As with nonpharmacological interventions, psychotropic medication has been explored in search of potential effects for core symptoms of autism. However, existing studies have reported that currently available medications are not effective for the treatment of these core diagnostic symptoms, including social communication difficulties as well as repetitive and restricted behaviors and interests (Howes et al., 2018; King et al., 2009).

In contrast, research has supported the effectiveness of pharmacotherapy for psychiatric conditions that occur in autistic individuals (McGuire et al., 2016). These conditions include anxiety, depression, inattention, hyperactivity-impulsivity, aggression and irritability, self-injurious behavior, obsessive compulsive disorder, and sleep difficulties (Simonoff et al., 2008). Therefore, current expert consensus on the role of psychopharmacotherapy in autistic individuals is to address co-occurring psychiatric problems/disorders (Howes et al., 2018).

While difficult to capture formally, it is not unreasonable to posit that improvement in psychiatric co-occurring conditions could also positively impact core autistic symptoms. To the extent that anxiety could be a setting event for repetitive behaviors, or depression could impact the desire for social interaction, successful treatment of these conditions could be particularly important in autism. Studies have not been specifically designed to address these questions, but such outcomes are commonly observed in clinical practice.

Initiating Pharmacotherapy

Although co-occurring psychiatric conditions can be treatment targets for pharmacotherapy, not all autistic adults who have these psychiatric conditions require medication. As psychiatrists may not be the first clinicians who see autistic adults, it is important for other professionals (psychologists, social workers, primary care providers) to be cognizant of when to refer these individuals to psychiatrists. However, there are currently no practice guidelines determining the optimal timing to initiate pharmacological treatment in autism. Therefore, we suggest that, similar to autistic children and adolescents, the necessity of psychotropic medication use is determined by clinicians based on the severity of co-occurring psychiatric conditions, the level of functional impairment due to autism-associated symptoms, and treatment response to nonmedication treatment, such as behavioral therapy and psychotherapy (McGuire et al., 2016).

Nonpharmacological interventions, including individual therapy and parent behavioral training, are the mainstays for addressing mild symptoms. These interventions are also essential for moderate and severe symptoms, but some individuals may not be able to fully benefit from these evidence-based interventions due to the severity of symptoms. While no medication will substitute for the need to study to pass an exam, treating a headache may improve the effectiveness of studying for that calculus test. Similarly, adults with severe social anxiety may have difficulty attending cognitive behavioral therapy (CBT) sessions. In such a case, the reduction of some degree of anxiety with pharmacotherapy could improve treatment adherence. As exemplified in these two scenarios, the severity of psychiatric conditions supports the combination of therapy and medication rather than therapy alone. In fact, studies involving nonautistic individuals have reported the superiority of combined medication and therapy for psychiatric conditions to therapy alone or medication alone (March et al., 2004; Piacentini et al., 2014). A common misconception about pharmacotherapy in autistic individuals is that medication is a last resort. However, as described previously, pharmacotherapy can be judiciously combined with nonpharmacological interventions.

PATIENTS' AND CLIENTS' PERSPECTIVES INTO PHARMACOTHERAPY

Clinicians need to acknowledge patients' reservations and concerns about pharmacotherapy. There may be concerns about side-effects, particularly in the setting of a history of sensitivities to dietary or other environmental changes. They may feel that medication is a confirmation that they are mentally ill or that it will fundamentally change who they are or how they think. Such concerns can be attributable to multiple factors, and the current psychotropic nomenclature may well be one of the critical ones (Sultan et al., 2018). For example, autistic adults may feel confused if their online search reveals that the psychiatrist is proposing an "antipsychotic medication" for mitigating their irritability. Although antipsychotic medications can be indicated for a variety of symptoms unrelated to psychosis (tics, irritability, and aggression) through their effects on dopamine receptors, the current name "antipsychotics" does not account for how medications act in our central nervous systems at all, potentially leading to confusion and stigma. This disease-based psychotropic nomenclature issue also applies to other medications, such as antidepressants and stimulants.

Providing the neuroscience-based mechanism of action nomenclature alone instead of traditional psychotropic classification names (e.g., "dopamine antagonists" instead of "antipsychotics") in this chapter may lead to confusion to readers who are familiar with traditional nomenclature. Therefore, in order to assist readers in furthering their understandings of commonly used medication in this population, we will provide descriptions of each medication class using both traditional and mechanism-of-action medication nomenclature as much as possible (see Table 18-1).

PSYCHIATRIC CONDITIONS THAT CO-OCCUR IN AUTISTIC ADULTS

There are many reasons to support the clinical importance of addressing co-occurring problems in autism. The presence of co-occurring disorders is associated with poor prognosis, greater functional impairment, lower quality of life, and increased family burden (Chiang & Gau, 2016; Joshi et al., 2010, 2013). As noted earlier, co-occurring problems potentially exacerbate core autistic symptoms (e.g., exacerbations of repetitive behaviors due to anxiety; Duvekot et al., 2018).

In autistic children and adolescents, methodologically sound epidemiological studies have revealed high co-occurring psychiatric conditions in this population, where attention deficit/hyperactivity disorder (ADHD), behavioral disorder, and anxiety disorder are the most prevalent (Simonoff et al., 2008).

Research on the trajectory of these co-occurring psychiatric problems from childhood into adulthood is limited. One study using the Australian longitudinal cohort of autistic individuals revealed that rates of emotional and behavioral problems decreased over time (Gray et al., 2012). However, the rate of these problems in adulthood (mean age 24.8 years) remained higher in the autistic group than that in the comparison sample of adults with intellectual disability. A recently published study that examined trajectories of emotional, behavioral/conduct, and ADHD symptoms using the Strengths and Difficulties Questionnaire from childhood to adulthood among autistic individuals in the UK revealed similar findings (i.e., a decrease in these symptoms over time; Stringer et al., 2020).

The prevalence of co-occurring psychiatric conditions in autistic adults has a wide variation depending on study populations (age, sex, presence of intellectual disability), study settings (a total population sample versus clinically referred sample, different countries), measurements for autistic, and measurements for

Disease-based category	Medication	Pharmacology domain/ neurotransmitter	Mechanism of action	Other names	Side effects
Antidepressant	fluoxetine fluvoxamine sertraline escitalopram	5-HT	reuptake inhibitor	SSRI	Gastrointestinal symptoms, insomnia, activation, sexual dysfunction
	venlafaxine	5-HT, NE	reuptake inhibitor	SNRI	Same as above
	clomipramine	5-HT, NE	reuptake inhibitor	TCA	Dry mouth, constipation
	mirtazapine	NE, DA	multimodal		Sedation, appetite increase
	trazodone	5-HT, H	multimodal		Sedation, dry mouth
Antipsychotic	aripiprazole	DA, 5-HT	partial agonist and antagonist	atypical, SGA	Extrapyramidal symptoms, sedation, weight gain, galactorrhea, tardive dyskinesia
	risperidone	D, 5-HT, NE	antagonist		
	olanzapine	DA, 5-HT	antagonist		
	quetiapine	DA, 5-HT, NE	multimodal		
	loxapine	DA, 5-HT	antagonist		
	haloperidol	DA	antagonist	typical, FGA	
Psychostimulant	methylphenidate amphetamine derivative	DA, NE	multimodal		Appetite suppression, insomnia
Anxiolytic	lorazepam	GABA	positive allosteric modulator	benzodiazepine	Sedation, muscle relaxation, memory deficit
	hydroxyzine	H	antagonist		Sedation
Antiepileptic	valproate	glutamate	unclear		Weight gain, sedation, elevated liver enzyme
	lamotrigine	glutamate	channel blocker		Rash

	Drug	Target	Mechanism		Side effects
Hypnotic	melatonin ramelteon	melatonin	agonist		Sedation, muscle relaxation, memory deficit
	zolpidem	GABA	positive allosteric modulator		
Others	propranolol	NE	antagonist	beta-blocker	Sedation, bradycardia
	guanfacine clonidine	NE	agonist	alpha agonist	Sedation, hypotension, fatigue
	atomoxetine	NE	reuptake inhibitor		Headache, decreased appetite
	lithium carbonate	lithium	enzyme modulator		Hand tremor, diarrhea
	naltrexone	opioid	antagonist		Gastrointestinal symptoms

ABBREVIATIONS: DA = dopamine, FGA = first-generation antipsychotic, GABA = gamma-aminobutyric acid, H = histamine, NE = norepinephrine, SGA = second-generation antipsychotic, SNRI = serotonin noradrenaline reuptake inhibitor, SSRI = selective serotonin reuptake inhibitor, TCA = tricyclic antidepressant, 5-HT = serotonin psychiatric conditions (in-person assessment via semi- or structured interview vs. questionnaire alone).

To provide a better understanding of co-occurring psychiatric disorders in autistic adults, we list findings from a quantitative synthesis of 24 studies included in a systematic review (Lugo-Marín et al., 2019) in Table 18-2. As seen in Table 18-2 and reported from other studies, anxiety disorder, ADHD, and mood disorder are common in adulthood (Croen et al., 2015; Hofvander et al., 2009; Joshi et al., 2013).

Other important psychiatric conditions that are not included in Table 18-2 are suicidality, disruptive behaviors, tics, and catatonia, all of which can be indications for pharmacotherapy. Suicidality among autistic individuals has recently gained substantial attention. An epidemiological study showed high frequencies of suicide plans (66%) and suicide attempts (35%) in adults with Asperger syndrome (Cassidy et al., 2014), underpinning the importance of recognizing suicidality in this population. Disruptive behaviors, including aggression and self-injurious behaviors, have been extensively studied in autistic youth. However, these problems also occur at higher rates in autistic adults than those with no disability or other developmental disabilities (McCarthy et al., 2010). Lastly, catatonia is a syndrome characterized by a group of symptoms that usually involve a lack of movement and communication and can also include agitation, confusion, and restlessness (Rasmussen et al., 2016), the co-occurrence of which is more frequent in autistic individuals than that in non-autistic individuals (Kakooza-Mwesige et al., 2008).

Taken together, results from studies in autistic adults support the clinical imperative to further our understanding of co-occurring psychiatric conditions in this population. Additionally, these findings highlight the necessity for adequate

Table 18-2 PREVALENCE OF CO-OCCURRING PSYCHIATRIC DISORDERS IN ADULTS WITH AUTISTIC

Psychiatric disorders	Prevalence (%)	95% CI (%)	N of studies included for meta-analyses	Sample size
Any psychiatric	54.8	46.6–62.7	18	3400
ADHD	25.7	18.6–34.3	18	24511
Mood	18.8	10.6–31.1	14	21797
Anxiety	17.8	12.3–25.2	17	23082
Schizophrenia spectrum	11.8	7.7–17.6	17	22176
Substance use	8.3	4.1–16.1	16	21661
Eating disorders	3.6	2.1–6.1	8	678

NOTE: Obsessive compulsive disorder (OCD) was included in the anxiety disorder category in this meta-analytic study.

Modified from Lugo-Marín et al. (2019).

interventions to prevent negative outcomes. As pharmacotherapy is an important treatment option, we will review available evidence for psychopharmacotherapy in adults with autistic in the next section.

MEDICATIONS FOR CO-OCCURRING PSYCHIATRIC PROBLEMS/DISORDERS

In this section, psychotropic medications used for autistic adults are summarized in Table 18-1. Medication names are listed with their pharmacology (neurotransmitter targeted) and mechanism of action to facilitate readers' understandings of the neuroscience-based nomenclature (NbN) of medications, as discussed previously and obtained from the platform for the NbN managed by the International College of Neuropsychopharmacology (https://www.cinp.org/nomenclature). Common side-effects are also listed. Clinical indications are described in the following section.

When it comes to describing how medications work, it is common to identify which neurotransmitter system or domain in the brain they primarily interact with and also the nature of that interaction. The neurotransmitter is like a common currency with which a system communicates. Serotonin, dopamine, norepinephrine, glutamate, GABA, and others each function in this way. Many medications interact with more than one neurotransmitter system, as highlighted in Table 18-1. Some medications essentially act like counterfeit neurotransmitters and are called "agonists," and some medications get in the way of neurotransmitters and reduce their effects. Medications that reduce or block activity are called "antagonists." Still other medications may affect the synthesis or natural recycling mechanisms for neurotransmitters in the brain.

Antidepressants

The largest subgroup of antidepressants are serotonergic agents, which refer to drugs that affect serotonin (5-HT) systems. These agents can be categorized into serotonin reuptake inhibitors, serotonin receptor agonists, and serotonin receptor antagonists.

SELECTIVE SEROTONIN REUPTAKE INHIBITORS (SSRIs)
SSRIs bind to the serotonin transporter (SERT) which is a transmembrane protein embedded in the presynaptic terminal. Normally, a fraction of 5-HT binds to SERT after it is released into the synaptic cleft and this triggers a conformational change in SERT allowing for 5-HT to move into the neuron. The SSRI is the first-line medication for the treatment of anxiety and depression in neurotypical individuals.

Although antidepressants are the most frequently prescribed class of psychotropics among autistic adults (Buck et al., 2014; Cvejic et al., 2018), there have been only a limited number of placebo-controlled randomized controlled trials (RCT's) examining the efficacy and safety of SSRIs in this population. Two studies were with fluoxetine and one study was with fluvoxamine. In these studies, SSRIs were superior to placebo in reducing repetitive behaviors. Only one study, with a very small sample size (n = 6), revealed the efficacy of fluoxetine in anxiety based on the improvement of the Hamilton rating scales for anxiety, but not on the depression scale, indicating potential effects of this medication on anxiety. However, this needs to be replicated in studies with larger sample sizes.

A lower level of evidence for the use of SSRIs in autistic adults is also available from noncontrolled trials, case series, and case reports. In these studies, SSRIs (fluoxetine, fluvoxamine, and sertraline) were effective for the reduction of repetitive and aggressive symptoms (Koshes, 1997; McDougle et al., 1990; McDougle, Brodkin, et al., 1998), but not in treating depression (Fontenelle et al., 2004).

Taken together, a systematic review of existing studies does not support the efficacy of SSRIs in autistic adults for core diagnostic features of autism (Williams et al., 2013); however, it remains unknown if this finding extends to treatment for indications for which ample evidence of efficacy exists in the general population.

Serotonin Noradrenaline Reuptake Inhibitor (SNRI)
Like SSRIs, SNRIs also inhibit SERT, but SNRIs additionally inhibit the norepinephrine transporter by binding allosterically. Venlafaxine, in a retrospective review of 10 autistic adults, was associated with improvements in repetitive behaviors and interests, social deficits, communication, inattention, and hyperactivity (Hollander et al., 2000); however, neither anxiety nor depressive symptoms were measured in this study.

Tricyclic Antidepressant (TCA)
Tricyclic antidepressants take their name from the chemical structure of the drug molecule. Their mechanism of action is complex but they bind to specific receptor sites and mimic the action of endogenous neurotransmitters like serotonin.

Although nearly half of the 33 autistic adults showed good response to the TCA clomipramine, with reductions of repetitive thoughts and behaviors and aggression in an open-label trial (Brodkin et al., 1997), this medication failed to improve stereotypy in a controlled study including autistic adults (Remington et al., 2001). This controlled study also revealed poor tolerability of clomipramine; nearly 40% of participants prematurely dropped out from the study due to side effects, including exacerbations of behavioral problems. Due to their side effects (see Table 18-1), particularly the potential to lower seizure threshold in individuals with epilepsy, TCAs are not commonly prescribed in autism.

OTHER SEROTONERGIC DRUGS

As noted previously, in addition to inhibiting neurotransmitter reuptake, there are also serotonergic medications that act directly on 5-HT receptors. Among them, buspirone is a serotonin partial agonist. It also has a slight affinity for dopamine receptors in the brain. Buspirone showed some benefits with reductions of challenging behaviors, including self-injurious behaviors in autistic individuals and intellectual disabilities (Brahm et al., 2008) and in anxiety in adults with Williams syndrome (Dratcu et al., 2007).

Combining aspects of many serotonergic agents, mirtazapine is both pharmacologically unique and complex. Mirtazapine is an antagonist of α2-adrenergic, 5-HT, and histamine receptors, and thus may target anxiety, depression, and even insomnia, the effects of which is supported only in a case report (Posey et al., 2001).

Trazodone is another common serotonin modulator that exerts antidepressant effects principally by blocking the 5-HT2A receptors present throughout the neocortex. Trazodone also possesses considerable H1 and α-adrenergic receptor antagonism and is thus used for the treatment of insomnia.

Antipsychotics

Antipsychotics are divided into two classes: typical (or first-generation) and atypical (or second-generation) depending on their pharmacology. Currently, two atypical antipsychotics, risperidone and aripiprazole, are the only medications that have U.S. FDA approval for the treatment of behaviors associated with autism, specifically irritability and aggression. While these medications are approved only for autistic children and adolescents, they are widely prescribed for autistic adults (Alfageh et al., 2020; Buck et al., 2014).

ATYPICAL ANTIPSYCHOTICS

Only one placebo-controlled study examined the efficacy and safety of atypical antipsychotic medication in autistic adults, where risperidone, a D2 receptor antagonist, effectively reduced repetitive behavior, irritability and aggression, anxiety, and depression (McDougle, Holmes, et al., 1998). Participants tolerated risperidone well in this trial, only with mild transient sedation. Evidence of other atypical antipsychotics, including aripiprazole and olanzapine, was only supported by case series; both of these medications mitigated challenging behaviors (Jordan et al., 2012; Potenza et al., 1999). Appetite increase and weight gain were problematic in patients with olanzapine.

TYPICAL ANTIPSYCHOTICS

A placebo-controlled trial of haloperidol in autistic adults demonstrated the efficacy of this typical antipsychotic medication in reducing irritability and hyperactivity (Remington et al., 2001). However, nearly one third of participants prematurely discontinued the study due to side effects, including but not limited to fatigue, lethargy, and dystonia.

Antiepileptics and Mood Stabilizers

Many antiepileptic (anticonvulsant) medications, including valproate, are also used as mood stabilizers. No controlled studies have been conducted using antiepileptics in autistic adults. Although one noncontrolled study demonstrated that autistic adult patients with valproate reported improvement in aggression and impulsivity (Hollander et al., 2001), a meta-analysis of existing controlled trials with antiepileptics in autistic youth did not support the superiority of antiepileptics, including valproate, over placebo (Hirota et al., 2014).

Lithium is a nonantiepileptic mood stabilizer. Despite a wealth of empirical evidence supporting its efficacy in stabilizing mood, specific mechanisms by which lithium exerts its mood-stabilizing effects are not well understood. The evidence level of the efficacy of lithium for behavioral problems in autism is limited to a retrospective chart review (Mintz & Hollenberg, 2019).

Psychostimulants

As neurodevelopmental disorders typically persist into adulthood, autistic adults and ADHD may require ongoing treatment for their ADHD, including pharmacotherapy. However, there have been no controlled trials on stimulants, alpha adrenergic drugs, or atomoxetine conducted in this population. Instead, studies in autistic adults are limited to one case report (Roy et al., 2009). Due to the paucity of data, it is recommended that providers follow the pharmacology guidelines issued by national or international organizations.

Anxiolytics/Benzodiazepine (BZP)

Benzodiazepines (BZPs) have also been found to be efficacious in the treatment of generalized anxiety disorder (GAD) in adults without autism, generally leading to a reduction of emotional and somatic symptoms within minutes to hours. The use of BZPs should generally be limited to the short-term and tapered off gradually due to concerns about risks of dependence and tolerance.

In clinical practice, short-term use of BZPs can be beneficial for some individuals with and without autism to ease their fear and anxiety before procedures (for example, dental procedures). However, the use of BZPs requires some caution, particularly in autistic adults, given that it is anecdotally reported that these individuals are more likely to have paradoxical reactions to GABA-promoting agents, including BZPs, compared to nonautistic individuals. Paradoxical reactions are characterized by increased talkativeness, emotional release, excitement, and excessive movement.

The use of BZPs in autism is mostly reported in cases with catatonia. Although no controlled studies have been conducted, experts in this field recommend lorazepam as the first-line medication for catatonia (Fink et al., 2006).

OTHER MEDICATIONS THAT ARE USED
FOR AUTISTIC ADULTS IN CLINICAL PRACTICE

Naltrexone

Based on a hypothesis that self-injurious behaviors may be due to overactivity in opioid systems, researchers have examined the efficacy of naltrexone, an opioid antagonist, in autistic individuals; however, two small sample-sized controlled trials failed to show the superiority of naltrexone in reducing aggression and self-injury over placebo in autistic adults (Willemsen-Swinkels et al., 1995; Zingarelli et al., 1992).

Alpha-2 Agonists

Clonidine and guanfacine stimulate presynaptic autoreceptors that dampen adrenergic tone. This property accounts for their usefulness in severe hypertension, opiate withdrawal, and pain syndromes. In clinical psychiatry, these agents are used for ADHD (note that extended-release form of clonidine and guanfacine are approved for ADHD), tic disorders, anxiety, and impulsive aggression. A controlled trial of the extended-release guanfacine reported its efficacy for ADHD in autistic children and adolescents (Scahill et al., 2015). Despite the persistence and progression of the symptoms and disorders described previously from childhood into adulthood, there is a paucity of evidence in the use of these medications in adult populations.

Beta Blockers

Propranolol can be used for reducing emotional and behavioral dysregulation (Sagar-Ouriaghli et al., 2018). In a controlled trial of propranolol in autistic adults, the primary outcome was a change in performance on the conversational reciprocity task (Zamzow et al., 2016). In this study, however, neither autonomic activity nor anxiety was significantly associated with drug response.

CHALLENGES IN PHARMACOTHERAPY

Polypharmacy, defined as the concurrent use of multiple medications, is common in autistic adults, with as many as half taking two or more psychotropic drugs (Buck et al., 2014; Esbensen et al., 2009). In particular, studies have reported the trend toward increasing the use of more than one antipsychotic in the treatment of behavioral problems in autistic individuals (Schubart et al., 2014). This is concerning, considering the risks of adverse effects associated with these medications, including extrapyramidal symptoms, weight gain, and metabolic risks. Furthermore, the effectiveness of polypharmacy is minimally supported by evidence.

Although no regulations are placed on autistic individuals specifically, the use of antipsychotics and other psychotropic medications in individuals with intellectual disability is strictly regulated in institutional settings by federal and state agencies in the United States (Janowsky et al., 2005). The guidelines include periodic case reviews to determine the necessity of psychotropic medications and use of the lowest effective dose or minimally effective doses needed. Thus, psychotropic medication reductions and discontinuations are routine in institutions for individuals with intellectual disabilities (Janowsky et al., 2005). However, relapse of aggressive and other target symptoms during medication withdrawal trials is common and can be clinically severe in individuals with intellectual disabilities as well as autism (Haessler et al., 2007; Research Units on Pediatric Psychopharmacology Autism Network, 2005). For an individual who was treated with a medication for symptoms of irritability, who is no longer actively symptomatic after a lengthy period of time, it is absolutely appropriate to determine if the drug is still necessary. However, for an individual with well-documented bipolar disorder, whose mood stabilizing medication is meant to prevent the recurrence of episodes, the decision to withdraw an effective treatment (measured by the absence of illness), is much more complicated.

In clinical practice, it can often be challenging to assess whether autistic adults benefit from polypharmacy on psychotropics or not and to determine medication reductions and discontinuations. This is particularly common when we see adult patients whose caregivers do not have good recollections of reasons for polypharmacy (whether medication withdrawal was previously attempted, how patients responded to monotherapy of psychotropic medication before). Abrupt medication reductions or discontinuations may lead to relapses of behavioral problems in autistic individuals. Additionally, as reported in some studies, these procedures can result in the development of withdrawal dyskinesia (defined as involuntary movements after the discontinuation of or the reduction in the dosage of antipsychotics; Kumar et al., 2018). Whether individuals with neurodevelopmental disorders, including autism, are more vulnerable to these negative consequences or not remains unknown.

CASE STUDY

Ben is a 28-year-old autistic man who was diagnosed with generalised anxiety disorder. Although he improved somewhat after the completion of 12-session psychotherapy, his anxiety persisted and unfortunately deteriorated a few months ago. This prompted a visit with a psychiatrist who recommended a trial of fluoxetine (one of the SSRIs).

Ben initially declined a medication trial, as he was concerned about possible suicidal ideation as a side effect of fluoxetine, which he found while searching this medication on the internet. The psychiatrist provided information on this medication and assisted him in comparing the benefits and risks of the medication treatment (and of not taking medication for anxiety). The psychiatrist also gave Ben clear instructions on how to monitor his anxiety and behaviors after the start of fluoxetine, how frequent he required psychiatric clinic visits, when to expect to see improvement, and what to look for as signs of recovery. Following this thorough psychoeducation on medication treatment, Ben provided informed consent to fluoxetine treatment.

He started with a low dose of fluoxetine, which the psychiatrist gradually increased while carefully monitoring his anxiety as well as neurovegetative symptoms, including sleep and appetite. Three weeks after he started fluoxetine, the psychiatrist observed notable improvement in Ben's anxiety symptoms, as captured by the General Anxiety Disorder-7 scale.

CONCLUSIONS AND FUTURE DIRECTIONS

Despite the high prevalence of co-occurring psychiatric conditions, evidence specifically informing psychopharmacotherapy among autistic adults is scarce. Many existing studies are open-label trials, and the sample size of existing RCTs is small, leading to the lack of power to determine the efficacy and safety of psychotropics in this population. Large-scale controlled studies and long-term follow-up studies are clearly needed. Taken together, at this point, we recommend that providers follow currently available guidelines (albeit not developed exclusively for autistic individuals) for treating these psychiatric conditions in autism.

Polypharmacy is pervasive in this population, reflecting challenges that physicians face both in the assessment and treatment of these conditions. This phenomenon is concerning as these individuals can be sensitive to psychotropics. A dearth of physicians specializing in pharmacological interventions for co-occurring psychiatric conditions in this population may contribute to polypharmacy. It is clear that more training programs providing adequate education and clinical experiences in this field, and clinical systems allowing primary care providers or general psychiatrists to consult specialists, in this field could be impactful.

Lastly, more discussions about optimal outcomes in clinical trials in the autistic population are needed. Although existing studies have mostly focused on improvements in psychopathology, capturing changes in life satisfaction and well-being could be alternative and important measures of success for autistic adults in future intervention studies.

REFERENCES

AACAP Autism Parents' Medication Guide Work Group. (2016). *Autism spectrum disorder: Parents' medication guide*. American Academy of Child and Adolescent Psychiatry.

Alfageh, B. H., Man, K. K. C., Besag, F. M. C., Alhawassi, T. M., Wong, I. C. K., & Brauer, R. (2020). Psychotropic medication prescribing for neuropsychiatric comorbidities in individuals diagnosed with autism spectrum disorder (ASD) in the UK. *Journal of Autism and Developmental Disorders, 50*(2), 625–633.

Brahm, N. C., Fast, G. A., & Brown, R. C. (2008). Buspirone for autistic disorder in a woman with an intellectual disability. *Annals of Pharmacotherapy, 42*(1), 131–137.

Brodkin, E. S., McDougle, C. J., Naylor, S. T., Cohen, D. J., & Price, L. H. (1997). Clomipramine in adults with pervasive developmental disorders: A prospective open-label investigation. *Journal of Child and Adolescent Psychopharmacology, 7*(2), 109–121.

Buck, T. R., Viskochil, J., Farley, M., Coon, H., McMahon, W. M., Morgan, J., & Bilder, D. A. (2014). Psychiatric comorbidity and medication use in adults with autism spectrum disorder. *Journal of Autism and Developmental Disorders, 44*(12), 3063–3071.

Cassidy, S., Bradley, P., Robinson, J., Allison, C., McHugh, M., & Baron-Cohen, S. (2014). Suicidal ideation and suicide plans or attempts in adults with Asperger's syndrome attending a specialist diagnostic clinic: A clinical cohort study. *The Lancet Psychiatry, 1*(2), 142–147.

Chiang, H.-L., & Gau, S. S.-F. (2016). Comorbid psychiatric conditions as mediators to predict later social adjustment in youths with autism spectrum disorder. *Journal of Child Psychology and Psychiatry, 57*(1), 103–111.

Croen, L. A., Zerbo, O., Qian, Y., Massolo, M. L., Rich, S., Sidney, S., & Kripke, C. (2015). The health status of adults on the autism spectrum. *Autism, 19*(7), 814–823.

Cvejic, R. C., Arnold, S. R. C., Foley, K.-R., & Trollor, J. N. (2018). Neuropsychiatric profile and psychotropic medication use in adults with autism spectrum disorder: Results from the Australian Longitudinal Study of Adults with Autism. *BJPsych Open, 4*(6), 461–466.

Dratcu, L., McKay, G., Singaravelu, V., & Krishnamurthy, V. (2007). Aripiprazole treatment of Asperger's syndrome in the acute psychiatric setting: Case report. *Neuropsychiatric Disease and Treatment, 3*(1), 173–176.

Duvekot, J., Ende, J. van der, Verhulst, F. C., & Greaves-Lord, K. (2018). Examining bidirectional effects between the autism spectrum disorder (ASD) core symptom domains and anxiety in children with ASD. *Journal of Child Psychology and Psychiatry, 59*(3), 277–284.

Esbensen, A. J., Greenberg, J. S., Seltzer, M. M., & Aman, M. G. (2009). A longitudinal investigation of psychotropic and non-psychotropic medication use among adolescents and adults with autism spectrum disorders. *Journal of Autism and Developmental Disorders, 39*(9), 1339–1349.

Fink, M., Taylor, M. A., & Ghaziuddin, N. (2006). Catatonia in autistic spectrum disorders: A medical treatment algorithm. *International Review of Neurobiology, 72*, 233–244.

Fontenelle, L. F., Mendlowicz, M. V., Bezerra de Menezes, G., dos Santos Martins, R. R., & Versiani, M. (2004). Asperger syndrome, obsessive-compulsive disorder, and major depression in a patient with 45,X/46,XY mosaicism. *Psychopathology, 37*(3), 105–109.

Gray, K., Keating, C., Taffe, J., Brereton, A., Einfeld, S., & Tonge, B. (2012). Trajectory of behavior and emotional problems in autism. *American Journal on Intellectual and Developmental Disabilities, 117*(2), 121–133.

Haessler, F., Glaser, T., Beneke, M., Pap, A. F., Bodenschatz, R., Reis, O., & Zuclopenthixol Disruptive Behaviour Study Group. (2007). Zuclopenthixol in adults with intellectual disabilities and aggressive behaviours: Discontinuation study. *The British Journal of Psychiatry: The Journal of Mental Science, 190*, 447–448.

Hirota, T., Veenstra-Vanderweele, J., Hollander, E., & Kishi, T. (2014). Antiepileptic medications in autism spectrum disorder: A systematic review and meta-analysis. *Journal of Autism and Developmental Disorders, 44*(4), 948–957.

Hofvander, B., Delorme, R., Chaste, P., Nyden, A., Wentz, E., Stahlberg, O., Herbrecht, E., Stopin, A., Anckarsater, H., Gillberg, C., Rastam, M., & Leboyer, M. (2009). Psychiatric and psychosocial problems in adults with normal-intelligence autism spectrum disorders. *BMC Psychiatry, 9*(1), 35.

Hollander, E., Dolgoff-Kaspar, R., Cartwright, C., Rawitt, R., & Novotny, S. (2001). An open trial of divalproex sodium in autism spectrum disorders. *The Journal of Clinical Psychiatry, 62*(7), 530–534.

Hollander, E., Kaplan, A., Cartwright, C., & Reichman, D. (2000). Venlafaxine in children, adolescents, and young adults with autism spectrum disorders: An open retrospective clinical report. *Journal of Child Neurology, 15*(2), 132–135.

Howes, O. D., Rogdaki, M., Findon, J. L., Wichers, R. H., Charman, T., King, B. H., Loth, E., McAlonan, G. M., McCracken, J. T., Parr, J. R., Povey, C., Santosh, P., Wallace, S., Simonoff, E., & Murphy, D. G. (2018). Autism spectrum disorder: Consensus guidelines on assessment, treatment and research from the British Association for Psychopharmacology. *Journal of Psychopharmacology (Oxford, England), 32*(1), 3–29.

Janowsky, D. S., Barnhill, L. J., Shetty, M., & Davis, J. M. (2005). Minimally effective doses of conventional antipsychotic medications used to treat aggression, self-injurious and destructive behaviors in mentally retarded adults. *Journal of Clinical Psychopharmacology, 25*(1), 19–25.

Jordan, I., Robertson, D., Catani, M., Craig, M., & Murphy, D. (2012). Aripiprazole in the treatment of challenging behaviour in adults with autism spectrum disorder. *Psychopharmacology, 223*(3), 357–360.

Joshi, G., Petty, C., Wozniak, J., Henin, A., Fried, R., Galdo, M., Kotarski, M., Walls, S., & Biederman, J. (2010). The heavy burden of psychiatric comorbidity in youth with autism spectrum disorders: A large comparative study of a psychiatrically referred population. *Journal of Autism and Developmental Disorders, 40*(11), 1361–1370.

Joshi, G., Wozniak, J., Petty, C., Martelon, M. K., Fried, R., Bolfek, A., Kotte, A., Stevens, J., Furtak, S. L., Bourgeois, M., Caruso, J., Caron, A., & Biederman, J. (2013). Psychiatric comorbidity and functioning in a clinically referred population of adults with autism spectrum disorders: A comparative study. *Journal of Autism and Developmental Disorders, 43*(6), 1314–1325.

Kakooza-Mwesige, A., Wachtel, L. E., & Dhossche, D. M. (2008). Catatonia in autism: Implications across the life span. *European Child & Adolescent Psychiatry*, *17*(6), 327–335.

King, B. H., Hollander, E., Sikich, L., McCracken, J. T., Scahill, L., Bregman, J. D., Donnelly, C. L., Anagnostou, E., Dukes, K., Sullivan, L., Hirtz, D., Wagner, A., Ritz, L., & STAART Psychopharmacology Network. (2009). Lack of efficacy of citalopram in children with autism spectrum disorders and high levels of repetitive behavior: Citalopram ineffective in children with autism. *Archives of General Psychiatry*, *66*(6), 583–590.

Koshes, R. J. (1997). Use of fluoxetine for obsessive-compulsive behavior in adults with autism. *American Journal of Psychiatry*, *154*(4), 578.

Kumar, M., Mattison, R., & Baweja, R. (2018). Withdrawal-emergent dyskinesia after acute discontinuation of risperidone in a child with autism spectrum disorder. *Journal of Clinical Psychopharmacology*, *38*(6), 640–642.

Lugo-Marín, J., Magán-Maganto, M., Rivero-Santana, A., Cuellar-Pompa, L., Alviani, M., Jenaro-Rio, C., Díez, E., & Canal-Bedia, R. (2019). Prevalence of psychiatric disorders in adults with autism spectrum disorder: A systematic review and meta-analysis. *Research in Autism Spectrum Disorders*, *59*, 22–33.

March, J., Silva, S., Petrycki, S., Curry, J., Wells, K., Fairbank, J., Burns, B., Domino, M., McNulty, S., Vitiello, B., Severe, J., & Treatment for Adolescents With Depression Study (TADS) Team. (2004). Fluoxetine, cognitive-behavioral therapy, and their combination for adolescents with depression: Treatment for Adolescents With Depression Study (TADS) randomized controlled trial. *JAMA*, *292*(7), 807–820.

McCarthy, J., Hemmings, C., Kravariti, E., Dworzynski, K., Holt, G., Bouras, N., & Tsakanikos, E. (2010). Challenging behavior and co-morbid psychopathology in adults with intellectual disability and autism spectrum disorders. *Research in Developmental Disabilities*, *31*(2), 362–366.

McDougle, C. J., Brodkin, E. S., Naylor, S. T., Carlson, D. C., Cohen, D. J., & Price, L. H. (1998). Sertraline in adults with pervasive developmental disorders: A prospective open-label investigation. *Journal of Clinical Psychopharmacology*, *18*(1), 62–66.

McDougle, C. J., Holmes, J. P., Carlson, D. C., Pelton, G. H., Cohen, D. J., & Price, L. H. (1998). A double-blind, placebo-controlled study of risperidone in adults with autistic disorder and other pervasive developmental disorders. *Archives of General Psychiatry*, *55*(7), 633–641.

McDougle, C. J., Price, L. H., & Goodman, W. K. (1990). Fluvoxamine treatment of co-incident autistic disorder and obsessive-compulsive disorder: A case report. *Journal of Autism and Developmental Disorders*, *20*(4), 537–543.

McGuire, K., Fung, L. K., Hagopian, L., Vasa, R. A., Mahajan, R., Bernal, P., Silberman, A. E., Wolfe, A., Coury, D. L., Hardan, A. Y., Veenstra-VanderWeele, J., & Whitaker, A. H. (2016). Irritability and problem behavior in autism spectrum disorder: A practice pathway for pediatric primary care. *Pediatrics*, *137 Suppl 2*, S136–148.

Mintz, M., & Hollenberg, E. (2019). Revisiting lithium: Utility for behavioral stabilization in adolescents and adults with autism spectrum disorder. *Psychopharmacology Bulletin*, *49*(2), 28–40.

Mohiuddin, S., & Ghaziuddin, M. (2013). Psychopharmacology of autism spectrum disorders: A selective review. *Autism: The International Journal of Research and Practice, 17*(6), 645–654.

Piacentini, J., Bennett, S., Compton, S. N., Kendall, P. C., Birmaher, B., Albano, A. M., March, J., Sherrill, J., Sakolsky, D., Ginsburg, G., Rynn, M., Bergman, R. L., Gosch, E., Waslick, B., Iyengar, S., McCracken, J., & Walkup, J. (2014). 24- and 36-week outcomes for the Child/Adolescent Anxiety Multimodal Study (CAMS). *Journal of the American Academy of Child & Adolescent Psychiatry, 53*(3), 297–310.

Posey, D. J., Guenin, K. D., Kohn, A. E., Swiezy, N. B., & McDougle, C. J. (2001). A naturalistic open-label study of mirtazapine in autistic and other pervasive developmental disorders. *Journal of Child and Adolescent Psychopharmacology, 11*(3), 267–277.

Potenza, M. N., Holmes, J. P., Kanes, S. J., & McDougle, C. J. (1999). Olanzapine treatment of children, adolescents, and adults with pervasive developmental disorders: An open-label pilot study. *Journal of Clinical Psychopharmacology, 19*(1), 37–44.

Rasmussen, S. A., Mazurek, M. F., & Rosebush, P. I. (2016). Catatonia: Our current understanding of its diagnosis, treatment and pathophysiology. *World Journal of Psychiatry, 6*(4), 391–398.

Remington, G., Sloman, L., Konstantareas, M., Parker, K., & Gow, R. (2001). Clomipramine versus haloperidol in the treatment of autistic disorder: A double-blind, placebo-controlled, crossover study. *Journal of Clinical Psychopharmacology, 21*(4), 440–444.

Research Units on Pediatric Psychopharmacology Autism Network. (2005). Risperidone treatment of autistic disorder: Longer-term benefits and blinded discontinuation after 6 months. *American Journal of Psychiatry, 162*(7), 1361–1369.

Roy, M., Dillo, W., Bessling, S., Emrich, H. M., & Ohlmeier, M. D. (2009). Effective methylphenidate treatment of an adult Aspergers syndrome and a comorbid ADHD: A clinical investigation with fMRI. *Journal of Attention Disorders, 12*(4), 381–385.

Sagar-Ouriaghli, I., Lievesley, K., & Santosh, P. J. (2018). Propranolol for treating emotional, behavioural, autonomic dysregulation in children and adolescents with autism spectrum disorders. *Journal of Psychopharmacology (Oxford, England), 32*(6), 641–653.

Scahill, L., McCracken, J. T., King, B. H., Rockhill, C., Shah, B., Politte, L., Sanders, R., Minjarez, M., Cowen, J., Mullett, J., Page, C., Ward, D., Deng, Y., Loo, S., Dziura, J., McDougle, C. J., & Research Units on Pediatric Psychopharmacology Autism Network. (2015). Extended-release guanfacine for hyperactivity in children with autism spectrum disorder. *American Journal of Psychiatry, 172*(12), 1197–1206.

Schubart, J. R., Camacho, F., & Leslie, D. (2014). Psychotropic medication trends among children and adolescents with autism spectrum disorder in the Medicaid program. *Autism: The International Journal of Research and Practice, 18*(6), 631–637.

Simonoff, E., Pickles, A., Charman, T., Chandler, S., Loucas, T., & Baird, G. (2008). Psychiatric disorders in children with autism spectrum disorders: Prevalence, comorbidity, and associated factors in a population-derived sample. *Journal of the American Academy of Child and Adolescent Psychiatry, 47*(8), 921–929.

Stringer, D., Kent, R., Briskman, J., Lukito, S., Charman, T., Baird, G., Lord, C., Pickles, A., & Simonoff, E. (2020). Trajectories of emotional and behavioral problems from childhood to early adult life. *Autism: The International Journal of Research and Practice, 24*(4), 1011–1024.

Sultan, R. S., Correll, C. U., Zohar, J., Zalsman, G., & Veenstra-VanderWeele, J. (2018). What's in a name? Moving to neuroscience-based nomenclature in pediatric psychopharmacology. *Journal of the American Academy of Child and Adolescent Psychiatry, 57*(10), 719–721.

Willemsen-Swinkels, S. H., Buitelaar, J. K., Nijhof, G. J., & van England, H. (1995). Failure of naltrexone hydrochloride to reduce self-injurious and autistic behavior in mentally retarded adults. Double-blind placebo-controlled studies. *Archives of General Psychiatry, 52*(9), 766–773.

Williams, K., Brignell, A., Randall, M., Silove, N., & Hazell, P. (2013). Selective serotonin reuptake inhibitors (SSRIs) for autism spectrum disorders (ASD). *Cochrane Database of Systematic Reviews, 8.*

Zamzow, R. M., Ferguson, B. J., Stichter, J. P., Porges, E. C., Ragsdale, A. S., Lewis, M. L., & Beversdorf, D. Q. (2016). Effects of propranolol on conversational reciprocity in autism spectrum disorder: A pilot, double-blind, single-dose psychopharmacological challenge study. *Psychopharmacology, 233*(7), 1171–1178.

Zingarelli, G., Ellman, G., Hom, A., Wymore, M., Heidorn, S., & Chicz-DeMet, A. (1992). Clinical effects of naltrexone on autistic behavior. *American Journal of Mental Retardation: AJMR, 97*(1), 57–63.

19

Ensuring Accessible and Acceptable Service Delivery for Adults With Autism

DEBBIE SPAIN, SUSAN W. WHITE, AND FRANCISCO M. MUSICH ■

KEY CONSIDERATIONS

- There are multiple systemic and individual barriers to service access for adults with autism.
- Engaging the client, and their family, in discussion about possible obstacles prior to beginning therapy can be helpful in sustaining services.
- Inquiring about the client's preferences regarding terminology, gender orientation, and other qualities can help reduce isolation and unintentional harm.
- Arranging the physical space for therapy, including waiting room, to feel safe and supportive can facilitate engagement.
- It is important that clinicians consider the client's voice and personally held goals in designing treatment programs and in measuring outcomes.

BARRIERS TO ACCESSIBLE PSYCHOLOGICAL THERAPY FOR ADULTS WITH AUTISM

Despite high rates of co-occurring conditions, individuals with autism routinely experience difficulties accessing physical and mental health services (for review, see

Adams & Young, 2020; Doherty et al., 2020; Mason et al., 2019; Walsh et al., 2020). Barriers to accessing psychological therapies for adults with autism may include:

- Service-related factors, such as a lack of services available locally, individuals not seeming to meet service eligibility criteria, referrals being "bounced" between services, long waiting times, and inflexible models/ packages of care that are unsuited to or insufficient for the needs of individuals with autism.
- Provider-related factors, such as poor knowledge of autism, failure to recognize need or underestimating the extent of an individual's difficulties, lack of expertise in working with this client group, stigma, perceptions that individuals with autism do not benefit from psychological therapy, and limited understanding of how to appropriately adapt communication style and interventions.
- Client-related factors, such as not knowing how to ask for support or lack of confidence to do so, feeling overwhelmed by the help-seeking process, limited satisfaction with or trust in services and clinicians, insufficient time, social communication difficulties, sensory sensitivities, cognitive rigidity, difficulties tolerating change and uncertainty, and therapy "burn out" following years of receiving a myriad services from many providers.
- A paucity of funding for services.

Taken together, adults with autism can experience multiple barriers to accessing psychological therapy. There is, therefore, an impetus to understand barriers at both individual and systemic levels, so as to increase therapy accessibility, accept-ability and, in turn, effectiveness.

TAILORING INTAKE AND SERVICE PROVISION

Beginning with a new mental health provider is anxiety provoking for most clients. It is likely amplified for adults with autism. Even though they often have prior experience of working with providers from a range of disciplines, it may be their first experience of independently securing services or in being expected to complete forms and actively engage (rather than relying on their parent or care-giver) in the process. Likewise, they may be accompanied to appointments by a guardian, sibling, or other familiar person.

Clinical Practice Implications

- Service providers are likely to benefit from knowledge and understanding of autism in order to be able to develop autism-friendly and autism-specific services.

- When possible, adults with autism (and their families, as appropriate) should be involved in discussions and decision-making about developing services they might access.
- If possible, intake forms/materials should be proofread by clients with autism, to ensure clarity. Avoid use of jargon.
- New clients may prefer to complete intake paperwork remotely, prior to the first session, to reduce time in the waiting room and so they can secure help from others, as needed.
- Some clients may need assistance to complete intake paperwork by their caregivers or the provider, in particular, when if they also have an intellectual disability or impaired language skills.
- Clients' expectations for the involvement of guardians/others in sessions should be clarified. Privacy rules should be explained.
- It can be important to accommodate sensory sensitivities. This may include setting up the waiting area and office to be calming, reducing distractions, and avoiding perfumes, strong scents and bright lights. Explicitly asking clients if there is anything they find distracting or irritating can be helpful, as they may not think to mention this or may feel nervous to do so.
- Clients' preferences for communicating with others, such as using email, text messages or the phone, should be clarified at the outset.

ENHANCING COMMUNICATION

In setting up accessible services, providers must be attentive to what communication modalities are used and the language used within. In our collective experience, being very clear in spoken and written language is important in therapeutic work with adults with autism. Using jargon, colloquialisms, or nonspecific and undefined terms can cause confusion and stress. Rather than being related to cognitive or even verbal ability, this unneeded confusion is more likely a function of a tendency toward literal interpretation and limited automaticity in using context cues to aid interpretation. Additionally, even well-intentioned providers can unknowingly conduct microaggressions (Williams, 2020) and risk alienating a new client if assumptions (e.g., about gender identity, orientation, or preference for caregiver involvement) are made without first checking the client's preferences. Related to this and the growing body of research indicating heightened gender diversity within autism (Strang et al., 2020), we find it helpful to use nongendered pronouns in paperwork and ask clients at intake about preferred pronouns and names. Clarity and respect also apply to this domain when considering the ongoing and lively debate about terminology about autism itself (see chapter 1).

Clinical Practice Implications

- Preferences for language used (e.g., person first or disability first language, pronouns) should be established.

- Social communication and language skills can be assessed during the first couple of sessions. This may be formally via a screening questionnaire or speech and language therapy assessment, or informally, in the context of interaction. It may understandably take clients time to feel more comfortable within the therapy context.
- Providers may need to adapt their communication style. This might involve using shorter sentences, asking about one construct at a time (e.g., about anxiety and then low mood, rather than about how the client is feeling), using a combination of closed rather than open-ended questions, and recapping frequently.
- Operationalizing terminology used (e.g., anxiety, anger, worry) may be appropriate; definitions may change over time as clients become more emotionally literate.
- Individuals with autism may seem less emotionally expressive, which may either be part of autism, or result from alexithymia or mental health symptoms (e.g., depression). Clarifying how clients are feeling is important if there seems to be an incongruence between verbal and nonverbal communication (e.g., their facial expressions may be flat when discussing traumatic events).
- Using visual means alongside discussion, such as diagrams and mini-formulations, may be appropriate. Some clients may benefit from a written session summary.

ACCOMMODATING HYPO- AND HYPERSENSORY SENSITIVITIES AND AVERSIONS

Most individuals with autism experience sensory sensitivities and aversions (APA, 2013), with some evidence to suggest links between sensory processing and mental health symptoms, including anxiety, mood disturbance, and agitation (for review, see Glod et al., 2015). Sensory experiences can be heightened for individuals with autism, and it is unsurprising that anticipatory worry about, and avoidance of, salient cues can become learned responses.

Clinical Practice Implications

- Formal or informal assessment of hypo and hyper sensory sensitivities may be prudent. Sensory profile assessments are available but may incur cost. Informal discussion about this can be perfectly adequate on the proviso that a broad range of sensory experiences are explored. The assessment may also focus on what coping strategies the client has employed to manage these.
- Consideration of factors that appear to heighten sensory experiences, such as during pregnancy or when tired, can also be helpful to elicit.

- Sensory preferences should be accommodated during sessions; for example, by checking if clients prefer the lights off or on or whether the sound of the air conditioning is bothersome.
- Sensory issues may be relevant for the treatment formulation. These may be causally implicated in the development or maintenance of mental health symptoms.
- Some psychological therapies, notably CBT, emphasize reducing safety behaviors as part of the treatment plan. These are behaviors and responses designed to keep the person "safe," but that indirectly perpetuate mental health symptoms, with avoidance being a good example of this. If sensory sensitivities and aversions contribute to avoidance, conversation can focus on the degree to which avoidance may be an adaptive and helpful response in some contexts (e.g., not going to the supermarket on Christmas Eve) versus less helpful in others (e.g., not going to a supermarket early in the morning when it is quiet).

DEVELOPING A THERAPEUTIC ALLIANCE

A strong therapeutic alliance—comprising agreement and collaboration on therapy goals and tasks, and a reciprocal bond between a client and provider (Borden, 1979)—is found to be predictive of treatment outcomes (Baier et al., 2020; Horvath et al., 2011). Both provider- and client-related factors can mediate successful development of a therapeutic alliance. Pooled (meta-analytic) findings from neurotypical samples suggest that, on average, clients do better when seen by providers who are more adept at developing an alliance (Del Re et al., 2012).

Scant research has focused on the therapeutic alliance in psychological therapy for individuals with autism. However, preliminary evidence indicates this may be similarly important when examined in studies about CBT (Kerns et al., 2018; Klebanoff et al., 2019), mindfulness (Brewe et al., 2021) and social skills interventions for children, adolescents, and/or young adults with autism. A consistent theme in this burgeoning area of research is that the therapeutic alliance is dynamic (i.e., this may become stronger or weaker during therapy); for example, factors including autism symptom severity, affective symptoms, and emotion regulation can influence development and strength of the therapeutic alliance (Brewe et al., 2021; Kerns et al., 2018; Klebanoff et al., 2019).

Clinical Practice Implications

- Providers may wish to consider factors that impact development of a therapeutic alliance. This could include core autism traits (e.g., social motivation, capacity for reciprocity, quality and amount of social overtures), mental health symptoms (e.g., social anxiety, low mood, negative symptoms of psychosis), negative beliefs about others (e.g., that others cannot be trusted, concerns about abandonment), negative beliefs about self (e.g., about being inept or different), adverse life events (e.g., victimization, exploitation) or a lack of opportunities to engage in social relationships and learn the skills integral to this.

- Clarification of clients' preferences for social interaction with others, within the boundaries of therapy, can be explored; for example, do they enjoy or dislike small talk, are they aware that personal questions they ask of providers may be unanswered.
- Providers can role model norms and conventions inherent to social relationships.
- Clients should have time to talk about their hobbies and interests. They may find these easier and more engaging topics than conventional small talk.
- Clarity should be provided about the parameters of interaction during therapy and once this has ended; for example, confirming preferred methods of communication between sessions and the speed with which clients might expect a reply, whom to contact when if there are more urgent concerns, and whether contact ceases at the point of discharge from therapy.
- It can be useful to find out about the types of situations that can contribute to misunderstandings and disagreements and how these are typically resolved. There may be a standing agenda item at the end of sessions to confirm if the provider has made any comments that have led to upset or concern.

GENERAL PRINCIPLES FOR ADAPTING THERAPY

As is exemplified in chapters 2 to 17, many adults with autism can benefit from adaptations to the session structure and content, irrespective of the therapeutic modality, to accommodate core autism traits, impairments in facets of executive functioning (EF; e.g., information processing style, difficulties with generativity and attention), impaired theory of mind, and alexithymia. It is often not possible to undertake formal assessment of cognitive functioning within a psychological therapy service; this is usually considered to be beyond the remit of the service and there may be a lack of appropriately qualified clinicians to conduct this. Additionally, many adults, and especially those diagnosed with autism in adulthood and who have been able to complete formal education without substantial problems, are presumed to have an intelligence quotient (IQ) in at least the average range. They are, therefore, unlikely to have had cognitive assessment elsewhere.

Adults with autism may not feel comfortable telling providers about their preferences and needs spontaneously. Alternatively, they may not tend to initiate many social overtures (which is characteristic of autism), or it may not occur to them that they can do this. They may be prone to acquiescing in conversation with others, particularly if they are in a novel, unfamiliar, or anxiety-provoking situation. It is also important to bear in mind that many adults with autism have had therapy before, with varying degrees of success. For some, this may have been a useful and suitably adapted series of sessions, and what they are now looking for is a "top up." Yet for others, this may have been a confusing, overwhelming, or distressing experience, resulting in worries about failing, getting it wrong or being beyond help. Worries such as these can increase anxiety about further sessions, hopelessness about ability to reach therapeutic goals, and ultimately reduce propensity to be assertive.

Clinical Practice Implications

- As part of the initial assessment session(s), it is important to find out about a client's capabilities and strengths. This might involve asking them to walk the provider through "a typical day," prompting for information about their autonomy and independence to complete activities of daily living, and clarifying who else in the system offers support, if at all. When possible, focus on the here-and-now and one or two junctures in the past, perhaps when their circumstances were different, such as at college or in a prior job, as this can illustrate the trajectory of functioning or impairment.
- Specific activities that can be helpful to ask about—in order to develop rapport, enhance reciprocity in interaction, and find out more about the individual—include how able they are to follow a sequence of events from start to finish (e.g., grocery shopping for the week, planning and cooking a meal, going on a trip to an unfamiliar location), completing nonroutine tasks at work (e.g., preparing and delivering a presentation, first week at a new job), and managing unexpected social situations (e.g., a surprise party, a disagreement with a friend or colleague).
- Attention should also be given to establishing the degree to which mental health symptoms, such as anxiety or low mood, impact on volition to engage in tasks, and completion of these. It may be that as mental health starts to improve during therapy, functioning may also improve.
- Clients may be able to say what could make the structure, timing, and duration of sessions more manageable for them. If they find it difficult to generate examples, providers may need to offer suggestions. Providing a checklist of aspects of sessions that can be adapted and asking clients to reflect on this between sessions might feel easier for some.
- Related to this, "rules" and expectations for therapy should be contracted, which may include between-session practice and assignments, as problems with EF can often lead to difficulty with homework completion.

MEASURING OUTCOMES

Determining whether psychological therapy has gleaned favorable outcomes for clients, and how so, is clearly important. Choice of outcome measurement can vary according to the service setting and therapeutic modality, with perhaps stronger emphasis placed upon this for evaluating the effectiveness of behavioral therapy and CBT.

Some adults with autism struggle to complete self-report questionnaires, such as those that focus on mental health symptoms, distress, or emotional well-being. This can be due to a range of factors, including poor ecological validity of questions, alexithymia, amotivation, and perseveration over responses. There are also wider considerations associated with using standardized mental health outcome measures with individuals with autism, notably that psychometric properties (e.g., normative thresholds) and validity and reliability are largely unknown (Brugha et al., 2015). This means scores above or below the indicative threshold on a questionnaire may require further exploration rather than being taken at face value.

Asking clients to complete questionnaires is fairly standard practice in child and adolescent mental health contexts. However, discrepancies between self- and informant ratings are not uncommon, especially for symptoms of internalizing conditions (De los Reyes et al., 2015). There are advantages and considerations with asking family, friends, or colleagues to complete questionnaires when working with adults with autism. On the one hand, this can provide a wider perspective about how things are outside the therapy room, in terms of symptoms, well-being and functioning. Additionally, family in particular, may be well placed to comment on the stability and trajectory of symptoms over time. On the other hand, some adults with autism may understandably not want others to be aware that they are having therapy. Additionally, adults with autism may perceive that their opinions are not valid or that these are being quashed by others, potentially impacting their engagement and propensity to be assertive.

Clinical Practice Implications

- Responses on self-report screening questionnaires should be discussed with clients. If they score below the indicative threshold on a measure that is used to determine eligibility for services, it may be worthwhile taking into account other available information that could help to contextualize presenting problems, instead of declining support.
- After assessment, decisions about which questionnaires to use should be informed by the treatment formulation.
- Constructs assessed on questionnaires (e.g., emotional well-being), terminology used (e.g., feeling down, hopeless) and directionality of statements (e.g., straightforward versus reverse-scored items) may warrant explanation.

- Clients may benefit from support to complete questionnaires. They may need more time than is usual but may feel uncomfortable about asking for help.
- If using more than one self-report questionnaire, choose those that focus on the same time period if feasible (e.g., symptoms during the last week or month).
- Clients' thoughts about an informant (e.g., parent or partner) completing questionnaires should be elicited. Scores should be discussed in a sensitive manner.
- Completing questionnaires at each session may be too onerous, and this can be a factor for clients disengaging with therapy.
- It can be useful to develop idiosyncratic scales. These may incorporate special interests.
- Measuring change via subjective units of distress (SUDS) ratings represents an alternative or complementary option to formal questionnaires.

CONSIDERATIONS FOR PROVIDERS

Research to date indicates that health professionals working in non-autism services can lack knowledge about autism and related conditions (for review, see Corden et al., 2021), partly as there is typically minimal formal teaching about autism in core professional (clinical) training (Maddox et al., 2020). Providers may also have limited confidence or skills around adapting standard interventions for individuals with autism (Adams & Young, 2020).

Attitudes towards autism, and working with clients with autism, can also influence practice (Corden et al., 2021). In a sample of 100 providers delivering CBT, for example, participants had more favorable attitudes and higher descriptive normative pressure (i.e., that others would like them to offer therapy) about working with people without, rather than with, autism (Maddox et al., 2019).

Treatment fidelity, defined as the degree to which a treatment is delivered as intended, is understandably deemed important within psychological therapy (Fonagy & Luyten, 2019). However, as implementation science has grown in recent years, clinical researchers have grown more aware of the need for flexibility in implementation, sometimes at the cost of fidelity in order to optimize the effectiveness of the treatment (Cohen et al., 2008). Ensuring treatment fidelity in routine practice can be more complex when working with adults with autism. For instance, clients may well present with more than one condition, meaning that the treatment approach may need to incorporate aspects of several protocols. Alternatively, it may be that providers need to adopt a more didactic or directive style during sessions and when setting homework, even if a more Socratic manner is integral to the therapeutic approach (e.g., CBT or EMDR).

Taken together, it seems possible that some providers may feel uncomfortable about deviating from manualized interventions or they may decide not to deliver a protocolized therapy. This thereby potentially limits the treatment options available to adults with autism. Providers or trainees may also fail therapy fidelity scales when their practice is assessed on these, even if they are providing good quality therapy and when some points are less relevant for working with some adults with autism.

Clinical Practice Implications

- Service managers should ensure all professionals working in clinical services have access to robust autism training programs. Training may comprise elements of general awareness (e.g., what is autism), as well as more specific topics for providers (e.g., how to adapt standard psychological approaches). Training should be co-produced with adults with autism and families, in so far as is possible.
- Providers can benefit from having regular clinical supervision or consultation with someone with experience and expertise in working with adults with autism. Augmenting individual supervision with group/peer meetings may enhance options for shared learning.
- Opportunities to reflect on assumptions about autism (e.g., whether anxiety is part of or separate to autism, whether adults with autism can engage in cognitive interventions, how far one can deviate from a protocolized treatment, what types of outcomes are realistic to work towards), can be an important aspect of clinical supervision.
- Providers should attempt to manage a balance between fidelity (integrity) to the manual or therapeutic approach they are deploying, with sufficient flexibility to "meet the client where they are," so to speak.

CONCLUDING REMARKS

Contributing authors to this edited book provide comprehensive and informative overviews of psychological therapies that can be effective for treating co-occurring symptoms and conditions in adults with autism, with case vignettes exemplifying theory in practice. We hope that providers will feel inspired to consider offering adults with autism a broader range of interventions, depending on presenting need, the treatment formulation, and goals for therapy.

Overall, the evidence base for several psychological therapies for adults with autism is limited, but growing. Further research focusing on which approaches are beneficial, when, for whom, and why, seems key. Concurrently, more research examining how service provision can be better tailored for autistic individuals, and what additional knowledge and skills providers can benefit from in order to work more effectively with this client group, seems warranted.

REFERENCES

Adams, D., & Young, K. (2020). A systematic review of the perceived barriers and facilitators to accessing psychological treatment for mental health problems in individuals on the autism spectrum. *Review Journal of Autism and Developmental Disorders*, 1–18.

American Psychological Association. (2013). *Diagnostic and statistical manual of mental disorders* (5th ed.). American Psychological Association.

Baier, A., Kline, A. C., & Feeny, N. (2020). Therapeutic alliance as a mediator of change: A systematic review and evaluation of research. *Clinical Psychology Review*.

Bordin, E. (1979). The generalizability of the psychoanalytic concept of the working alliance. *Psychotherapy: Theory, Research & Practice, 16*(3), 252.

Brewe, A., Mazefsky, C., & White, S. (2021). Therapeutic alliance formation for adolescents and young adults with autism: Relation to treatment outcomes and client characteristics. *Journal of Autism and Developmental Disorders, 51*(5), 1446–1457.

Brugha, T., Doos, L., Tempier, A., Einfeld, S., & Howlin, P. (2015). Outcome measures in intervention trials for adults with autism spectrum disorders; a systematic review of assessments of core autism features and associated emotional and behavioural problems. *International Journal of Methods in Psychiatric Research, 24*(2), 99–115.

Cohen, D., Crabtree, B., Etz, R., Balasubramanian, B., Donahue, K., Leviton, L., Clark, E. C., Isaacson, N. F., Stange, K. C., & Green, L. (2008). Fidelity versus flexibility: Translating evidence-based research into practice. *American Journal of Preventive Medicine, 35*(5), S381–S389.

Corden, K., Brewer, R., & Cage, E. (2021). A systematic review of healthcare professionals' knowledge, self-efficacy and attitudes towards working with autistic people. *Review Journal of Autism and Developmental Disorders*, 1–14.

De Los Reyes, A., Augenstein, T., Wang, M., Thomas, S., Drabick, D., Burgers, D., & Rabinowitz, J. (2015). The validity of the multi-informant approach to assessing child and adolescent mental health. *Psychological Bulletin, 141*(4), 858.

Del Re, A, Flückiger, C., Horvath, A., Symonds, D., & Wampold, B. (2012). Therapist effects in the therapeutic alliance–outcome relationship: A restricted-maximum likelihood meta-analysis. *Clinical Psychology Review, 32*(7), 642–649.

Doherty, A., Atherton, H., Boland, P., Hastings, R., Hives, L., Hood, K., James-Jenkinson, L., Leavey, R., Randell, E., Reed, J., Taggart, L., Wilson, N., & Chauhan, U. (2020). Barriers and facilitators to primary health care for people with intellectual disabilities and/or autism: an integrative review. *BJGP Open, 4*(3), 1–10.

Fonagy, P., & Luyten, P. (2019). Fidelity vs. flexibility in the implementation of psychotherapies: Time to move on. *World Psychiatry, 18*(3), 270–271.

Glod, M., Riby, D., Honey, E., & Rodgers, J. (2015). Psychological correlates of sensory processing patterns in individuals with autism spectrum disorder: A systematic review. *Review Journal of Autism and Developmental Disorders, 2*(2), 199–221.

Horvath, A., Del Re, A., Flückiger, C., & Symonds, D. (2011). Alliance in individual psychotherapy. *Psychotherapy, 48*(1), 9–16.

Kerns, C., Collier, A., Lewin, A., & Storch, E. (2018). Therapeutic alliance in youth with autism spectrum disorder receiving cognitive-behavioral treatment for anxiety. *Autism, 22*(5), 636–640.

Klebanoff, S., Rosenau, K., & Wood, J. (2019). The therapeutic alliance in cognitive-behavioral therapy for school-aged children with autism and clinical anxiety. *Autism, 23*(8), 2031–2042.

Maddox, B., Crabbe, S., Beidas, R., Brookman-Frazee, L., Cannuscio, C., Miller, J., Nicolaidis, C., & Mandell, D. (2020). "I wouldn't know where to start": Perspectives from clinicians, agency leaders, and autistic adults on improving community mental health services for autistic adults. *Autism, 24*(4), 919–930.

Maddox, B., Crabbe, S., Fishman, J., Beidas, R., Brookman-Frazee, L., Miller, J., Nicolaidis, C., & Mandell, D. (2019). Factors influencing the use of cognitive-behavioral therapy with autistic adults: A survey of community mental health clinicians. *Journal of Autism and Developmental Disorders, 49*(11), 4421–4428.

Mason, D., Ingham, B., Urbanowicz, A., Michael, C., Birtles, H., Woodbury-Smith, M., Brown, T., James, I., Scarlett, C., Nicolaidis, C., & Parr, J. R. (2019). A systematic review of what barriers and facilitators prevent and enable physical healthcare services access for autistic adults. *Journal of Autism and Developmental disorders, 49*(8), 3387–3400.

Strang, J., van der Miesen, A., Caplan, R., Hughes, C., daVanport, S., & Lai, M. (2020). Both sex-and gender-related factors should be considered in autism research and clinical practice. *Autism, 24*(3), 539–543.

Walsh, C., Lydon, S., O'Dowd, E., & O'Connor, P. (2020). Barriers to healthcare for persons with autism: A systematic review of the literature and development of a taxonomy. *Developmental Neurorehabilitation, 23*(7), 413–430.

Williams, M. (2020). *Managing microaggressions: Addressing everyday racism in therapeutic spaces*. Oxford University Press.

For the benefit of digital users, indexed terms that span two pages (e.g., 52–53) may, on occasion, appear on only one of those pages.

Tables and figures are indicated by *t* and *f* following the page number.